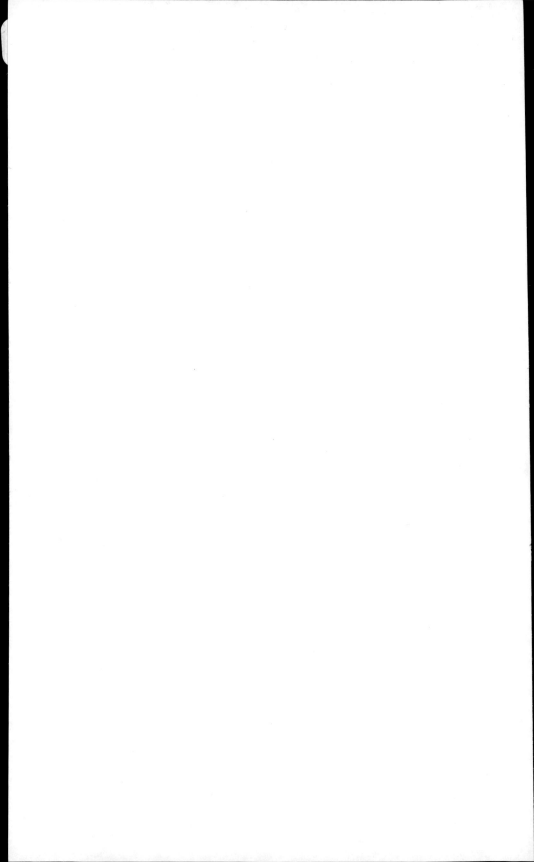

ANNUAL REVIEW OF NURSING RESEARCH

Volume 3, 1985

ANNUAL REVIEW OF NURSING RESEARCH

Volume 3, 1985

Harriet H. Werley, Ph.D.
Joyce J. Fitzpatrick, Ph.D.

Editors

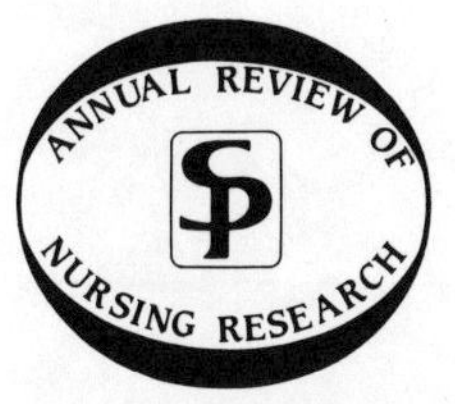

SPRINGER PUBLISHING COMPANY
New York

Order ANNUAL REVIEW OF NURSING RESEARCH, Volume 4, 1986, prior to publication and receive a 10% discount. An order coupon can be found after the index.

Springer Publishing Company, Inc.
536 Broadway
New York, New York 10012

85 86 87 88 89 / 10 9 8 7 6 5 4 3 2 1

ISBN 0-8261-4352-0
ISSN 0739-6686

Annual Review of Nursing Research is indexed in *Cumulative Index to Nursing and Allied Health Literature*.

Printed in the United States of America

Contents

Preface

Judging from the response to the publication of the first volume—as reflected in verbal comments, letters, and references to individual chapters or the volume generally—the *Annual Review of Nursing Research (ARNR)* series is welcomed, valued, and needed, as the founding editor (Werley) had envisioned. This attitude toward the series also has been reflected by the audiences in attendance at several symposia, conducted by the editors, when chapter authors and Advisory Board members were featured at national research conferences and the American Nurses' Association Convention. In these symposia, the process and the end product were highlighted, so authors for the first volumes could acquaint the audiences with what was involved in developing and writing a review chapter. Authors commissioned for chapters for later volumes, potential authors planning to volunteer to write a chapter, and potential users of this reference series found the content of interest and raised questions.

As indicated in the preface for Volume 1, the chapters under Nursing Practice for Volume 3 generally pertain to the community, while those for Volume 1 dealt with human development along the life span, and for Volume 2, the family. In keeping with the idea that there would be repeat chapters in the same areas over time as indicated by the volume of research, the chapters under Nursing Practice in Volume 4 again will pertain to human development. Volume 5 chapters will pertain to patient or client responses related to health problems, while those for Volume 6 will deal with human processes related to health and nursing interventions. In the initial volumes, an effort has been made to be inclusive in the selection of chapter topics, while at the same time working toward the nursing framework that is stated in the American Nurses' Association (1980) social policy statement.

The purpose of the *ARNR* series is to assess the state of the art as it pertains to nursing research. The chapters are critical, integrative reviews of published research, thus providing a base from which to recognize gaps and to project future research directions. Although the first volume of the *ARNR* appeared in December 1983 (copyright, 1984), an effort has been made to have subsequent volumes published earlier in the year. Volume 4 is scheduled to appear in spring of 1986.

Research reviewed for Volume 3 again follows the established format of five major parts: Nursing Practice, Nursing Care Delivery, Nursing Education, the Profession of Nursing, and Other Research. In the nursing practice area, Grayce M. Sills and Jean Goeppinger examine the community as a field of inquiry in nursing; Shu-Pi C. Chen and Judith A. Sullivan review research on school nursing; Ramona T. Mercer examines teenage pregnancy as a community problem; and Toni Tripp-Reimer and Molly C. Dougherty review cross-cultural nursing research. In the nursing care delivery area, Sherry L. Shamansky deals with the topic of nurse practitioners and primary care, and Marjory Gordon covers nursing diagnosis. The area of nursing education includes reviews of continuing education research by Alice M. Kuramoto and doctoral education of nurses by Juanita F. Murphy. Research on the profession of nursing is represented by Susan R. Gortner's review of ethical inquiry and the Claire M. Fagin and Barbara S. Jacobsen chapter on cost-effectiveness analysis in nursing research, while other research includes the work on philosophy of science and the development of nursing theory by Frederick Suppe and Ada K. Jacox.

We acknowledge most gratefully the work of the authors, the advice of the Advisory Board members, the critiques of anonymous reviewers, and the secretarial assistance provided by Margaret M. Sprung at the University of Wisconsin-Milwaukee School of Nursing, as well as the staff at the Case Western Reserve University Schools of Nursing, respectively.

We welcome readers' reactions to the volumes and specific chapters, as well as expressions of interest in contributing a critical review chapter on a relevant area of research.

REFERENCE

American Nurses' Association. (1980). *Nursing: A social policy statement*. Kansas City, MO: Author.

Contributors

Shu-Pi C. Chen, Dr.P.H.
College of Nursing
University of Illinois at Chicago
Chicago, Illinois

Molly C. Dougherty, Ph.D.
College of Nursing
University of Florida
Gainesville, Florida

Claire M. Fagin, Ph.D.
School of Nursing
University of Pennsylvania
Philadelphia, Pennsylvania

Jean Goeppinger, Ph.D.
School of Nursing
University of Virginia
Charlottesville, Virginia

Marjory Gordon, Ph.D.
School of Nursing
Boston College
Chestnut Hill, Massachusetts

Susan R. Gortner, Ph.D.
School of Nursing
University of California
San Francisco
San Francisco, California

Barbara S. Jacobsen, M.S.Ed.
School of Nursing
University of Pennsylvania
Philadelphia, Pennsylvania

Ada K. Jacox, Ph.D.
School of Nursing
University of Maryland
Baltimore, Maryland

Alice M. Kuramoto, Ph.D.
School of Nursing
University of Washington
Seattle, Washington

Ramona T. Mercer, Ph.D.
School of Nursing
University of California
San Francisco
San Francisco, California

Juanita F. Murphy, Ph.D.
College of Nursing
Arizona State University
Tempe, Arizona

Sherry L. Shamansky, Dr.P.H.
School of Nursing
Yale University
New Haven, Connecticut

Grayce M. Sills, Ph.D.
College of Nursing
The Ohio State University
Columbus, Ohio

Judith A. Sullivan, Ed.D.
College of Nursing
University of Illinois at Chicago
Chicago, Illinois

Frederick Suppe, Ph.D.
Program in History and Philosophy of Science, School of Nursing
University of Maryland
College Park, Maryland

Toni Tripp-Reimer, Ph.D.
College of Nursing
University of Iowa
Iowa City, Iowa

Forthcoming

ANNUAL REVIEW of
NURSING RESEARCH, Volume 4

Tentative Contents

PART I

Research on Nursing Practice

CHAPTER 1

The Community as a Field of Inquiry in Nursing

GRAYCE M. SILLS
COLLEGE OF NURSING
THE OHIO STATE UNIVERSITY
AND
JEAN GOEPPINGER
SCHOOL OF NURSING
UNIVERSITY OF VIRGINIA

CONTENTS

We acknowledge the assistance of Louise Anderson and Nikki Polis in the collection of the bibliographic material and of Nikki Polis in the editing.

Presented in this review is a discussion of the emergence of a perspective on community nursing. The basic concepts of this perspective are described. The criteria and procedures for conducting the review are discussed. Relevant nursing research is then analyzed. Questions are raised pertaining to research methodology, theory development, value orientations, and practice.

THE EMERGENCE OF THE FIELD OF COMMUNITY NURSING

It is likely that some would argue that community as a distinct perspective in nursing does not or should not exist. However, an examination of the nursing literature offers support for the position that the community is an appropriate phenomenological focus for the work of nurses and nursing. It is useful to speculate about the origins of this perspective.

Inasmuch as knowledge emerges in an historical context as well as a situation-specific context, it is instructive to consider briefly the period during which this perspective on nursing came into view, the 1960s and 1970s. In that time period, American communities were experiencing marked social unrest. Large segments of the citizenry were concerned with the basic inequities perceived to exist in society. The dominant theme was disenchantment with institutions and institutionalized ways of dealing with human problems. There were great societal pressures for change—change in ways of thinking about old problems and change in ways of responding to problems, old and new.

Nurses, too, felt those pressures. Public health nursing was challenged. Was it any longer relevant? Had public health nursing become so mandated and bureaucratized that it was unable to respond flexibly? Psychiatric nurses also were pushed by the political, legal, and social activism of the times to reexamine their focus and locus. The movement toward community-based mental health programs was reflected in the changes in locus and focus of psychiatric nursing practice. Nurses in other specialities also rediscovered the ambulatory patient in the community setting. Thus, nursing, especially public health nursing and psychiatric nursing, was on the cutting edge of societal change. A new focus, that is, a perspective on community, both different from and similar to earlier perspectives, emerged. It is this emerging synthesis that presently guides some research and provides great promise for the continued development of nursing knowledge.

The research reviewed reflected the lack of conceptual clarity in the field. This was to be expected. Nowhere was this dilemma better exemplified than in the use of the term *client* as community. While the term client was, as commonly understood, connotative of a person, it had been used in the perspective of community to denote the setting of practice, the unit of practice, and the target of practice. Thus, nurses, as well as persons in other disciplines such as history, philosophy, sociology, community psychology, and architecture, are developing their perspectives on the community.

THE COMMUNITY CLIENT: A CONCEPTUAL OVERVIEW

The various interpretations of the term *community client* have been recognized by some (Archer, 1976; Archer & Fleshman, 1975). Few attempts have been made, however, to delineate them systematically. Current thinking is summarized here to provide a conceptual overview.

The Setting of Practice

The distinctiveness of public health nursing traditionally has been attributed to the practice setting. Thus, the term community client was first understood as a practice site. Homes, schools, and industries were the practice environments. With the creation and institutionalization of the nurse practitioner role in neighborhood health centers and medical offices, and the changed locus of psychiatric nursing practice, the community sites of practice were extended even further. In these instances, the community was identified as the client primarily because nursing care occurred outside of the hospital.

The Unit of Practice

In this approach to the community, the client has been defined in two ways: as an aggregate or in interactional terms. First, with the aggregate approach the investigator used a group of individuals who possessed common personal or environmental characteristics. Research reflecting this definition of community has been categorized as epidemiological, needs assessment, and program planning studies. Second, when the conceptual approach to the research has been interactional, the work typically has been categorized as social support or community competence. In both approaches the community has been considered the means through which healthful community change can be planned and realized.

The Target of Practice

The community has been considered as the target of practice when nurses, regardless of the setting or unit of practice, have been community oriented. Community-oriented nursing practice implied that healthful change was sought for the common good. The setting might be the hospital, home, school, industry, or city hall. The units of service or instruments of change might be individuals, families and other interacting groups, aggregates, institutions, communities, and even societies. The concept of community as the target of practice has meant that the focus was neither on the settings nor on the units, but rather on the entity that they compose—the community in its essence of wholeness. This is the most current meaning.

These initial attempts to delineate a nursing perspective on the community only recently have been used to guide research. Thus, the impact of nursing practice with the community client was inadequately documented to a large extent. Some scholarly work has occurred. This work has been exemplified by the modest research efforts of a few community health nurse researchers.

CONDUCT OF THE REVIEW

Given the recent state of conceptual development in the field, particular attention was paid to the conceptual fit between the research problem and the emerging phenomenological focus of the field. The major criterion for inclusion of a study was whether it reflected a definition of the community client. Review of research related to the community as practice setting has been done by Highriter (1984). Therefore, the research reviewed here relates only to the community client defined as a unit and target of practice.

Additional criteria utilized in the screening of studies for inclusion were the notation of a nurse investigator among the authors, and publication in a community health journal, a nursing research journal, or *Dissertation Abstracts*. Studies meeting these criteria were reviewed. The unevenness of the analysis to follow reflects the wide range of quality in the research, undoubtedly a result of the rudimentary development of the field.

Manual reviews were done of all issues of the following nursing journals: *Nursing Research* (1952 to 1983), *Advances in Nursing Science* (1978 to 1983), *Research in Nursing and Health* (1978 to 1983), *International Journal of Nursing Studies* (1963 to 1983), *Topics in Clinical Nursing* (1979 to 1983), *Journal of Advanced Nursing* (1976 to 1983), and

Image (1967 to 1983). Additionally, the *Journal of Psychosocial Nursing and Mental Health Services* (1970 to 1983), *Communicating Nursing Research* (1968 to 1979), and the *Western Journal of Nursing Research* (1980 to 1983) were reviewed. Appropriate dissertations also were located by using the Directory of Nurses with Earned Doctoral Degrees (1969) and the 1970, 1971, and 1972 supplements published in *Nursing Research,* as well as by reviewing the "Recent Doctorates" section of the Sigma Theta Tau newsletter, *Reflections*. This method of search was done in order to limit the reviewed studies to those completed by nurse researchers. Given the nature of this topic, the *American Journal of Public Health* (1972 to 1983) and the *American Journal of Epidemiology* (1972 to 1983) also were searched for appropriate studies that included nurse investigators.

THE COMMUNITY AS THE UNIT OF PRACTICE

Epidemiological, Needs Assessment, and Program Planning Studies

These categories reflect the conception of the community as a unit of practice. The community is considered, explicitly or implicitly, as a service unit and principally as an object for assessment. The sophisticated epidemiological studies that guide public policy at the federal and state level are most often carried out by governmental agencies or interdisciplinary teams in universities with academic departments of epidemiology. Conceptually, the work done by nurse researchers is related more closely to needs assessment and program planning studies.

Three studies characterized by needs assessment and identification of target communities were identified (Carey & Rogers, 1973; Murphy & Landsberger, 1980; Selwyn, 1978). In their survey of health studies, health knowledge, and health decision-making skills Carey and Rogers (1973) revealed that students in an urban community college were at high health risk because of such factors as reported morbidity from at least one of nine major diseases, lack of health insurance, and an impaired ability to deal realistically with health and illness needs. This study was, like most needs assessments, atheoretical. The study also had several methodological weaknesses. The investigators did not use a random sample, although the sample "proved to correspond quite closely" to the student population (p. 127). They did not attempt to correlate any of the demographic and epidemiological variables with disease risk. This would have enabled the investigators to identify more precisely those groups of students at high risk. The investigators did not compute the age-adjusted morbidity rates. To have done so would have allowed more explicit comparisons with a standard. The practical implications of the study were not described and, without these, the purposes of a needs assessment were not fully achieved.

The Murphy and Landsberger study (1980) was a secondary analysis of health status data gathered by the health service agencies of North Carolina and was aimed at identifying the health needs of infants in three counties proximate to the University of North Carolina at Chapel Hill School of Nursing. This study was noteworthy for three reasons. First, the investigators used existing data, a source often overlooked by nurse researchers. Second, they conducted the study for the explicit purpose of developing a data base relevant to the School's research and service missions. And, finally, the investigators recognized as an implication of the findings the importance of intervention strategies ranging from a curative approach to primary prevention and the betterment of the socioeconomic status of disadvantaged population groups.

Selwyn (1978) used a case-comparison design to determine the characteristics of users and nonusers of child health services in one barrio of Cali, Colombia, and thus avoided the shortcomings of the needs assessment study conducted in a community college. The investigative approaches of Selwyn (1978) and Carey and Rogers (1973) were similar; both studies were atheoretical, and the investigators failed to identify and discuss the nursing implications of the findings. Consequently, although these findings may be depended upon for programming decisions when the population is similar to these samples, such studies are not likely to advance the knowledge base of nursing. This is a serious drawback.

Four studies were identified that were focused on the older adult as a target group in the community (Franck, 1979; Hain & Chen, 1976; Johnson, Cloyd, & Wer, 1982; Managan et al., 1974). The Managan et al. study (1974) was done in DuPage County, Illinois. The sample, noninstitutionalized adults over 65 years of age ($N = 1{,}446$), was sufficient to draw significant conclusions about health problems defined by five major indices: health condition, physical functioning, accessibility to medical care, social isolation, and service needs. The findings indicated that functional impairment, lack of a family physician, and social isolation were major problems. The Nursing Division of the Health Department served 4.2% of the older adults in 1971, while the study indicated a 15% need for service. Implications for nursing practice and further research were presented. No follow-up studies to this work were found, although the method was replicated in two studies (Franck, 1979; Hain & Chen, 1976).

Hain and Chen (1976) studied persons 65 years of age and over (*N* = 137) living in two high-rise apartment dwellings. One housed a low-income group and the other a moderate-income group. However, the samples were not matched. They also compared couples with men living alone and women living alone. The instruments were the same as those used in the DuPage County study (Managan et al., 1974). These investigators (Hain & Chen, 1976) found a higher prevalence of health-related problems than did the investigators of the DuPage County study. Even though the investigators chose to use age-segregated housing sites for the collection of data, they did not give major emphasis to this aspect of the community as an explanation for the findings. They identified many implications for appropriate nursing interventions. No follow-up study was discovered to indicate whether or not the findings were implemented and evaluated. This study was an excellent example of the replication process needed in nursing research to build on the work of other investigators. Hain and Chen utilized the methods of Managan et al. (1974) and looked at a different sample.

Franck (1979) also used the methods of the DuPage County study in an investigation of a rural population in Iowa (*N* = 82). Since the DuPage County sample was largely urban, it was thought that a comparison of the rural-urban dimension would be useful. The results demonstrated a striking similarity in needs of the elderly in midwestern rural and urban settings. Franck (1979), however, raised questions about the adequacy of the instruments to delineate effectively the differences in the ways in which the residents of the two communities defined their experience.

Johnson, Cloyd, and Wer (1982) examined life satisfaction among a sample of poor, black, urban aged (*N* = 45). The sex of the sample was not reported by the investigators. The instrument used was the Life Satisfaction Index—Z Scale (Wood, Wylie, & Sheaford, 1969). Both institutionalized (*N* = 22) and noninstitutionalized (*N* = 23) subjects were used. The major findings were that noninstitutionalized subjects exhibited higher life satisfaction than institutionalized subjects. Perceived health and freedom to make independent choices were highly correlated with life satisfaction. This study raised many important questions with respect to the community of the elderly. While many of the findings were interpreted in terms of the culture of the black experience, further study could demonstrate whether or not these findings also are likely to pertain to other urban, poor, elderly communities.

The final set of studies reviewed related to illness absence behavior (Basco, Eyres, Glasser, & Roberts, 1972), intent to utilize disease prevention and health promotion services (Pender & Pender, 1980), and knowledge about illness among members of Hispanic and Appalachian cultures

(Ailinger, 1982; Flaskerud, 1980). The epidemiological analysis of the absence behavior in school-age children (Basco et al., 1972) was done to direct changes in school nursing practice and to derive hypotheses to be tested in experimental studies. In many ways this study was an excellent example of high-quality research. Care and precision with concepts, terms, and methods were readily apparent. Findings included a profile of the high-absentee child, the population group at risk.

Program evaluation studies have been reported that related to the work of Basco and colleagues. A nursing program targeted at school children with high absence records has been evaluated (Long, Whitman, Johansson, Williams, & Tuthill, 1975; Tuthill, Williams, Long, & Whitman, 1972). These studies were supported by a U.S. Department of Health, Education, and Welfare Division of Nursing contract to the School of Public Health, University of North Carolina at Chapel Hill. They were aimed at developing the program-evaluation skills of nurses in local health agencies, and ascertaining the ways in which community nursing skills were utilized best. The studies were carried out in the Palm Beach County Health Department (Long et al., 1975; Tuthill et al., 1972). The greatest strength of these studies was the methodological awareness of the investigators. For example, when racial integration of the schools was introduced as an intervening variable, biases were acknowledged. However, the lack of a theoretical perspective seriously weakened the contributions such studies could make to a body of knowledge. As an outcome of the study conducted in Palm Beach, the school health services were reorganized (Long et al., 1975).

Pender and Pender (1980) provided a prospective analysis of consumers' intentions to utilize illness-prevention and health-promotion services provided by nurse practitioners. Noteworthy in this study was its prospective nature and the complexity of the design. Sixty-one percent of the cross-sectional telephone-surveyed sample ($N = 388$) indicated intention to use services provided by a nurse practitioner. Intentions to use services did not differ significantly ($p < .05$) between subjects who had a regular personal physician and those who did not. Major life change emerged as a significant predictor of intention to use the services of a nurse practitioner. A major limitation of the study was the unknown relationship between intention and actual behavior. The prospective method used by these investigators would serve well as a pretest measure for a nursing intervention study within a community analysis framework.

Ailinger (1982) used the Hypertension Knowledge Interview Schedule (HKIS), developed for a national survey (Harris, 1973), with a specific target population, an Hispanic community from which the sample was drawn ($N = 330$). Additional items were included to reflect Hispanic cultural beliefs and practices. There were methodological problems with this investigation, including use of telephone interviews and the low reliability of the HKIS (.70, using Cronbach's alpha). Nonetheless, this study represented an effort to isolate some important variables, such as the culture of the Hispanic community, and provide a base for program planning. Ailinger's (1977) interest in the Spanish-speaking community also was evidenced in an anthropological study of illness referral in a Spanish-speaking community, largely Latin-American in background. As more efforts such as this are undertaken, they will provide fertile ground for hypothesis testing and theory development.

Similar to the Ailinger (1977) work was the study of Flaskerud (1980). This research was distinguished by the use of a framework including the concepts of cultural relativism and social labeling. The investigator compared two cultural groups—Appalachian and non-Appalachian. The non-Appalachian group was divided into two groups: mental health professionals and laypersons. Findings included significant differences between the Appalachian subjects and the other two groups on the labeling of mental illness and the appropriate management for such behaviors. Such findings require further testing with samples from other populations to build the body of research-based information for community nursing practice.

The value assumptions underlying many of the studies reported in this section have not been analyzed. However, such analysis might offer students of research methodology an example of such inquiry. Thus, for these purposes, the values of two studies are compared. The first was the pioneering work of Milio (1967) in which she directly examined the value assumptions of the dominant middle classes with respect to maternity behavior, cultural orientation, and social class. This work was based on concepts derived from the work of Parsons (1958), Parsons and Shils (1962), Kluckhohn (1950), and Merton (1957). Milio reframed the question of appropriate maternity care for the lower-class population into a question of what the values of that population were which deemphasized the dominant view. In so doing, she demonstrated the extent to which shared values between practitioners and clients were important determinants of health attitudes and health practices. Milio did what Myrdal (1968) instructed. Myrdal maintained that science is never value free and scientists are obligated to make explicit their value premises. He stated that when values are implicit and unconscious, they allow biases to enter investigative work.

Contrast, then, Milio's (1967) work with a study by Triplett (1970) to determine whether there were demographic or personal characteristics that differentiated good from poor users of preventive health services. The categorization of good users and poor users of preventive health services was made by public health nurses. The constructs of threat and disparity were used to examine self-perceptions of medically indigent women's interactions with health workers, the women's utilization of health care services, the women's perceptions of themselves, and the relationships among these variables and certain demographic characteristics. Triplett raised numerous questions about possible biases in the study. However, the researcher failed to make explicit the underlying value premise that lower-class women defined as poor users were problems since they did not share the dominant values of the existing health care delivery system. This comparison was not meant to be invidious, but to stimulate thoughtful consideration of the very important issue of the relationship of the investigator's value premises to the research methods, procedures, and data analyses.

A final note of some import to this section of the review is in order. The recent innovation of health risk appraisal as a strategy for health needs assessment based on aggregate data was discussed in two reports (Doerr & Hutchins, 1981; Goetz & McTyre, 1981). These should be read by anyone considering the use of health risk appraisal (HRA) tools. Doerr and Hutchins (1981) provided an excellent summary of the available instruments, as well as a thorough discussion of the models underlying the instruments. Further, they raised appropriate methodological concerns with the work in this field. Goetz and McTyre (1981) presented an equally compelling discussion of the reliability of HRA data. They suggested caution in the application of the HRA results on the basis that the equation was set with the premise of all other things being equal. All other things are not equal. Very different genotypes and different exposures to the environment are of equal or greater concern. It is the latter issue, the environment, especially the social environment, that community nurse researchers need to address in a way that will add to the efficacy of health risk appraisal instruments.

In summary, the research reviewed was characterized by its atheoretical nature; it was focused on assessment and exploration with little mention of intervention, experimentation, or program planning and education; and it used an uneven, generally unsophisticated methodology. The research was recast within the conceptual structure of the community client as unit of service. Such reinterpretation suggested the potential of continued research for the development of nursing knowledge and the design of nursing practice. In the next section the second cluster of studies reflecting the community client as the unit of service is considered.

Social Support and Community Competence Studies

Social climate or environment long has been recognized by health professionals as a determinant of health–illness as well as a buffer against stress and disease. This assertion was recognized in the spate of research produced in the past two decades. In the middle 1970s several influential review articles (Cassel, 1976; Cobb, 1976; Kaplan, Cassel, & Gore, 1977) were published that included analyses of the rapidly accumulating research findings of a relationship between social support and health. Further, in these reviews investigators helped to disentangle the important concepts of social support and social network. They also identified questions for further research. The guidance provided by these reviews undoubtedly resulted in the subsequent increase in quantity and diversity of published research. In the early 1980s in two additional reviews (Broadhead et al., 1983; Thoits, 1982) investigators provided updates to the previous reviews.

Nurses contributed to this area of research, principally by developing instruments to assess family competence, as well as a variety of social support and social network variables (Benoliel, McCorkle, & Young, 1980; Boardman, Zyzanski, & Cottrell, 1975; Brandt & Weinert, 1981; Norbeck, Lindsey, & Carrieri, 1981; Nuckolls, Cassel, & Kaplan, 1972). At least two of these investigators, Boardman and Nuckolls, conducted their research while studying with the social epidemiologists who were among the first scholars in the area, Kaplan and Cassel.

Other nurse investigators pursued a related line of inquiry, that of community competence (Goeppinger & Baglioni, 1983; Goeppinger, Lassiter, & Wilcox, 1982; Kaswan, Schwebel, & Sills, 1975–1976; Schwebel, Kaswan, Sills, & Hackel, 1976). These investigators conceptualized social support as community competence, that is, the ability of a community to problem solve effectively. First, social support research will be analyzed. A review of studies relating to community competence will follow.

Brandt and Weinert (1981) developed and tested the validity and reliability of a multidimensional social support measure, the Personal Resource Questionnaire (PRQ). They based their work on the Weiss (1974) model of relational functions. Instrument development was part of a larger effort to examine relationships among the stress of long-term illness, social support of the well spouse, and family functioning.

Attempts to develop measures of family competence and psychosocial assets, such as social support, were also part of the larger studies. These investigators explored the extent to which social-psychological strain, as represented by level or degree of family competence, were related to the number of illness-related school absences among family members (Boardman et al., 1975), and the degree to which psychosocial assets and multiple life changes were protective of or detrimental to health (Nuckolls et al., 1972). Boardman and associates developed a questionnaire to measure family competence; Nuckolls et al. developed a measure of the adaptive potential for pregnancy (TAPPS). Unlike Boardman et al. (1975) and Brandt and Weinert (1981), Norbeck and colleagues (1981) reported only on the construction of an instrument to measure social support. They developed and tested the Norbeck Social Support Questionnaire (NSSQ).

Each of these studies was based on knowledge extant at the time they were conducted. Each of the research teams used somewhat different theoretical approaches. Three of the four (Boardman et al., 1975; Brandt & Weinert, 1981; Nuckolls et al., 1972) viewed social support as a potential buffer against life stress.

Brandt and Weinert (1981) relied heavily on the Weiss (1974) model of social support. The Weiss model delineated the functions of social support as intimacy, social integration, nurturance, worth, and assistance more clearly than the structure of social support, that is, social network variables. Kahn (1979) and Kahn and Antonucci's (1981) approach to social support, as used by Norbeck and her colleagues (1981), included the concepts of social support or function and social network or structure. Kahn (1979) proposed three components of supportive transactions—affect, affirmation, and aid—as well as the notion of convoy, that is, the mechanism or structure through which social support is provided.

The studies of Boardman et al. (1975) and Nuckolls et al. (1972) were grounded less strongly in theory. The social epidemiological approach from which they originated was more oriented toward the health consequences than toward the social precursors of health and illness. However, these studies were among the first conducted in this area. The theoretical antecedents were found in two sources, the early work by social behaviorists Mead (1934) and Cottrell (1976) used by Boardman et al. (1975) and by animal and stress researchers in the Nuckolls et al. work (1972).

The major theoretical issue in each of the three studies was the attribution of findings to the buffering hypothesis. Support for this hypothesis should be drawn with care, since several conceptual problems are unresolved. For example, in these studies social support was defined variously. Thus, the precise dimensions of social support that might mitigate the occurrence of distress cannot be ascertained. Brandt and Weinert (1981) and Norbeck et al. (1981) acknowledged support as a multidimensional concept, and Norbeck et al. attempted to measure both types and sources of social support. Neither Boardman et al. (1975) nor Nuckolls et al. (1972) measured social network variables. These conceptual inadequacies need resolution, especially since they pose serious methodological concerns.

A different tool to assess social support was developed in each of the above investigations (Boardman et al., 1975; Brandt & Weinert, 1981; Norbeck et al., 1981; Nuckolls et al., 1972). Each tool was multidimensional and self-administered. All elicited reliable responses. The tools were redundant, however; later research failed to build on earlier work. This problem was particularly serious because much work remained to be done on the psychometric properties of all the instruments. Both Brandt and Weinert (1981) and Norbeck et al. (1981) failed to establish the construct validity of their instruments. Boardman et al. (1975) and Nuckolls et al. (1972) did not address this issue adequately.

Another methodological problem, present even in the Nuckolls et al. longitudinal study (1972), was that the possible direct effects of undesirable events in the respondent's past on the social network were ignored. Thus, the effects of social support, social network, and stressful events were confounded. In the Nuckolls et al. study, the network was not assessed. Social support was measured only at prenatal clinic registration when one stressful event, pregnancy, may be presumed to have occurred. The impact of other stressful events was noted during the 32nd week of pregnancy and following delivery.

A final issue is that all of the investigators used small samples and one team (Norbeck et al., 1981) used a sample composed of students whose norms likely were appreciably different from those of clinical populations. Each instrument would profit from additional tests and refinement, both to extend the population to which results may be generalized and to improve the psychometric properties.

Although the implications for practice seem rather clear, none of the instruments, as presently developed, is ready for clinical application. Both Boardman et al. (1975) and Nuckolls et al. (1972) suggested the utility of the instruments in identifying families-at-risk so appropriate interventions could be designed. This is, of course, essential for practice. Norbeck (1981) developed intervention strategies in another article; she did not base the discussion on her research.

A study by Turner (1979) is worthy of note due to the prevalence of deinstitutionalized mental patients in communities. The major focus of this study was the extent of disability in a sample of former mental patients living in a rural community. Findings were that social support and social networks in the community were correlated significantly ($p < .05$) with measured functional capacity. Further, Turner noted the essentially rural nature of the population from which the sample was drawn. Social support was measured by an index of "self reported specific assets claimed or denied by the respondent and more general expressions of satisfaction" (Turner, 1979, p. 154). The sample size was small ($N = 103$); thus the findings must be viewed in a tentative light. Further testing of the reliability and validity of the social support measures and replication in another community context might add to the understanding of community networks.

Two approaches were evident in the research on community competence. One approach, like the research on social support, was centered on the development of a tool or procedure to assess community competence (Goeppinger & Baglioni, 1983). The second approach reflected a commitment to action research, usually in the form of case studies of intervention in small communities (Goeppinger et al., 1982; Kaswan et al., 1975–1976; Schwebel et al., 1976). This research typically was conducted by interdisciplinary groups that included community developers, psychologists, and nurses. Each approach had a similar theoretical base; each, unfortunately, had serious methodological shortcomings. Each was instructive, not prescriptive, for practice.

Each approach was grounded in the concepts of competence or efficacy and self-help. The value premise underlying these concepts was that persons can use their available resources and capabilities to problem solve. Applied to the community level, this premise suggested that communities can recognize and manage their collective needs when they identify strengths and difficulties in the community process and act to strengthen the interactions. This principle had its theoretical origins in the work of Mead (1934). The research in the area, except for that aimed at construction of assessment procedures, was linked loosely with the relevant theory. This was a notable problem related to development of a knowledge base.

The generation of theory and methods for the study of community is of major importance in the development of knowledge. Wilson's (1977) study of community at the microlevel yielded the concept of limiting intrusion as a subset of the larger construct of social control in communities. The setting for the Wilson study was an experimental treatment community for diagnosed schizophrenics. However, the adequacy of the concept seems to have generalizability for other community settings and for macrolevels of community. Theory generating work of this nature augurs well for the future.

A contribution to methods was presented in the work of Cohen, Sills, and Schwebel (1977). The investigators demonstrated a two-stage process for the development of a community needs-assessment measure. The rationale was demonstrated by first asking randomly selected community residents about their perceptions of needs. The second step was to construct the survey instrument from the data collected in the first stage. Such a process avoided the bias of professionals with respect to perceptions of needs of others.

Descriptive research, such as that represented by case studies, was an essential point of departure for the study of community processes. When, however, the researchers implied that observed changes in community competence were caused by the "facilitating orientation" of professional helpers (Kaswan et al., 1975–1976), the drawbacks became obvious. In two of the case studies reviewed here, investigators had this orientation (Goeppinger et al., 1982; Kaswan et al., 1975–1976).

Another issue identified is that research methods necessary to develop and test an instrument are very sophisticated and demanding of the investigator's time and financial resources. The one measure developed had been tested in only five communities, and that process required two years (Goeppinger & Baglioni, 1983). A long-term plan is needed, but the research to date does not reflect such planning.

Research in this area is worthy of continued investment since the impact of nursing on community health status has not been substantiated yet. The influence of nurses on outcome measures, especially in the area of nurse–community interaction where many community nursing efforts are concentrated, must be determined.

THE COMMUNITY AS THE TARGET OF PRACTICE

In only two studies (Anderson, 1983; Cruise & Storfjell, 1980) investigators attempted to delimit the community as the target of practice. Cruise and Storfjell identified three dimensions of community-focused nursing: client-oriented services, aggregate needs identification, and aggregate planning and intervention. Client-oriented services were described as "direct services to clients and families within the context of the community" (p. 10); aggregate needs identification dealt with "community information-gathering and awareness of community needs and problems" (p. 10); and aggregate planning and information was defined as "active involvement in planning and intervention at the community level and community outreach, or advocacy" (p. 11). Community health nursing educators were consistently in most agreement with the community focus. Community health nursing staff were most apt to disagree with the community focus. Responses of nurse administrators exhibited the greatest variation. Anderson (1983) also compared the perceived importance of community-focused functions among the three groups. Although she clustered the functions differently, that is, by using the steps of the nursing process, like Cruise and Storfjell (1980) she found that educators attached the greatest importance to community-oriented functions. Administrators, however, viewed community-oriented functions as more important than did staff respondents.

These studies (Anderson, 1983; Cruise & Storfjell, 1980) were pioneering efforts to develop a theoretical basis for viewing the community as the target of service. Despite the fact that most textbooks in public health and community health nursing and many leaders in the field emphasize the importance of orienting care to the community, the theoretical and research bases remain underdeveloped. These investigators made a beginning contribution to the development of the theoretical base for community nursing practice. By the construction of instruments to describe the community client as the target of service and further by examination of the extent to which community health nursing administrators, educators, and practitioners agree with the description, they initiated the process needed for the development of a theoretical base. This was their greatest achievement.

The methods used in the studies were divergent. Anderson (1983) identified 50 community-focused functions from a review of community public health nursing textbooks; Cruise and Storfjell (1980) developed their list of 41 functions during brainstorming sessions with community health nursing practitioners, educators, and students. Reliance on experts in the field to identify community-focused nursing behaviors was certainly an appropriate technique for instrument development. Other experts acted as respondents, again an appropriate use of sampling. Neither Cruise and Storfjell (1980) nor Anderson (1983) discussed the psychometric properties of their instruments. Efforts in this area are vital to continued development of the instruments and, eventually, to the construction of theory for community-oriented nursing. This was the greatest weakness of these studies.

The researchers' reports were rich in practice implications, even though these must be qualified by the relatively unsophisticated methodology of one (Anderson, 1983) and the absence of psychometric data on the instruments. As a basic step in circumscribing the realm of community-oriented nursing practice, the findings may lead one to suggest ways of investigating critical questions such as: To what extent are community-focused functions actually performed by community health nurses, educators, and/or administrators? The instruments used in these studies (Anderson, 1983; Cruise & Storfjell, 1980) also could be used as a basis for quality-assurance studies and could assist in clarification of community-focused functions for job descriptions.

SUGGESTED RESEARCH DIRECTIONS

In the review of the research in this chapter theory, methods, practice, and values questions were emphasized. More questions were raised than were answered, which is as it should be, given the nascent state of the field. Other observations are in order to round out this discussion. First, issues related to the preparation of nurses for work as community nurses were discussed. Anderson, Gottschalk, Grimes, Ives, and Skrovan (1977), in an excellent report, detailed the development and implementation of a curriculum model for community nurses. The investigators provided guidelines for nurse educators to consider in preparing competent practitioners to develop this "new-old" approach to the achievement of health of communities.

Second, although all international journals were not searched, it was noted that nurse investigators in the United Kingdom (Dawe, 1980; Griffith & Mangen, 1980; Mangen & Griffith, 1982) appeared to have joined community nursing practice and evaluation studies, specifically in the instance of community psychiatric nursing. The model for the health care delivery system in the United Kingdom is very different from that of the United States. Hence, generalizability is an issue. Nonetheless, these reports were provocative. Noteworthy was the Mangen and Griffith (1982) study, in which investigators compared community psychiatric nursing care to psychiatric follow-up care. Findings indicated a greater patient satisfaction with the modality of nurse-given care. The random assignment of the patients to the two groups gave the study the rigor of a prospective nature and reduced sample bias. Both factors added to the credibility of the findings.

Third, Allor (1983) and Spratlen (1982) developed community assessment tools for the primary purpose of assisting students in skill development in this area. Neither tool was tested in a systematic study. It seems likely that this could be done in the future.

Fourth, work has been done by nurses (Hamilton, 1983; McLaughlin, 1982) to create models that might serve as bases for community theory development and testing by researchers. Hamilton (1983) focused on the use of community nursing diagnosis by nurses in their practice in communities. She developed a typology different from that used in this review. She suggested that as the concept of nursing diagnosis is used by community nurses, it would "become clear if nursing of individuals in the community, nursing of individuals influenced by the community, and nursing of the community are real or artificial distinctions" (p. 34).

Whether or not the posing of such questions is seen as facilitative to the future work of nurse researchers remains to be determined. Thus, in part, the above comments support the earlier conceptual discussion of client community in this chapter.

McLaughlin (1982), on the other hand, presented a model for community health program service delivery based on tested theory of health beliefs and health behavior. She acknowledged that much further work should be done with respect to standardization of psychological and situational troubles in community-based studies. The perspective expressed in this chapter, however, is clear: McLaughlin sensed the enormous societal pressures for cost-effective health care delivery, for social accountability for those costs, and for adaptive measures on the part of community nursing services. This would seem a realistic perception and a realistic model. Given the above statement the authors of this review would still argue for the profession of nursing to remain open to the idea of community in its essence of wholeness as it develops its disciplinary domain.

Fifth, the deinstitutionalization of the mentally ill by means of community placement has created a significant societal issue. The best presentation of this issue in all of its complexity is found in the work of Krauss and Slavinsky (1982). The authors synthesized the research of others and presented case studies to offer a coherent whole with respect to this issue. Thus, while the work is not research per se, it demonstrated the use of research in this area and did so in a critically thoughtful and exemplary way.

In summary, we presented a review and analysis of research in the area of client community. Methods, issues, and methodological concerns were discussed. Further, attention was given to emerging work in theory building and nursing education that shows promise for a good fit with the concept of client community.

American society in its present state seems less likely than it was in the 1970s to be willing to invest in the research needed to develop this field. The underlying premises for this focused work clearly reflect a value orientation based on the principles of distributive justice. Thus, the long-term perspective about the future must contain the hope for healthy communities. Communities, then, are places where people learn and grow. Communities, then, are places where the common good is the goal, and health is a cherished right and responsibility, not a privilege. Community as a field of inquiry holds much promise to assist in the understanding of the complex phenomena that create the place, the space, and the matrix of persons that the human family call home.

REFERENCES

Ailinger, R. L. (1977). A study of illness referral in a Spanish speaking community. *Nursing Research, 26,* 53–56.

Ailinger, R. L. (1982). Hypertension knowledge in a Hispanic community. *Nursing Research, 31,* 207–210.

Allor, M. T. (1983). The "community profile." *Journal of Nursing Education, 22,* 12–17.

Anderson, E. T. (1983). Community focus in public health nursing: Whose responsibility? *Nursing Outlook, 31,* 44 – 48.

Anderson, E. T., Gottschalk, J., Grimes, D., Ives, J., & Skrovan, C. (1977). *The development and implementation of a curriculum model for community nurse practitioners* (DHEW Publication No. HRA 77-24). Washington, DC: U.S. Government Printing Office.

Archer, S. E. (1976). Community nurse practitioners: Another assessment. *Nursing Outlook, 24,* 499–503.

Archer, S. E., & Fleshman, R. P. (1975). Community health nursing: A typology of practice. *Nursing Outlook, 23,* 358–364.

Basco, D., Eyres, S., Glasser, J. H., & Roberts, D. E. (1972). Epidemiologic analyses in school populations as a basis for change in school-nursing practice—Report of the second phase of a longitudinal study. *American Journal of Public Health, 62,* 491– 497.

Benoliel, J. A., McCorkle, R., & Young, K. (1980). Development of a social dependency scale. *Research in Nursing and Health, 3,* 3–10.

Boardman, V., Zyzanski, S., & Cottrell, L. S. (1975). School absences, illness, and family competence. In B. H. Kaplan & J. C. Cassel (Eds.), *Family health: An epidemiological approach* (pp. 63–87). Chapel Hill, NC: University of North Carolina.

Brandt, P. A., & Weinert, C. (1981). The PRQ —A social support measure. *Nursing Research, 30,* 277–280.

Broadhead, W. E., Kaplan, B. H., James, S. A., Wagner, E. H., Schoenbach, V. J., Grimson, R., Heyden, S., Tibblin, G., & Gehlbach, S. H. (1983). The epidemiologic evidence for a relationship between social support and health. *American Journal of Epidemiology, 117,* 521–537.

Carey, J., & Rogers, E. L. (1973). Health status and health knowledge of the student in the changing community college. *American Journal of Public Health, 63,* 126 –133.

Cassel, J. C. (1976). The contribution of the social environment to host resistance. *American Journal of Epidemiology, 104,* 107–123.

Cobb, S. (1976). Social support as a moderator of life stress. *Psychosomatic Medicine, 38,* 300–314.

Cohen, M. W., Sills, G. M., & Schwebel, A. I. (1977). A two-stage process for survey in community needs. *Journal of the Community Development Society, 8,* 54–61.

Cottrell, L. S. (1976). The competent community. In B. H. Kaplan, R. N. Wilson, & A. H. Leighton (Eds.), *Future exploration in social psychiatry* (pp. 195–209). New York: Basic Books.

Cruise, P., & Storfjell, J. (1980). *The Storfjell-Cruise community focus model of community health nursing*. Unpublished master's thesis, The University of Michigan, Ann Arbor, MI.

Dawe, A. (1980). A case for community psychiatric nurses. *Journal of Advanced Nursing, 5,* 485– 490.

Directory of nurses with earned doctoral degrees. (1969). *Nursing Research, 18,* 465– 480.

Doerr, B. T., & Hutchins, E. B. (1981). Health risk appraisal: Process, problems, and prospects for nursing practice and research. *Nursing Research, 30,* 299–306.

Flaskerud, J. H. (1980). Perceptions of problematic behavior by Appalachians, mental health professionals, and lay non-Appalachians. *Nursing Research, 29,* 140 –149.

Franck, P. (1979). A survey of health needs of older adults in Northwest Johnson County, Iowa. *Nursing Research, 28,* 360 –364.

Goeppinger, J., & Baglioni, A. J. (1984). *Assessing community competence.* Manuscript submitted for publication.

Goeppinger, J., Lassiter, P. G., & Wilcox, B. (1982). Community health is community competence. *Nursing Outlook, 30,* 464 – 467.

Goetz, A. A., & McTyre, R. B. (1981). Health risk appraisal: Some methodologic considerations. *Nursing Research, 30,* 307–313.

Griffith, J. H., & Mangen, S. P. (1980). Community psychiatric nursing—A literature review. *International Journal of Nursing Studies, 17,* 197–210.

Hain, M. H., & Chen, S. C. (1976). Health needs of the elderly. *Nursing Research, 25,* 433– 439.

Hamilton, P. (1983). Community nursing diagnosis. *Advances in Nursing Science, 5*(3), 21–36.

Harris, L. (1973). *The public and high blood pressure* (DHEW Publication No. 77-356). Washington, DC: U.S. Government Printing Office.

Highriter, M. E. (1984). Public health nursing practice evaluation, education, and professional issues: 1977–1981. In H. H. Werley & J. J. Fitzpatrick (Eds.), *Annual Review of Nursing Research* (Vol. 2). New York: Springer Publishing Co.

Johnson, F., Cloyd, C., & Wer, J. (1982). Life satisfaction of poor urban black aged. *Advances in Nursing Science, 4*(3), 27–34.

Kahn, R. L. (1979). Aging and social support. In M. W. Riley (Ed.), *Aging from birth to death: Interdisciplinary perspectives*(pp. 77–91). Boulder, CO: Westview Press.

Kahn, R. L., & Antonucci, T. C. (1981). Convoys over the life course: Attachment, roles, and social support. In P. B. Battes & O. C. Brim, Jr. (Eds.), *Life span development and behavior*. New York: Academic Press.

Kaplan, B. H., Cassel, J. C., & Gore, S. (1977). Social support and health. *Medical Care, 15,* 47–57.

Kaswan, J. W., Schwebel, A. I., & Sills, G. M. (1975–1976). Community problem solving through an urban extension program. *Journal of Mental Health Administration, 4,* 36 – 45.

Kluckhohn, F. R. (1950). Dominant and substitute profiles of cultural orientations: Their significance for the analysis of social stratification. *Social Forces, 28,* 376 –393.

Krauss, J. B., & Slavinsky, A. T. (1982). *The chronically ill psychiatric patient and the community*. Boston: Blackwell.

Long, G. V., Whitman, C., Johansson, M. F., Williams, C. A., & Tuthill, R. W. (1975). Evaluation of a school health program directed to children with history of high absence: A focus for nursing intervention. *American Journal of Public Health, 65,* 388 –393.

Managan, D., Wood, J., Heinichen, C., Hoffman, M., Hess, G., & Gillings, D. (1974). Older adults: A community survey of health needs. *Nursing Research, 23,* 426 – 432.

Mangen, S. P., & Griffith, J. H. (1982). Patient satisfaction with community psychiatric nursing: A progressive controlled study. *Journal of Advanced Nursing, 7,* 477– 482.

McLaughlin, J. S. (1982). Toward a theoretical model for community health programs. *Advances in Nursing Science, 5*(1), 7–28.

Mead, G. H. (1934). *Mind, self, and society*. Chicago: The University of Chicago Press.

Merton, R. K. (1957). *Social theory and social structure* (rev. ed.). New York: Free Press.

Milio, N. (1967). Values, social class, and community health services. *Nursing Research, 16,* 26–31.

Murphy, N., & Landsberger, B. (1980). A data-based approach to reducing infant mortality in three rural counties of a southern HSA. *Advances in Nursing Science, 2*(2), 97–109.

Myrdal, G. (1968). *Asian drama: An inquiry into the poverty of nations* (Vol. 1). New York: Pantheon.

Norbeck, J. S. (1981). Social support: A model for clinical research and application. *Advances in Nursing Science, 3*(4), 43–59.

Norbeck, J. S., Lindsey, A. M., & Carrieri, V. L. (1981). The development of an instrument to measure social support. *Nursing Research, 30,* 264 –269.

Nuckolls, K. B., Cassel, J. C., & Kaplan, B. H. (1972). Psychosocial assets, life crises and the prognosis of pregnancy. *American Journal of Epidemiology, 95,* 431– 441.

Parsons, T. (1958). Definitions of health and illness in the light of American values and social structure. In G. Jaco (Ed.), *Patients, physicians and illness: Sourcebook in behavioral science and medicine* (pp. 165–187). Glencoe, IL: Free Press.

Parsons, T., & Shils, E. A. (Eds.). (1962). *Toward a general theory of action.* New York: Harper & Brothers.

Pender, N. J., & Pender, A. R. (1980). Illness prevention and health promotion service provided by nurse practitioners: Predicting potential consumers. *American Journal of Public Health, 70,* 798–803.

Schwebel, A. I., Kaswan, J. W., Sills, G. M., & Hackel, A. S. (1976). University extension in urban neighborhoods. *Journal of Higher Education, 47,* 205–215.

Selwyn, B. J. (1978). An epidemiological approach to the study of users and non-users of child health services. *American Journal of Public Health, 68,* 231–235.

Spratlen, L. P. (1982). Strategies for teaching nursing research: Community assessment as a basis for nursing intervention. *Western Journal of Nursing Research, 4,* 240 –243.

Thoits, P. A. (1982). Conceptual, methodological, and theoretical problems in studying social support as a buffer against life stress. *Journal of Health and Social Behavior, 23,* 145–159.

Triplett, J. L. (1970). Characteristics and perceptions of low-income women and use of preventive health services. *Nursing Research, 19,* 140 –146.

Turner, S. L. (1979). Disability among schizophrenics in a rural community: Services and social support. *Research in Nursing and Health, 2,* 151–161.

Tuthill, R. W., Williams, C. A., Long, G., & Whitman, C. (1972). Evaluating a school health program focused on high absence pupils. A research design. *American Journal of Public Health, 62,* 40 – 42.

Weiss, R. (1974). The provision of social relationships. In Z. Rubin (Ed.), *Doing unto others* (pp. 17–26). Englewood Cliffs, NJ: Prentice-Hall.

Wilson, J. S. (1977). Limiting intrusion—social control of outsiders in a healing community. *Nursing Research, 26,* 103 –111.

Wood, V., Wylie, M., & Sheaford, B. (1969). An analysis of a short self report measure of life satisfaction: Correlation with rater judgments. *Journal of Gerontology, 24,* 465– 469.

CHAPTER 2

School Nursing

Shu-Pi C. Chen and Judith A. Sullivan
College of Nursing
University of Illinois at Chicago

CONTENTS

In this chapter, significant advances in research on school nursing are described and evaluated. It is not a comprehensive review of all published articles on school nursing. Articles were selected on the basis of their contribution to clarifying knowledge, adding new knowledge, or increasing understanding of existing knowledge.

This chapter includes studies of the health of children from kindergarten through 12th grade, evaluation of the state of the art in research, and future directions for school nursing services. Articles related to college students were excluded, because these students generally were regarded as adults in terms of caring for their own health. Sources of the articles selected included the authors' collections, computer searches, and citations of published articles. To be included, articles must have been (a) within the defined subject area since 1960, (b) data based, and (c) widely accessible. This chapter is organized into three sections: review of research methodology, content review by subject areas, and discussion and future research directions.

REVIEW OF RESEARCH METHODOLOGY

A total of 82 articles was reviewed to describe the relative research sophistication of the field. The process of reviewing an article included (a) assigning each article to its primary subject area and (b) analyzing the article by preestablished guidelines. Assignment of each article to its primary subject area was to avoid duplication of reviews within the same chapter. The preestablished guidelines contained eight criteria: presence of a nurse as author, adequacy of the literature review, type of study design, sampling method, indication of informed consent, type of instrumentation, presence of reliability and validity data, and type of statistics used in the analysis.

Half of the studies had nurse authors, 23 as first authors and 18 as other authors, while the remaining 41 studies had no nurses as authors. This fact was surprising in light of the prominent role of the nursing program in virtually all of the studies reviewed. Only seven authors published more than one study, and the majority of these were not nurses. However, five of these seven authors had continued publishing and had published within the last ten years; a third of these were nurses.

Three categories were developed by the chapter authors to describe the adequacy of the literature reviews upon which each study was based. Adequate, the midpoint, referred to articles in which investigators clearly developed the definition and conceptualization for the research. Thorough and inadequate were used to express the two extremes of the continuum. While 30% (25 studies) had a thorough literature review, as many as 26% (21 studies) had inadequate literature reviews. The remaining 44% of the 82 (36 studies) had adequate literature reviews for the particular content area of school nursing studied. It is by building on prior investigations that refinements in applied theory and practice are made; thus, at least adequate literature reviews are required to contribute to the cumulative nature of developing a knowledge base.

The two elements of sustained nurse authorship and adequacy of literature review for investigations set the tone for the state of the art in school nursing research. With sustained effort by clinicians and researchers devoted to an area of study, the fullest development of the literature supporting practice and improved methods used in its study will be achieved. While 82 studies represent a considerable amount of attention to research in this area, an additional four articles (Yankauer, Frantz, Drislane, & Katz, 1962; Yankauer & Lawrence, 1955; Yankauer & Lawrence, 1956; Yankauer, Wendt, Eichler, Fry, & Lawrence, 1961) were reviewed that did not include nursing per se, but provided good background for the understanding of the nurse practitioner role.

Judging on the basis of the remaining six criteria, the research in school health nursing was at a beginning level. First, the predominant research approach was descriptive (80% of the 82 studies), which was appropriate for the initial studies in a field to determine the relevant variables. Only 16 studies were categorized beyond the descriptive level: 11 were correlational and 5 were causal association studies.

Second, convenience sampling, rather than other less biased methods, was the prevailing sampling method used. In five studies, the sampling method was not mentioned. In terms of informed consent, the majority of the investigators dealt appropriately with the subjects. Only one investigator of the 82 studies did not report obtaining informed consent when it appeared necessary.

Among the various methods of data collection used, structured questionnaires comprised the greatest number. Substantial use also was made of structured interviews, health records, physical examinations, and other forms of data collection, such as standardized tests, referral forms, encounter forms, and clinical logs. Although a variety of methods were used to collect data, relatively few investigators reported on the reliability and validity of the data (17% and 29%, respectively). This represented an understandable weakness in the beginning level, descriptive studies, but a necessary component of the work to be strengthened. Replication of selected studies with attention to establishing the validity and reliability of the tools was noted as a critical step in the further development of research in this field.

As would be expected, the statistics applied to the data were largely descriptive in nature. However, about half of the studies also included a component of inferential statistics. The implications of the studies were drawn appropriately (90% of the 82 studies), with only eight investigators describing findings beyond the data. On the whole, while there is much to be done in school nursing research, the studies reviewed in this chapter represent much of the groundwork in its initial stages.

CONTENT REVIEW BY SUBJECT AREA

Subject areas for this review are those in which a school nurse contributed to the development of knowledge or its application to clinical practice. The subject areas included in this chapter are school nursing services; health screening and periodic examinations performed by nurses; school health services involving nurses; referrals and follow-up by nurses; visits to school nurses; knowledge, role, and functions of school nurses; nurse practitioners in schools; views and attitudes of children; health education programs related to nursing; school health team; health aides; and a survey of school health programs.

School Nursing Services

In this area, six articles containing clearly delineated nursing interventions were selected for review (Basco, 1963; Basco, Eyres, Glasser, & Roberts, 1972; Brophy, 1970; Bryan & Cook, 1967; Long, Whitman, Johansson, Williams, & Tuthill, 1975; Roberts, Basco, Slome, Glasser, & Handy, 1969). Basco (1963) measured specified nursing activities in a generalized public health nursing program. The nurse–pupil ratio ranged from about 1:900 to 1:11,300 among the study schools, and the accomplishment of nursing activities was higher in the schools with lower nurse–pupil ratios. Basco (1963) also identified health appraisal, prevention and care of illness, and follow-up of children with special health problems as activities frequently performed by the nurses, whereas program development, operations, and health education were performed less frequently by the nurses.

Roberts et al. (1969) and Basco et al. (1972) identified the school population groups at risk for absence and illness and intended to design new patterns of health services for these high-risk groups. High absence was associated with low grade point average, being overage for one's grade, low socioeconomic status, broken homes, and urban schools, especially among 10th graders and in groups of nonwhites. Absence in the prior year was highly predictive of absence behavior in later years.

Effects of assigning a public health nurse to work with children having a history of high absence were evaluated. Children in an intervention group showed absence reduction averaging two days less than those in the control group during the 1970 to 1971 school year (Long et al., 1975). A planned program of personal contacts by the school nurse increased parental actions toward maintenance and promotion of the children's health (Bryan & Cook, 1967). When the school nurses conducted follow-up for 1,644 sixth graders, 3.8% of them had had a total of 63 medical defects (Brophy, 1970). As a result of the nurses' referrals, 46 of the 63 defects were corrected. Several recommendations were made by the above investigators, including the development of systematic approaches for assessing children and their families, documenting nursing actions, and establishing a range of nurse-to-pupil ratios.

In summary, very few research articles pertaining to school nursing services were reviewed and the interrelatedness of these studies was difficult to identify. This indicated the need for a new conceptualization of the nature of school nursing. Clarification of the concept of school nursing and identification of new knowledge and skills needed may serve as the beginning steps to establish a conceptual base for school nursing. It is evident in this review that research efforts of school nurses must be directed toward innovative nursing interventions. Some nurse researchers have done so. For instance, in the Long et al. (1975) study, investigators demonstrated that an innovative nursing program could reduce absenteeism. The Roberts et al. study (1969) was an epidemiological analysis of school absenteeism intended to serve as a base for an experimental study of nursing interventions. Unfortunately, the proposed intervention study was never undertaken because of the implementation of an integration plan at the particular school district that resulted in redistribution of the study students (D. Basco, personal communication, June 30, 1983).

Health Screening and Periodic Examination Performed by Nurses

Although health screening and periodic examination have been conducted in schools by physicians, nurses always have been involved in these activities. Recently, training of nurses in health assessment has made it possible for nurses to conduct health screening and periodic examinations for school-age children. Thus, an examination of the research findings in this area should increase further understanding of the school nurse role in early case finding and health promotion.

For this review, Henzell's (1977) definitions of both health screening and periodic examination were used. Health screening is the acquisition of preliminary information about characteristics that might be significant to the health, education, or well-being of the individual and are relevant to his or her life tasks. The means of data collection must be appropriate and reasonable with regard to the economics of time, money, and resources for dealing with large numbers of children. Periodic examination is a comprehensive physical examination performed by a physician for detecting any deviations from the normal health status for each child (Henzell, 1977); it is also called school physical examination and is required by law for children at selected grade levels. Recently, nurses have taken on greater responsibility for health screening and periodic examination, since the advent of the nurse practitioner movement in 1965. Fourteen articles are reviewed: eight in health screening and six in periodic examination in which nurses participated.

Health screening. Investigators of health screening studies assume that certain health conditions can be identified and should be corrected at the earliest possible time. Thus, the rationale for health screening activities or expected number of cases to be identified should be documented. For scoliosis screening, Abbott (1977) found that 34% of the 19,000 children screened for scoliosis in Scarborough, Ontario, Canada, were referred for a physician's examination. Of the 386 children seeing a physician, 58 received treatment and 5 had surgery for scoliosis. Benson, Wade, and Benson (1977) found that 17% of the 7,815 students screened were reexamined by the orthopedist and 1.5% were diagnosed to have scoliosis.

As the result of heart sound screening, an average rate of 13.8 per 1,000 children were referred for medical care (Dennison & Fenimore, 1971). The prevalence rate of abnormal forced expiratory flow rate was 3.1% among 7,063 grammar school children (Hyde, Bharani, Moore, Murray, & Haggerty, 1979). Screening for emotional disorders showed that 6% to 8% of the children were markedly maladjusted and 33.7% were somewhat maladjusted (Kolvin, Garside, Nicol, Leith, & MacMillan, 1977). A high prevalence rate of inflamed ears, perforated drums, and scarred drums was found among 5- to 17-year-olds, and the cost for ear screening by trained nurses was estimated at 53 cents per child (Stanhope, Aitchison, Swindells, & Frankish, 1978).

Kohler (1977a) reported that 186 of the 2,887 children screened needed further follow-up. Functionally, important health problems found among these children included visual defects, motor disturbances, obesity, bacterium, and hearing defects. About half of the identified health problems were known previously. Henzell (1977) revealed that 20 nurses identified 260 children as having heart murmurs. Medical officers confirmed a significant murmur in 15 of these 260 children, and 6 of these 15 had organic heart diseases. None of these 6 children had been missed by a nurse at the preliminary examinations. In summary, the investigators believed that referral would be a key factor to managing successfully the children's health problems.

Factors influencing the outcomes of referrals were suggested for further study. Cauffman's (1968) study of the factors affecting outcomes of referrals is discussed later in this chapter. Parent education and coordination of the efforts of nurses and other health professionals also were suggested for further study by the authors of these studies, but no specific research questions were posed.

Periodic examination. Because of the importance of their research on periodic examination of school children by physicians, four articles are discussed preliminary to the review of seven articles related to physical examinations conducted by nurse practitioners in schools. In the early 1950s, Yankauer and Lawrence (1955) conducted a study on physical examinations of school-age children. The overall purpose of the study was to define the value of periodic medical examinations in the school setting and to clarify the role of school physicians in the periodic examination. The population consisted of 6,906 first graders from 39 public and parochial schools in a single, medium-size city. Of the 1,056 children examined annually, 221 (21%) had adverse conditions. Of these, 78% already were receiving medical care. An additional 12% were known to the school as having health problems but were not receiving care. A total of 21 children (2%) had an adverse condition that could not have been observed by the classroom teacher.

In a further study, Yankauer and Lawrence (1956) found that less than 4% of the children with new adverse conditions were not receiving medical care nor were their conditions known to the school personnel. More health problems were found in younger children, and the number of problems decreased as the grade increased. Although general feelings about physicians, family doctors, and specialists were positive, the parents' knowledge of health care did not increase (Yankauer et al., 1961). The investigators recommended that the school health program should be tailored to meet the needs of individual school populations and not rely on periodic examinations as the prime element of the health program.

Because of the questionable value of the medical examinations as a case-finding method, four other methods of case finding were studied. Of these, teachers' observations and referrals and parent questionnaires were the most fruitful methods, while height–weight growth chart analysis and review of absenteeism records were not as productive (Yankauer, Frantz, Drislane, & Katz, 1962). A federally funded in-depth study of teacher observation and referral as a case-finding method is being conducted by the senior author of this chapter and colleagues. The project is entitled Health Awareness Program Conducted by School Nurses: Case Finding for Elementary School Personnel, and the final report was due in June 1984.

Seven additional articles were reviewed. Of the 849 children screened, 7% had mental, emotional, or behavioral problems, 24% had physical conditions, and 29% had developmental problems such as speech, language, or coordination disorders (Asbed, Schipper, Varga, & Marlow, 1977). About 13% of the 6,058 children examined had an abnormality previously undetected or inadequately followed (Grant, Fearnow, Hebertson, & Henderson, 1973). About 40% of 1,953 children from 12 elementary schools in a city in the southern United States had height and weight disproportions (Humphrey, 1979).

In another study, Kohler (1977b) reported that 15% of the 649 children examined had important health problems: 7.3% were newly detected and 7.7% were known previously. Kornfalt, Jonsson, and Roslund (1979) reported that more than 50% of 410 children had slight deviations from normal, most commonly of the spine and the skin. The nurses detected more deviations than the doctors. The nurses' assessments showed good agreement with those of the physicians concerning functionally important deviations. About 60% of the medical defects causing the rejection of young men for military service were recorded on the documents of the school health service (Lee, 1958). Screening of children from medically indigent families revealed that two thirds of abnormalities found were judged not significant by the examining physicians and the cost was $40 per visit (Sweeney, 1981).

For further studies, validation of screening tools for clinical observation is needed (Asbed et al., 1977). Although trained paramedical personnel or volunteers may be used in screening visual acuity, hypertension, albuminuria, and obesity, evaluation studies are needed to determine the accuracy of paramedical personnel or volunteers in conducting the screening. Because of the high cost of screening and the relatively small number of conditions found, alternative methods of screening should be considered, such as identifying high-risk populations or the use of parents and teachers as the first-line screeners. Intervention studies should be developed by the nurses to seek alternative ways for better coordinated programs of health screening and follow-up.

School Health Services Including Nurses

Sixteen articles were reviewed in this category: twelve were in general areas of school health services, two in mental health, and two in evaluation of school health services. To improve health services to the targeted populations, adequate nursing time for pupil evaluation, referral, and follow-up on health problems was needed (Bourne, 1971). The follow-up of children with health defects by school nurses through telephone and home visits significantly improved the rate of defect corrections (Callan & McCray, 1972; Campbell, Garside, & Frey, 1970). Illnesses of the respiratory system contributed to 64.4% of all illnesses among the school-age children (MacCarthy & Morison, 1972). Chinn (1973) argued that since a healthy child more likely would achieve adequately in the classroom regardless of socioeconomic standing, school health services aimed at general health promotion should be provided. The school attendance rates were determined by complex factors, particularly race and sex (Kaplan, Lave, & Leinhardt, 1972). Families with a low need for medical and dental services used more health care than those families with a high need for services (Leopold, 1974).

Utilization of services within the school programs was demonstrated in five studies. When a comprehensive high school clinic was established, the use of the clinic increased by two thirds over the previous year equally for boys and girls (Edwards, Steinman, & Hakanson, 1977). Nader, Gilman, and Bee (1980) indicated that visits to the school health room accounted for 85% of all contacts between pupils and health personnel. A school health pilot project on delivery of services through a neighborhood health center was developed by Nader, Emmel, and Charney (1972). Comparison of this pilot project with a traditional school health program indicated a need for further program development and evaluation.

According to C. E. Lewis, M. A. Lewis, Lorimer, and Palmer (1977), children's patterns of using health services were similar to those of adults. Rates of utilization were associated with those variables known to affect adult patterns of use: sex (female), social class (more affluent), ordinal position (only child or youngest child), and health orientation. The pattern of use was not associated with the presence of known medical problems. Children who had used the health service system placed greater emphasis on their own responsibilities for maintaining their health. To analyze cost and benefit of health service activities, Newman, Newman, and Martin (1981) reported that the cost for the school was $7,460 to provide health services for 294 students for the 36 weeks of the school year. This cost equaled $43.12 per school day for all students, or $1.89 per student contact with a school health team member.

Several authors offered suggestions for further studies. These included (a) the development of school health programs to assist children in learning the appropriate use of health resources and in taking responsibility for one's own health care (Lewis et al., 1977; Nader et al., 1980), (b) a further cost and benefit analysis of health programs provided in various school settings (Newman et al., 1981), and (c) a determination of the relationships among specific health problems and school achievements (Chinn, 1973).

For mental health services, two articles were reviewed. Crosby and Connelly (1970) found that learning stress was the most common manifestation of mental health problems. Cvejic and Smith (1979) found that 80% of the students referred for mental health problems were from grades seven to nine, and the majority of them were followed by a nurse.

Two articles were reviewed in relation to the evaluation of school health services. Gilman and Nader (1979) reported that (a) 84% of 622 children contributed to the 2,409 episodes of health care during the first year of the study and (b) of the 505 children involved in a preventive school health program, 90% had their immunizations up to date, were screened for vision and hearing, and had defects corrected. Howell and Martin (1978) described the implementation of health policies in the local schools in the State of Virginia.

The investigators cited above had diverse views of school health services and, thus, many approaches to research in this area were observed. Some believed the school health service should be a generalized health service. Some believed school health service should be oriented to health problems, while others believed that it should be targeted for specific population groups. The investigators also differed in their views of the relationship between school health services and community health services. Thus, to discuss a general model of school health services for all school districts would be unrealistic. Nader et al. (1972) piloted a model in Rochester, New York, and concluded that different types of health problems were handled in school health services and community health care systems. Lewis et al. (1977) advocated another model, which placed the responsibility for seeking health care on the children, but did not mention the relationship between school health services and community health services. While the model of school health services may differ in various settings, the relationship between school health services and community health services remains a central issue for further research.

School nurses play an essential role in school health services, particularly in follow-up on health problems (Bourne, 1971). School nurses must come to a consensus about their role in school health services and define the scope of their services to guide research in this area. Most importantly, the nurses must specify the measurable outcomes of their services. If the nursing services are a part of the community health care system, to what extent does the school nursing service contribute to this larger system? On a more philosophical level, if primary health care is a right of everyone, should the school be a primary health care site for children? What can the school nurses do to provide primary health care? Research on school nursing is needed to answer these questions.

Referrals and Follow-up by Nurses

Eleven articles were reviewed in this section. A large-scale study conducted by Cauffman and associates was reported in six papers between 1967 and 1969; five of these reports dealt with referral. Several important findings specific to the study questions were reported (Cauffman, 1968; Cauffman, Affleck, Warburton, & Shultz, 1969; Cauffman, Petersen, & Emrick, 1967; Cauffman, Roemer, & Shultz, 1967; Cauffman, Warburton, & Shultz, 1969). The three best independent estimators of outcome of referral were methods of notification, social rank, and parents' urgency rating. Insurance coverage was associated with a greater likelihood of corrective care. For all six ethnic groups, having a family dentist was associated with receiving attention. Naming a family physician and the use of medical clinics were associated with receiving care. The optimal referral pattern was a written notice by a physician and a telephone call by a nurse. The potency of this pattern was linked with two notifications and two contact techniques. Central to these notifications and techniques was the personal contact between school personnel and parents. In an additional study, Cauffman, Casady, Randall, Warburton, and Shultz (1969) investigated whether the nurses' personal attributes affected the children's receipt of care. The marital status, age, religion, education, ethnicity, absenteeism, and length of services of the nurses were not associated with the referral outcomes.

In summary, the findings from the Cauffman et al. studies cited above gave clear direction for referral and follow-up of children in need of health care. They demonstrated that personal contact of school health personnel with the parents produced a beneficial effect on obtaining health care. The findings suggested that the school health service personnel should establish good interpersonal relationships with the parents. The communication and coordination skills of school health personnel, especially the school nurses, were the key to successful referral outcomes.

The remaining five studies in this section provided additional insights. The referral rates for children with health problems and defects were 72.8% and 66.7%, respectively (May Lan, Lowenstein, Sinnette, Rogers, & Novick, 1976). An average of 1.55 health problems per pupil were found among 109 second graders (Gabrielson, Levin, & Ellison, 1967). Students receiving nursing follow-up had a 32% higher rate of dental visits than those without nursing follow-up (Oda, Fine, & Heilbron, 1980). Effectiveness of follow-up of health referrals did not differ between health programs administered by the board of education and those administered by the health department (Patterson, 1969). Using school nurses to review immunization records and invite immunization-deficient children to a school-based clinic raised the level of immunization at school and decreased unnecessary immunizations (Vernon, Connor, Shaw, Lampe, & Doster, 1976).

Based on the suggestions of the above investigators, further areas for study include (a) determining the effects of concentrated health services for high-risk groups of children, (b) identifying ways to improve the health record system, and (c) using telephone calls extensively as a method of personal contact with parents.

Visits to School Nurses

Five articles were reviewed in this section. According to McKevitt, Nader, Williamson, and Berrey (1977), the average rate of visits to the school nurse was 602 visits per 1,000 pupils per school year for elementary schools, 607 for middle schools, and 466 for high schools. Girls visited the sickroom more often than boys (Newman & Newman, 1979). High users of the sickroom in a given semester tended to be the high users in the following semester, and the same trend was true for the low users. Children visiting school nurses frequently were black, from broken families, from families in which mothers had been hospitalized for illness during the previous year, low in academic achievement, highly dependent on their teacher, and less accepted by their peers (VanArsdell, Roghmann, & Nader, 1972). Peak numbers of visits to the school nurses occurred on Mondays and Fridays, with a minimum on Wednesdays.

The children making repeat visits to the nurse had a higher dependency on their teacher score than those children not making repeat visits (Stamler & Palmer, 1971). Most children initiated their own visits. However, three quarters of the visiting children discussed the problem with someone prior to the visit, and a quarter came with a friend (Snyder, Minnick, & Anderson, 1980). An exploration of means to meet the needs of these children and to identify the children needing assistance were suggested by the investigators.

Knowledge, Role, and Function of School Nurses

Seven articles were reviewed; six were related to role and function of school nurses, and one was related to knowledge level of the nurses. In 1963, the Illinois Association of School Nurses conducted a study of functions of school nurses as perceived by superintendents, principals, teachers, and school nurses. The opinions of elementary and secondary school principals corresponded well with those of the superintendents (Fricke, 1967).

The types of activities performed by school nurses vary by level of schools. Health counseling and conferences were given priority at elementary, junior high, senior high, and two-year college levels (Lowis, 1969). The time spent by the nurse in direct contact with the students and in parent interaction by phone increased as the school level increased (Gilman, Williamson, Nader, Dale, & McKevitt, 1979). The activities performed by the nurse in conjunction with the school staff varied little among school levels (Gilman et al., 1979).

In terms of role perception, Forbes (1967) indicated that teachers' perceptions of the school nurse role were affected by the administration of school health programs, level of the school, and the amount of time spent by the nurse in a given school. Three problem areas for the nurses were relations with teachers and school staff, relations with school administrators, and unessential duties (Grossman, 1956). Educators generally perceived the nurse as needing to care for the sick and injured (Greenhill, 1979).

The six articles on role and functions of school nurses are pieces of research conducted independently by various investigators. The findings often are unrelated to one another and too diversified to warrant a conclusion. The use of a conceptual framework for studying the school nurse role is indicated. Data-based articles are needed to provide evidence of the effectiveness of the role. Clearer specification of the nurse's role, instrument development for measuring role behaviors, and improvement of sampling for increasing generalizability of the results are essential steps in studying the role. Only one investigator reported the knowledge level of the nurses. When 129 high school nurses in Massachusetts were surveyed, only 32% of them had an adequate level of basic knowledge about syphilis and gonorrhea (McGrath & Laliberte, 1974). Obviously more studies are needed in determining the knowledge of nurses in various health areas.

Nurse Practitioners in Schools

Both school nurse practitioners and pediatric nurse practitioners work with school-age children. While school nurse practitioners work exclusively in school, pediatric nurse practitioners may work in schools as well as in other settings. Thus, both specialties of nurse practitioners were included in this review, if they were functioning in school health programs. Seven articles are reviewed in this area.

To compare the care provided, school nurse practitioners were less likely to exclude students from school and to refer them to physicians than traditionally prepared school nurses. Parents were able to recall school nurse practitioners' advice better than school nurses' advice (Hilmar & McAtee, 1973). School nurse practitioners spent more time with patients, saw more students per day, had more contacts with parents, and worked longer than did regular school nurses (McAtee, 1974).

Percentages of time allotted by school nurse practitioners were 12.8% for administration, 11.2% for history taking, 10.7% for physical examination, 13.7% for recording, 14.1% for health education, and the remaining time for other activities (Brink, Dale, Williamson, & Nader, 1981). Eight of the nine nurse practitioners used physician consultation by phone. For management procedures, both verbal and written standing orders were used. Five of the nine nurse practitioners examined 21 to 25 students per week (Dungy & Mullins, 1981). Better problem identification and improved access to community health care were cited as the result of instituting nurse practitioners in a traditional urban high school (Nader, Conrad, Williamson, McKevitt, & Berrey, 1978).

The cost for a Child Health Disability Prevention (CHDP) program for the 1977 to 1978 school year was reported as $11,036, and the cost per student physical averaged $43.44. The parents indicated overwhelming approval of the nurse practitioner services (Dungy, Knapper, Givner, & George, 1980). Evaluation of the impact of school nurse practitioners in a public school revealed that (a) teachers and principals were in favor of increasing nursing services for the students; (b) school nurse practitioners seemed promising in expanding the nursing services, although legal restriction in treatment must be considered; (c) children's attitudes and beliefs did not differ for nurse or nurse practitioners; and (d) parents were enthusiastic about the nurse practitioner services (Lewis, Lorimer, Lindeman, Palmer, & Lewis, 1974).

Questions for further study were raised. What is the impact of nurse practitioner services on the health status of school-age children and their learning behaviors? How do institutional factors such as assignment to several schools and availability of clerical assistance affect the productivity of the school nurse practitioner? What will be the cost documentation and cost effectiveness of nurse practitioner services beyond the physical assessment?

Views and Attitudes of Children

Five articles were reviewed on this topic. Brodie (1974) found that the views of healthy children toward illness differed from those of ill children and those of children with a high level of anxiety. The greatest concerns having health implications for the adolescents were school problems, drugs, sex, getting along with parents and adults, acne, depression, and obesity. The degree of these concerns for each individual was influenced by such factors as ethnic background, grade level, and sex of the individual (Parcel, Nader, & Meyer, 1977).

To study the effect of the drug education program on students' feelings toward drugs, the fifth graders could give reasons for taking drugs, but did not understand the complicated pharmacology of the drugs and distorted much of this information (Richardson, Nader, Roghmann, & Friedman, 1972). Adolescents' perceptions of sex education needs included such topics as marriage and parenthood, birth control and contraception, and strategies to understand themselves (Shirreffs & Dezelsky, 1979). Friends and media were important sources of sex information. For preschoolers and first graders, modeling of adult, peer, and sibling behaviors was associated with learning to smoke (Shute, St. Pierre, & Lubell, 1981). Exploration of alternative approaches to drug education, determination of effective means for sex education, and initiation of health education programs for smoking at kindergarten or first grade levels were suggested for further study.

Health Education Program Related to Nursing

Five articles were reviewed for this section. Health knowledge of 12th graders attending public schools was weak and their scores did not differ by sex, but differed by school (Conley & Jackson, 1978). For 50 children with asthma, their mean health locus of control and self-concept scores were comparable to those of healthy children (Green & Kolff, 1980). Giving health instructions in Grade 2 was most effective and in Grade 5 was least effective (Wantz & DuShaw, 1977). Teaching growth and development was most successful and teaching nutrition and family health was least successful.

The cardiovascular school health curriculum was successful in improving knowledge levels of ninth graders from two schools in the Southwest (Holcomb, Carbonari, Weinberg, & Nelson, 1981). In another study, 21% of the 95 students from two schools in the New York area had one or more measurements in cardiovascular health that appeared above optimal levels (Williams, Carter, Wynder, & Blumenfeld, 1979). To determine chronic disease risk factors for children, a full-scale controlled intervention study was suggested.

School Health Team

Three articles were reviewed. In studying role consensus, members of the school nurse, school physician, and health coordinator groups were found to have consensus on their roles. However, the consensus was highest in the nursing group (Chen, 1975). School nurses spent only about one third of their time on school nursing activities (Rosner, Pitkin, & Rosenbluth, 1970) and their major concerns were time and work load (Thomas, 1976). The need exists to delineate the roles of each member of the school health team, to increase the time spent by school nurses on direct health services, and to determine the effects of setting and educational background on the functions of an interdisciplinary team and its respective members.

Health Aides

The efforts of health aides were found to affect the use of time by the school nurses or nurse practitioners. The nurses readily delegated first aid and housekeeping activities to the health aide, but were slow in shifting the routine paper work (Dale et al., 1978).

Survey of School Health Programs

The status of state level school health programs including school nurse certification, school health educator certification, and state school health education programs was surveyed (Castile & Jerrick, 1976). Because of the lack of a universal standard and diversity in school nursing certification, the application of the results is limited. However, the responses from each state were tabulated.

DISCUSSION AND RESEARCH DIRECTIONS

The literature reviewed in this chapter shows a wide and diversified interpretation of the mission of school nursing, reflecting the range of characteristics of other health care delivery systems in this country. In effect, no specific form of service emerged as a prevailing pattern for offering and evaluating school nursing services. As an integral part of the school health program, direction for further research may be found in the description of overall school health program goals and services. This general literature must be reviewed in regard to its correspondence with the approaches and findings within the research in school nursing per se.

Four overall directions for the future of research in school nursing became apparent to the authors during this review. They are (a) the need for a conceptual framework upon which to base school nursing services and research, (b) the development and improvement of research methods to be used in the study of school nursing, (c) the provision of nursing leadership for school health services research, and (d) the relationship of school nursing with community health nursing.

Need for a Conceptual Framework

For school nursing to contribute to the scientific discipline of nursing, nurses must build a conceptual base upon which knowledge can be generated, modified, or advanced. It is difficult to determine the systematic development of research approaches among the 82 articles reviewed. A conceptual framework is needed to describe this knowledge base. Refinement of the mission of school nursing and development of a conceptual framework for practice and research becomes critically important for further development in this area.

Improvement in Research Methodology

Researchers in school nursing and school health must increase their levels of sophistication in research methodology. As mentioned previously, the overwhelming majority of studies were descriptive. While the descriptive study is important in understanding a phenomenon, a higher level of research design is more powerful in testing hypotheses or theories pertinent to the phenomenon described. Particularly lacking in the studies reviewed was the evidence of reliability and validity of instruments used in collecting data.

In addition, nursing intervention studies are needed urgently to evaluate approaches used in practice. To conduct such studies, efforts must be made to identify outcome measures related to the clients, the school children. The proof of the value of school nursing ultimately is based on the health status of the clients. Unfortunately, obtaining direct outcome measures is not always possible; the use of process measures also should be considered. A linkage between the process and outcome measures is essential in demonstrating the value of school nursing services. For example, an increased number of visits to school nurses by the children could be an indication of the need for school nursing. It would be far better, however, if one could demonstrate that the increased number of visits to school nurses would reduce the absenteeism due to illness. Thus, researchers in school health, both nurses and nonnurses, should be research-prepared and capable in the areas of experimental design, sampling, measurement, and data analysis and interpretation.

Nursing Leadership in School Health Services Research

A substantial contribution has been made by nurses in research on school nursing services. However, more nursing leadership is needed in this area. An examination of the literature revealed that school nursing services were influenced heavily by nonnurse researchers. For example, in the areas of health screening, periodic examination, referrals and follow-ups, and use of nurse practitioners, the most widely published researchers were not nurses.

The lack of nurse researchers has been a detriment to school nursing research in at least two ways. First, since nursing provides the bulk of the work force in school health services, this profession has a great deal to contribute to the study and improvement of its own practice. Although the research of other investigators can set goals for child health, and validate the general contribution of nursing, nurses must take responsibility for studying school nursing from a nursing perspective, investigating how the nursing process is to be carried out for maximal effectiveness. This involves study of the relevant variables identified by nurse clinicians and the integration of research findings into the education of school nurses.

The second way that the lack of nurse researchers has retarded progress in this field is in the dearth of systematic, sequential study. Nurses most familiar with this field of practice are likely to maintain a commitment to serious evaluation research over time. They also are most likely to select variables for study that are relevant to nursing practice and to contribute to the building of a conceptual framework upon which knowledge for practice and research is generated.

It is clear that more nurse researchers are needed for school nursing and these nurse researchers should be prepared at the doctoral level. The research training should include skills in conducting independent research and working with investigators from multidisciplinary areas. Some master's nursing programs may have included school nursing as a specialty area, but more emphasis is needed on research in school nursing by nurses at the doctoral level.

Relationships of School Nursing with Community Health Nursing

In the 82 articles reviewed investigators were generally vague on the relationships between community health and school health. Nurses must assume leadership in defining the relationships between community health nursing and school nursing. Is the practice of community health nursing and school nursing the same specialty, but in different settings? If so, in what way do these two specialties differ? Can the same conceptual framework be used for both community health nursing and school nursing? If school nursing is a part of community health nursing, how should these two services be coordinated to meet the needs of children both inside and outside the school programs?

SUMMARY

In summary, the relative sophistication of research in school nursing and analyses of the content of research by subject areas were presented. Suggested future directions include development of a conceptual framework for research and nursing interventions, an increase in the level of research methods sophistication, preparation of nurses at the doctoral level for clinical nursing research, and refinement of relationships between community health nursing and school nursing. Nurses must be prepared well to assume more leadership roles in school nursing services and related research.

REFERENCES

Abbott, E. V. (1977). Screening for scoliosis: A worthwhile preventive measure. *Canadian Journal of Public Health, 68,* 22–25.

Asbed, R. A., Schipper, M. T., Varga, L. E., & Marlow, III, E. S. (1977). Preschool roundup: Costly rodeo or primary prevention? *Health Education, 8*(1), 17–20.

Basco, D. (1963). Evaluation of school nursing activities. *Nursing Research, 12,* 212–221.

Basco, D., Eyres, S., Glasser, J. H., & Roberts, D. E. (1972). Epidemiologic analysis in school populations as a basis for change in school-nursing practice—Report of the second phase of a longitudinal study. *American Journal of Public Health, 62,* 491– 497.

Benson, K. D., Wade, B. A., & Benson, D. R. (1977). Results of school screening for scoliosis in the San Juan Unified School District, Sacramento, California. *The Journal of School Health, 47,* 483–484.

Bourne, I. B. (1971). A pilot project for improvement of school health services. *The Journal of School Health, 41,* 288–292.

Brink, S. G., Dale, S., Williamson, M. C., & Nader, P. R. (1981). Nurses and nurse practitioners in schools. *The Journal of School Health, 51,* 7–10.

Brodie, B. (1974). Views of healthy children toward illness. *American Journal of Public Health, 64,* 1156 –1159.

Brophy, H. E. (1970). "Project Pursuit": A health defect follow-up activity. *The Journal of School Health, 40,* 186 –189.

Bryan, D. S., & Cook, T. S. (1967). Redirection of school nursing services in culturally deprived neighborhoods. *American Journal of Public Health, 57,* 1164 –1176.

Callan, L. B., & McCray, A. (1972). Case studies on remediable health defects. *The Journal of School Health, 42,* 528–532.

Campbell, M. T., Garside, A. H., & Frey, M. E. C. (1970). Community needs and how they relate to the school health program: S.H.A.R.P.—the needed ingredient. *American Journal of Public Health, 60,* 507–514.

Castile, A. S., & Jerrick, S. J. (1976). School health in America: A summary report of a survey of state school health programs. *The Journal of School Health, 44,* 216 –221.

Cauffman, J. G. (1968). Factors affecting outcome of school health referrals. *The Journal of School Health, 38,* 333–339.

Cauffman, J. G., Affleck, M., Warburton, E. A., & Shultz, C. S. (1969). Health care of school children: Variations among ethnic groups. *The Journal of School Health, 39,* 296 –304.

Cauffman, J. G., Casady, L. L., Randall, H. B., Warburton, E. A., & Shultz, C. S. (1969). The nurse and health care of school children. *Nursing Research, 18,* 412– 417.

Cauffman, J. G., Petersen, E. L., & Emrick, J. A. (1967). Medical care of school children: Factors influencing outcome of referral from a school health program. *American Journal of Public Health, 57,* 60 –73.

Cauffman, J. G., Roemer, M. I., & Shultz, C. S. (1967). The impact of health insurance coverage on health care of school children. *Public Health Reports, 82,* 323–328.

Cauffman, J. G., Warburton, E. A., & Shultz, C. S. (1969). Health care of school children: Effective referral patterns. *American Journal of Public Health, 59,* 86–91.

Chen, S. C. (1975). Role relationships in a school health interdisciplinary team. *The Journal of School Health, 45,* 172–176.

Chinn, P. (1973). A relationship between health and school problems: A nursing assessment. *The Journal of School Health, 43,* 85–92.

Conley, J. A., & Jackson, C. G. (1978). Is a mandated comprehensive health program a guarantee of successful health education? *The Journal of School Health, 48,* 337–340.

Crosby, M. H., & Connolly, M. G. (1970). The study of mental health and the school nurse. *The Journal of School Health, 40,* 373–378.

Cvejic, H., & Smith, A. (1979). The evolution of a school-based mental health program using a nurse as a mental health consultant. *The Journal of School Health, 49,* 36 –39.

Dale, S., Gilman, S., McKevitt, R., Nader, P. R., Williamson, M., & Berrey, R. (1978, October). *Effects of health aides on school nurse/nurse practitioner activities.* Paper presented at the 106th Annual Meeting of American Public Health Association, Los Angeles.

Dennison, D., & Fenimore, J. A. (1971). A heart-sound screening program for elementary children. *The Journal of School Health, 41,* 349–351.

Dungy, C. I., Knapper, D., Givner, B., & George, J. (1980). Pediatric nurse practitioners in a school-based CHDP program. *The Journal of School Health, 50,* 76 –78.

Dungy, C. I., & Mullins, R. G. (1981). School nurse practitioners: Analysis of questionnaire and time/motion data. *The Journal of School Health, 51,* 475–478.

Edwards, L. E., Steinman, M. E., & Hakanson, E. Y. (1977). An experimental comprehensive high school clinic. *American Journal of Public Health, 67,* 765–766.

Forbes, O. (1967). The role and functions of the school nurse as perceived by 115 public school teachers from three selected counties. *The Journal of School Health, 37,* 101–106.

Fricke, E. B. (1967). The Illinois study of school nurse practice. *The Journal of School Health, 37,* 24 –28.

Gabrielson, I. W., Levin, L. S., & Ellison, M. D. (1967). Factors affecting school health follow-up. *American Journal of Public Health, 57,* 48–59.

Gilman, S., & Nader, P. R. (1979). Measuring the effectiveness of a school health program: Methods and preliminary analysis. *The Journal of School Health, 49,* 10 –14.

Gilman, S., Williamson, M. C., Nader, P. R., Dale, S., & McKevitt, R. (1979).

Task differentiation among elementary, middle, and high school nurses. *The Journal of School Health, 49,* 313–316.

Grant, W. W., Fearnow, R. G., Hebertson, L. M., & Henderson, A. L. (1973). Health screening in school-age children. *American Journal of Diseases of Children, 125,* 520 –522.

Green, K. E., & Kolff, C. (1980). Two promising measures of health education outcomes and asthmatic children. *The Journal of School Health, 50,* 332–336.

Greenhill, E. D. (1979). Perceptions of the school nurse's role. *The Journal of School Health, 49,* 368–371.

Grossman, J. (1956). The school nurse's perception of problems and responsibilities. *Nursing Research, 5,* 18–26.

Henzell, J. M. (1977). The expanded role of the school health nurse in paediatric screening. *Australia Paediatric Journal, 13,* 44 – 48.

Hilmar, N. A., & McAtee, P. A. (1973). The school nurse practitioner and her practice: A study of traditional and expanded health care responsibilities for nurses in elementary schools. *The Journal of School Health, 43,* 431– 441.

Holcomb, J. D., Carbonari, J., Weinberg, A., & Nelson, J. (1981). Evaluation of a comprehensive cardiovascular curriculum. *The Journal of School Health, 51,* 330 –335.

Howell, K. A., & Martin, J. E. (1978). An evaluation model for school health services. *The Journal of School Health, 48,* 433–442.

Humphrey, P. (1979). Height/weight disproportion in elementary school children. *The Journal of School Health, 49,* 25–29.

Hyde, J. S., Bharani, S. N., Moore, B. S., Murray, J., & Haggerty, N. (1979). Mass screening of children to detect obstructive pulmonary disease. *The Journal of School Health, 49,* 84–86.

Kaplan, R. S., Lave, L. B., & Leinhardt, S. (1972). The efficacy of a comprehensive health care project: An empirical analysis. *American Journal of Public Health, 62,* 924–930.

Kohler, L. (1977a). Physical health of 7-year-old children. *Acta Paediatrica Scandinavica, 66,* 297–305.

Kohler, L. (1977b). Physical mass examinations in the school health service. *Acta Paediatrica Scandinavica, 66,* 307–310.

Kolvin, I., Garside, R. F., Nicol, A. R., Leith, I., & MacMillan, A. (1977). Screening school children for high risk of emotional and educational disorder. *British Journal of Psychiatry, 131,* 192–206.

Kornfalt, R., Jonsson, B., & Roslund, I. (1979). Physical health screening of school children. *Acta Paediatrica Scandinavica, 68,* 879–885.

Lee, J. A. H. (1958). The effectiveness of routine examination of school children. *British Medical Journal, 1,* 573–576.

Leopold, E. A. (1974). Whom do we reach? A study of health care utilization. *Pediatrics, 53,* 341–348.

Lewis, C. E., Lewis, M. A., Lorimer, A., & Palmer, B. B. (1977). Child initiated care: The use of school nursing services by children in an "adult-free" system. *Pediatrics, 60,* 499–507.

Lewis, C. E., Lorimer, A., Lindeman, C., Palmer, B. B., & Lewis, M. A. (1974). An evaluation of the impact of school nurse practitioners. *The Journal of School Health, 44,* 331–335.

Long, G. V., Whitman, C., Johansson, M. S., Williams, C. A., & Tuthill, R. W. (1975). Evaluation of a school health program directed to children with history of high absence. *American Journal of Public Health, 65,* 388–393.

Lowis, E. M. (1969). An appraisal of the amount of time spent on functions by Los Angeles City School Nurses. *The Journal of School Health, 39,* 254 – 257.

MacCarthy, J., & Morison, J. (1972). An explanatory test of a method of studying illness among preschool children. *Nursing Research, 21,* 319–326.

May Lan, S. P., Loewenstein, R., Sinnette, C., Rogers, C., & Novick, L. (1976). Screening and referral outcomes of school-based health services in a low-income neighborhood. *Public Health Reports, 91,* 514–520.

McAtee, P. A. (1974). Nurse practitioners in our public schools? An assessment of their expanded role as compared with school nurses. *Clinical Pediatrics, 13,* 360 –362.

McGrath, P., & Laliberte, E. B. (1974). Level of basic venereal disease knowledge among junior and senior high school nurses in Massachusetts: A survey. *Nursing Research, 23,* 31–37.

McKevitt, R. K., Nader, P. R., Williamson, M. C., & Berrey, R. (1977). Reasons for health office visits in an urban school district. *The Journal of School Health, 47,* 275–279.

Nader, P. R., Conrad, J., Williamson, M., McKevitt, R., & Berrey, R. (1978). The high school nurse practitioner. *The Journal of School Health, 48,* 649–654.

Nader, P. R., Emmel, A., & Charney, E. (1972). The school health service: A new model. *Pediatrics, 49,* 805–813.

Nader, P. R., Gilman, S., & Bee, D. E. (1980). Factors influencing access to primary health care via school health services. *Pediatrics, 65,* 585–591.

Newman, I. M., & Newman, E. (1979). Utilization patterns of a rural elementary school health-sickroom. *The Journal of School Health, 49,* 322–326.

Newman, I. M., Newman, E., & Martin, G. L. (1981). School health services. *The Journal of School Health, 51,* 423–427.

Oda, D. S., Fine, J. I., & Heilbron, D. C. (1980). School nursing and dental referrals. *The Journal of School Health, 50,* 393–396.

Parcel, G. S., Nader, P. R., & Meyer, M. S. (1977). Adolescent health concerns, problems, and patterns of utilization in a triethnic urban population. *Pediatrics, 60,* 157–164.

Patterson, J. (1969). Effectiveness of follow-up of health referrals for school health services under two different administrative patterns. *The Journal of School Health, 39,* 687–692.

Richardson, D. W., Nader, P. R., Roghmann, K. J., & Friedman, S. B. (1972). Attitudes of fifth grade students to illicit psychoactive drugs. *The Journal of School Health, 42,* 389–391.

Roberts, D. E., Basco, D., Slome, C., Glasser, J. H., & Handy, G. (1969). Epidemiologic analysis in school populations as a basis for change in school nursing practice. *American Journal of Public Health, 59,* 2157–2167.

Rosner, L. J., Pitkin, O. E., & Rosenbluth, L. (1970). Improved use of health professionals in New York City schools. *American Journal of Public Health, 60,* 328–334.

Shirreffs, J. H., & Dezelsky, T. L. (1979). Adolescent perceptions of sex education needs: 1972–1978. *The Journal of School Health, 49,* 343–346.

Shute, R. E., St. Pierre, R. W., & Lubell, E. G. (1981). Smoking awareness and practices of urban pre-school and first grade children. *The Journal of School Health, 51,* 347–351.

Snyder, A. A., Minnick, K., & Anderson, D. E. (1980). Children from broken homes: Visits to school nurse. *The Journal of School Health, 50,* 189–194.

Stamler, C., & Palmer, J. O. (1971). Dependency and repetitive visits to the nurse's office in elementary school children. *Nursing Research, 20,* 254 – 255.

Stanhope, J. M., Aitchison, W. R., Swindells, J. C., & Frankish, J. D. (1978). Ear disease in rural New Zealand school children. *New Zealand Medical Journal, 88,* 5–8.

Sweeney, K. A. (1981, November). *School health screening: Experience and alternatives.* Paper presented at School Health Section of the 108th Annual Meeting of American Public Health Association, Detroit.

Thomas, B. (1976). The school nurse as a member of the school health team: Fact or fiction? *The Journal of School Health, 46,* 466 – 470.

VanArsdell, W. R., Roghmann, K. J., & Nader, P. R. (1972). Visits to an elementary school nurse. *The Journal of School Health, 42,* 142–148.

Vernon, T. M., Connor, J. S., Shaw, B. S., Lampe, J. M., & Doster, M. E. (1976). An evaluation of three techniques for improving immunization levels in elementary schools. *American Journal of Public Health, 66,* 457–460.

Wantz, M. S., & DuShaw, M. (1977). A cooperative project to evaluate health education at the elementary level. *The Journal of School Health, 47,* 462–465.

Williams, C. L., Carter, B. J., Wynder, E. L., & Blumenfeld, T. A. (1979). Selected chronic disease risk factors in two elementary school populations. *American Journal of Diseases of Children, 133,* 704–708.

Yankauer, A., Frantz, R., Drislane, A., & Katz, S. (1962). A study of case-finding methods in elementary schools. I. Methodology and initial results. *American Journal of Public Health, 52,* 656–662.

Yankauer, A., & Lawrence, R. A. (1955). A study of periodic school medical examinations. I. Methodology and initial findings. *American Journal of Public Health, 45,* 71–78.

Yankauer, A., & Lawrence, R. A. (1956). A study of periodic school medical examinations. II. The annual increment of new "defects." *American Journal of Public Health, 46,* 1553–1562.

Yankauer, A., Wendt, G. R., Eichler, H., Fry, C. L., & Lawrence, R. A. (1961). A study of periodic school medical examinations. IV. Education aspects. *American Journal of Public Health, 51,* 1532–1540.

CHAPTER 3

Teenage Pregnancy as a Community Problem

RAMONA T. MERCER
SCHOOL OF NURSING
UNIVERSITY OF CALIFORNIA, SAN FRANCISCO

CONTENTS

During the 1970s, the incidence of teenage pregnancies reached a peak along with increased sexual activity at earlier ages. One in every five births was to a teenager. The large teenage population of the 1970s resulted from

Appreciation is expressed to Dr. Virginia K. Saba, Nurse Consultant, Division of Nursing, Public Health Service, U.S. Department of Health and Human Services, for her assistance in conducting searches of several document retrieval systems that facilitated this review.

the increased birth rate during the World War II years. The total number of women aged 15 to 19 years will decrease by 20% from 10 million to 8 million during the 1980s to account for almost 70% of a projected decrease in the number of teenage births, with the rest attributed to decreasing fertility rates among teenagers (M. M. Adams, Oakley, & Marks, 1982). Although there was a 3.3% decline in the number of births among young women aged 15 to 19 years in 1981 (National Center for Health Statistics, 1982), others argue that pregnancy rates are increasing among teenagers and maintain that the continued decline in birth rates for this age-group is contingent on access to legal abortions (Alan Guttmacher Institute, 1981). Despite the decrease in birth rates projected, teenage pregnancy continues to be a multifaceted community problem because of the wide range of lives affected and the social circumstances related to the problem.

Societal responses to the pregnant teenager have changed over the past two decades, from early attitudes of punitiveness to more current attitudes of concern for providing improved health care and community help for the young woman and her child. During the 1960s, pregnant students were dismissed from school as soon as authorities became aware of their condition. Available maternity residencies frequently admitted only white, middle-, or upper-class adolescents, who were planning to relinquish their infants for adoption. The socially deprived, minority student expelled from school was left with little support from either the community or the health care system. Beginning in 1963 there was a significant change in the health care for pregnant teenagers as several demonstration programs became federally financed. Teenagers faced with an undesired pregnancy had an additional alternative to their problem in 1973 when the United States Supreme Court upheld a woman's right to obtain a first trimester abortion, holding that a state could not intervene in the decision-making process between a woman and her physician regarding abortion (*Roe v. Wade, Doe v. Bolton,* 1973). The adolescent's access to abortion was made easier by the Supreme Court decision in 1976 that prevented a third party from interfering with the decision of a consenting mature minor and her physician to terminate a pregnancy (*Danforth v. Planned Parenthood of Central Missouri,* 1976). In 1976, Title IX of the 1972 Education Amendments was implemented, making it illegal to expel pregnant or delivered teenagers from public schools.

During the years when a punitive climate prevailed toward the pregnant adolescent, little research was directed toward the problem. Prior to 1961, there were no citations in the *Cumulative Index to Nursing and Allied Health Literature* on teenage pregnancy. During 1961 to 1963 only one reference was made to the teenage mother. Since then research focused on the pregnant teenager has increased slowly, but steadily. In 1982 there were

22 references to pregnancy during adolescence. The present review is focused on the community problem of teenage pregnancy as reported by nurse researchers.

METHOD OF LITERATURE SEARCHES

The data base for this review of nursing research on teenage pregnancy as a community problem was the *Cumulative Index to Nursing and Allied Health Literature,* Volumes 1 through 27, 1956 to 1982, extensive searches of several document retrieval systems, "the invisible college" or informal exchange between scientists working on similar problems (Cooper, 1982), and additional searches through *Nursing Research,* Volumes 1 through 31, 1952 to 1982; *Communicating Nursing Research,* Volumes 1 through 15, 1968 to 1982; *Maternal-Child Nursing Journal,* Volumes 1 through 11, 1972 to 1982; *Journal of Obstetric, Gynecologic, and Neonatal (JOGN) Nursing,* Volumes 1 through 11, 1972 to 1982; *MCN, The American Journal of Maternal Child Nursing,* Volumes 1 through 7, 1976 to 1982; *Research in Nursing and Health,* Volumes 1 through 5, 1978 to 1982; *Advances in Nursing Science,* Volumes 1 through 4, 1979 to 1982; and *Western Journal of Nursing Research,* Volumes 1 through 4, 1979 to 1982. A limitation of missing data existed from two sources. Some of the articles cited were in journals that were neither readily available nor obtainable through interlibrary loan for review to determine whether they were research based. Research published in journals of other disciplines also may have been missed if the author was not identified as a nurse.

Because of the complexity of teenage pregnancy and the advantages of interdisciplinary involvement in the problem, when a nurse author was identifiable as one of any number of authors, that research was included. For a report to qualify as research based, the sample was described, and the method of data collection and analysis was mentioned, even if descriptions were missing or incomplete. Single case studies were included. The nursing literature has many papers based on either the author's clinical experiences with, or observations of, the pregnant adolescent, which are not presented as formal research, such as the B. N. Adams, Brownstein, Rennalls, and Schmitt (1976) description of a group approach for counseling pregnant adolescents and the Steinman (1979) guidelines for helping pregnant adolescents; these were excluded from the critical review. Theoretical papers such as Clark's (1964) discussion of the maturational crises facing the adolescent mother, Robbie's (1978) factors to consider in contraceptive counseling for adolescents, and the Panzarine, Elster, and McAnarney

(1981) conceptual model using systems theory for possible intervention in adolescent pregnancy were not included. Reviews of the literature such as Leppink's (1979) review of psychological factors affecting adolescent sexual behavior, or Schodt's (1982) review of adolescent grief following perinatal loss, also were not included.

Two or more references were found for seven of the research projects; different aspects of the project were emphasized in each of the papers. In these situations, the reports were reviewed for content and were considered as one study. An exception was a secondary theoretical analysis of a research project with a second author (Fischman & Palley, 1978) that was reported as two studies. Another research project conducted in two parts was considered as two studies since different populations were studied in each part (Reichelt & Werley, 1975a, 1975b).

METHODOLOGICAL FINDINGS AND ANALYSIS

Research Designs

Seventy-seven research projects were found and categorized by 10 types of research designs. Just over half (n = 39, 50.7%) of the research reports were at the descriptive level (case study and descriptive survey). Nine (11.7%) of the research reports were action research; the projects were undertaken to develop either new skills or new approaches to dealing with the problem of delivering quality health care to the pregnant adolescent Isaac & Michael (1971). The quality of the reported action research varied considerably; however, when the author described a program that was developed to solve a particular problem in meeting the needs of the child-bearing adolescent with some evaluative outcome, the report was included. Seven (9%) of the reports were categorized as evaluation research in which investigators evaluated the accomplishments of a special procedure or method designed to enhance health care for the pregnant adolescent (Treece & Treece, 1977). Fourteen (18%) were ex post facto or causal-comparative designs in which investigators compared two or more groups (Isaac & Michael, 1971). Only one research report was quasi-experimental and only one experimental. One study design had a prospective stage (Phase I in which an initial testing of all female students ages 13 to 15 years in six junior high schools was done) and a retrospective stage (Phase II in which a second test situation and interviews of a subsample who became pregnant during the year of study, a nonpregnant matched control group, a random sample of the total population, and an age-stratified random sample with the same age distribution as the pregnant sample were done).

Measures

Investigator-constructed measures or questionnaires were used in almost a third of the studies reported (n = 25, 32.5%). Of these investigator-constructed measures, only 6 (25%) investigators reported pretesting the tools. Over one fourth (n = 21, 27.3%) used interviews; often the interviews were not described by the type of interview or how the interview was evaluated. No mention was made of the measures in 17 (22%) of the reports. Record review was implied in the evaluation surveys, and observation was implied in some action research. Consequently, most of the measures reported in the 77 studies were used in only the one study. Only two of the instruments were used by more than one investigator. The Tennessee Self Concept Scale (Fitts, 1965) was used by Arnold (1980) and by Mercer, Hackley, and Bostrom (1982a, 1982b). The Broussard Neonatal Perception Inventories (Broussard & Hartner, 1971) were used by Mercer (1980) and Mozingo (1981). Fischman (1975, 1977) used the Rosenberg Self Esteem Scale (Rosenberg, 1965). Elster and Panzarine (1980) used the Offer Self-Image Questionnaire for Adolescents (Offer & Offer, 1972). In one study it was noted that the adolescent's personal appearance was a yardstick for self-esteem (Knight, 1965). With the egocentrism, self-preoccupation, and rapid body changes occurring during adolescence and pregnancy, more studies measuring a facet of self-perception were expected.

In 24 (31.2%) of the reports, the author reported attention to either validity or reliability. In many instances, only the validity of the questionnaire or measure was addressed. Thus, in over two thirds of the research reports, there was no report of validity and reliability of measures used to collect data.

Theoretical or Conceptual Framework

Authors in 44 studies (57.1%) reported a conceptual framework from which the research was approached, although it was not always labeled as such. Adolescent developmental theory alone, or in combination with other psychological changes of pregnancy, coping strategies, cultural impact, and interactional theories, was the framework for half (n = 22) of those studies in which frameworks were reported. In 13 of the reports (29.5%), literature relevant to the specific problem provided the conceptual framework. Investigators of three studies (6.8%) utilized role theory, three used both support theory and pregnancy psychological changes, and two (4.5%) used attachment theory. One researcher (Burbach, 1980) used a nursing theorist's (Orem, 1971) framework.

Sampling

Samples as a whole were convenience samples. Age, ethnicity, and socioeconomic status (SES) were almost always reported. Some samples were either all black or all white, or all lower or middle SES, severely limiting the external validity. Sample sizes were usually adequate for the analyses that were done.

SUBSTANTIVE FINDINGS AND ANALYSIS

The 77 research reports fall into six content categories; each category deals with a facet of the problem of adolescent pregnancy: (a) etiology or prevention, (b) reproductive decision making, (c) prenatal care, (d) intrapartum and postpartum care, (e) family relationships (adolescent mother-grandmother, and adolescent father-other family members), and (f) mothering. In this critique these categories are addressed in the order listed.

Etiology, Prevention

One fifth of the research efforts ($n = 16$) were directed toward preventing the problem of adolescent pregnancy. Only one report was a single case study; this illustrated a program for sex education for a blind, moderately retarded male adolescent (Smigielski & Steinmann, 1981), thus an effort to assist children with multiple handicaps. Seven (43.8%) of the studies were surveys. Three were ex post facto studies, two quasi-experimental, and there was one each with an action, evaluation, and correlational design. These reports focused on relationships with parents, poverty and culture, recreation and hobbies, stressful life events, inadequate knowledge, and psychosocial immaturity as etiological factors in teenage pregnancy.

The Bowns (1969) study stood out as an example of a research design with great potential to discriminate the adolescents who will get pregnant from those who will not. A total of 5,704 female junior high school students were tested in phase one. During phase two, the first 48 who became pregnant were matched with a control group (n = 48) for the variables of intelligence, age, race, grade, SES, place of birth, type of housing, marital status of the parents, ordinal position of the subject in the family, family size, and religious denomination. A second control group (n = 98) was selected randomly from all of those taking the tests during phase one. The major variable, the mother–daughter relationship as reported by the adolescents, failed to show differences between those who later became pregnant and the matched control group. There were differences between the pregnant subjects and the randomly selected control group. Pregnant subjects perceived less positive involvement with their mothers, felt that their mothers used hostile detachment as a means of control, and were less trusting. Since the randomly selected control group (n = 98) had a higher SES and overrepresentation of the younger ages, a third control group of 98 age-stratified, randomly selected subjects from phase one was selected. There were no differences between the pregnancy group and this third control group, indicating that the age factor did not make a difference. Higher SES girls had different perceptions of relationships with their mothers than lower SES girls.

Connell and Jacobson (1971) observed that poor family relationships was a common variable among 50 recently delivered adolescent mothers. Welches (1976/1977, 1978, 1979) surveyed 75 female high school students and observed that the percentage of those having had sexual intercourse differed by the type of relationship with both parents. When the relationship with both parents was good, only 6% reported having had intercourse. When the relationship with both parents was bad, 37% reported having intercourse. When the relationship with the mother was positive and the relationship with the father was negative, 44% reported having had intercourse. When a negative relationship with the mother and a positive relationship with the father was reported, 67% had had intercourse.

Fischman and Palley (1978) used a culture-of-poverty framework to argue that poverty leads to early childbearing, rather than the converse. Adolescents who chose to deliver rather than to have an abortion reflected an adaptive response to the inevitable; they received emotional support from their families for their decision, and some expressed feelings of fatalism.

Teenagers from three cultural groups tended to replicate their mothers' reproductive histories regarding teenage pregnancy (Speraw, 1982).

Blacks ($n = 19$) viewed pregnancy as a positive experience. Hispanics ($n = 10$) looked forward to nurturing and greater maturity, while whites ($n = 10$) were almost universally unhappy and reacted with guilt.

Sadly lacking among deprived groups was either sufficient opportunity for, or participation in, recreation which could provide an arena for achievement, social activities with peers, healthy competition, and expression of aggression. Curtis (1974) observed that 70% of 30 pregnant teenage subjects had no hobby compared to 20 nonpregnant teenage controls, all of whom had hobbies. Almost three fourths (73%) of the 30 pregnant teenagers spent most of their leisure time watching television or sleeping, while most of the nonpregnant teenagers were active in games and sports. Conception occurred in their own homes for one third of 100 subjects, and at two peak periods—Christmas holidays and summer months (Malo-Juvero, 1970).

The virgins in Welches' (1976/1977, 1978, 1979) study fell into two groups, one group with strong family ties, and another group with strong school ties, including many friends, hobbies, and extracurricular activities. The activities associated with school appeared to provide healthy outlets for the teenager.

Robbins (1981) failed to find a relationship between stressful life events among teenagers who were pregnant ($n = 20$) and those who were not ($n = 20$). No single stressful life event occurred more frequently in one of the two groups. Stressful events reported most frequently were hassling by parents, hassling by siblings, breaking up with a close boyfriend, and problems with acne or other body image concerns, such as being too short, too tall, too fat, or too thin. Importantly, Robbins had refined an Adolescent Life-Change Event Scale (Coddington, 1979), which merits further use and testing. Robbins' findings in part may have been due to the small sample size. A physician, using this Scale, observed that 121 pregnant adolescents reported more deaths of parents and grandparents, separations of parents, and illnesses of parents than 261 nonpregnant controls. However, Coddington's control sample differed from the pregnant sample by both ethnicity and SES, with the control sample being largely white with a higher SES.

Teenagers lacked basic knowledge of human anatomy and physiology (Gimpel, 1968; Inman, 1974; Sapala & Strokosch, 1981), as well as knowledge of contraception, abortion, and venereal disease (Reichelt & Werley, 1975a). Educational and counseling programs have the potential to bridge this gap. Rap sessions at a family planning clinic increased the teenager's knowledge of the pill, intrauterine device, diaphragm, and spermicides, but failed to dispel erroneous beliefs about condoms (Reichelt & Werley, 1975a, 1975b).

A potential barrier to effective contraceptive counseling for sexually active young people is the counselor or teacher who may not be comfortable in imparting this information to teenagers. In a survey of 264 student nurses, Elder (1976) found that two thirds did not support sex education for young teenagers. Further, they expressed reluctance to provide contraceptives for those teenagers who desired them. The student nurses were from six different schools in a North Central industrial city. The near-adolescent student nurse may not have been the most effective care provider for the teenager, in contrast to the suggestion by Kocinski (1965) that the student nurse who was viewed as a peer rather than an authoritarian adult may have been more effective with the teenage mother.

Although adolescent developmental theory was the major framework used for investigating adolescent pregnancy, in only one study was the relationship between development and sexual behavior or pregnancy tested. Howe (1981) found no relationship between psychosocial maturity as measured by the Psychosocial Maturity Scale (Greenberger, Josselson, Knerr, & Knerr, 1975) and sexual experience, contraceptive effectiveness, number of sexual partners, attitude toward abortion, birth control, and premarital sex among 95 male and female high school students. For male subjects lower trust scores predicted better contraceptive use. For female subjects better communication skills and resistance to change predicted better contraceptive use. Female subjects were generally more mature, expected a love commitment, had more negative feelings about pregnancy, and assessed their risk for pregnancy lower than did the male subjects. The roles scale of the Psychosocial Maturity Scale reflected knowledge and adherence to appropriate role behavior and discriminated 65.26% of the sample as virgins or nonvirgins. Those who were more skillful in role behavior had a higher rate of virginity. A decline of egocentrism occurred for achievement of role taking, which is also a function of higher cognitive development. Overall, sexual experience appeared to be a phenomenon of age, cultural background, tolerance, and role behavior; those who had sexual intercourse tended to be older, poorer, more often black, more tolerant, and less skillful in appropriate role behaviors than those who did not.

Summary. From the nursing research to date, there was agreement in the studies that teenagers who had negative relationships with their mothers and fathers were more likely to be nonvirgins and were more vulnerable to pregnancy. Adolescents with few hobbies, extracurricular activities, and outside interests also were at increased risk for pregnancy. There was agreement that the adolescent in general had inadequate and inaccurate contraceptive knowledge.

Although there was agreement among the research reports that the culture of poverty was an etiological factor in teenage pregnancy, further research is needed to control for family relationships across all SES levels. The tendency of the teenager to replicate her mother's history of teenage childbearing needs further study with larger samples. The variable, stressful life events, should be studied as a possible etiological factor in adolescent pregnancy, controlling for SES and ethnicity.

Only 3 of the 15 reports pertained to adolescent male subjects attitudes and knowledge tested about reproduction and contraception (Howe, 1981; Inman, 1974; Reichelt & Werley, 1975a). This is a serious gap, especially since Howe's work showed different predictors for male and female contraceptive behaviors. Male subjects were less accessible as research subjects at clinics, however. For example, Reichelt and Werley (1975a) had 1,190 female and 148 male subjects, a ratio of 9:1.

Extension or replication of studies such as Bowns' (1969) would have accelerated progress in identifying the etiology of teenage pregnancy. Bowns was not cited in any of the research reports, suggesting that other researchers were not aware of this important study. Lack of knowledge about this study may stem from the fact that it was not published in the scientific, periodic journals.

Reproductive Decision Making

Reproductive decision making involves a succession of decisions from the initial decision to have sexual intercourse to whether or not to use a contraceptive, whether or not to continue pregnancy if pregnancy occurs, whether or not to relinquish the child for adoption if pregnancy occurs, and whether or not to marry if pregnancy occurs. These decisions may be difficult for the early adolescent who has not reached the stage of formal operations in which she can problem solve and consider alternative possibilities. Six of the 77 research reports (7.8%) focused on reproductive decision making; four of these were descriptive and two were ex post facto designs.

Using an inductive approach Lindemann (1974, 1975) described three stages of problem solving to prevent unwanted pregnancy that young, unmarried women experience. The first was a natural stage during which the young woman did nothing to prevent pregnancy. The second was a peer stage in which the young woman obtained information from peers and experimented with various contraceptive methods. During the third, the expert stage, the young woman consulted a professional. Lindemann observed progression and retrogression among the 2,500 subjects, ages 13 to 26 years.

Burbach (1980) also observed that many pregnant teenagers had retrogressed from the expert stage to the natural stage. Since 94% had adequate knowledge of availability of contraceptives, and 59% had used contraceptives at some time, Burbach identified motivation for pregnancy and attitudes toward, and use of, contraceptives as variables for further research. Burbach's 51 pregnant 15- to 21-year-old subjects cited schools and parents as the most common source for their contraceptive information. A sample of 1,338 nonpregnant teenagers reported friends and the mass media as the two most common sources of sexual information (Reichelt & Werley, 1975a).

Cressy (1976) reported a positive correlation between low-income teenagers' quality of treatment by prenatal and intrapartum nurses and the use of family planning services postpartum in a sample of 235. However, less than one third (31.9%) accepted family planning at six weeks postpartum and returned for follow-up visits; another 34.5% accepted family planning services at six weeks postpartum but did not return for follow-up. This was the first study to show a relationship between subjects' reports of nursing care and the young woman's use of family planning services.

Fischman (1975, 1977) studied 229 black, pregnant teenagers and found differences between the teenager who chose to have her baby and the teenager who chose to have an abortion. Overall, 66% elected to deliver and 34% elected to have an abortion. The highest abortion rate was observed among the 13- to 15-year-olds, followed by the 17- to 18-year-olds. Teenagers with low self-esteem more often chose abortion. Those who chose to deliver had more positive relationships with their mothers; their mothers had less education and more often had unskilled jobs. Subjects had dropped out of school prior to pregnancy, rather than the converse. Age differences were observed in reported relationships with their mothers; 16-year-olds reported the most positive relationships.

Subsequent use of abortion by women who became mothers during their teen years appeared to be to control fertility (Jekel, Tyler, & Klerman, 1977). A follow-up of four groups who delivered a child before the age of 18 indicated that 80% of the women electing to have subsequent abortions had no subsequent term deliveries. Among the most recent group of largely poor, nonwhite school-age mothers, 34% had had one or more abortions.

Devaney and Lavery (1980) surveyed 50 young women who had made the decision to relinquish their infants for advice that they would give other young women, and to assess their impressions about their nursing care. The young women reported that seeing their infants helped in their decision to relinquish their infants; having a visual image to remember was important. Most of them wished that they had seen the infant more often during their hospital stay. Their nursing care did not take into account their needs; they reported that nurses did not come into their rooms very often, and that frequently, nurses forgot to bring their infants to them.

The paucity of research about adoption may reflect the infrequency of having encountered the adoption problem. Only 4% of the unmarried teenage mothers relinquished their children for adoption (Alan Guttmacher Institute, 1981). A decade earlier, 13% relinquished their children; the decrease is thought to be due to the availability of abortion (Alan Guttmacher Institute, 1981).

Summary. Important findings from these reports were the tendency of young women to do nothing to prevent pregnancy when they initially became sexually active, and the tendency to quit using contraceptives or to use them inconsistently once their use was begun. There was a lack of agreement on whether initial contraceptive information was obtained from friends, schools, parents, or the mass media. Importantly, if the nursing care received by the adolescent during her antepartum, intrapartum, and postpartum experience was perceived by the adolescent as sensitive to her needs, she was more likely to return for contraceptive planning and follow-up.

The fact that little research was focused on reproductive decision making points to the need to examine motivation for pregnancy and attitudes toward conception. The lower self-esteem and the poorer relationship with their mothers among those who opted for abortion points out a need to learn more about the teenagers' feelings about themselves in the area of reproductive decision making. Empirical data about factors involved in decision making regarding adoption are needed.

Prenatal Care

Twenty-one (27.3%) of the research reports were concerned with improving the quality of prenatal care for the pregnant teenager. Four were action research designs, four were evaluation, and four were ex post facto. Three were case studies, five were surveys, and one was a correlational study. The case studies illustrated both failures and successes (Anderson, 1976), hostility and distrust (Bomar, 1975), and developmental issues of adolescence in antepartum nursing care (Clark, 1967).

Early action research was important for two reasons; nurses were taking the initiative in setting up programs for pregnant students expelled from school (Day, 1965), and descriptions of the new programs provided models for nurses to emulate in other areas (J. E. Barnard, 1970; Knight, 1965). Russell (1975) developed a counseling record for use as a data-collection tool in providing sexuality counseling along with prenatal care.

Nurse researchers recognized early the importance of interdisciplinary planning of health education classes for unwed mothers (Burton & Holter, 1966), and resource materials for the pregnant unwed adolescent were found lacking (Burton & Holter, 1966; Townsend, 1967). Townsend (1967) extended the work of Burton and Holter (1966) and Knight (1965) in identifying educational needs for the pregnant teenager. In addition, emotional needs were stressed. A major concern of teenagers during the antepartum was the labor and delivery process, with less concern directed toward traditional prenatal class topics (Copeland, 1979; Schroeder, 1975). The majority (73%) of teenagers also were concerned with what would happen to their bodies during pregnancy (Copeland, 1979).

Planned group instruction was ineffectual for 90 students, with interest in topics presented by the students the most rewarding (Iungerich, 1967). In addition to attention to the pregnant teenager's immediate needs and problems, consideration of her life-style was important (Frye & Barham, 1975). Separate classes were suggested for antepartum and postpartum students, because the postpartum teen tended to be rebellious and frightening to her antepartum peers (Iungerich, 1967). Flexibility of objectives and two leaders were recommended because of the extensive energy required (Dickerson & Ovellette, 1982).

Innovative antepartum clinics were developed to encourage better attendance and better outcomes. Nurse-midwifery-directed antepartum programs demonstrated improved outcomes for the teenager receiving care in these clinics (Abbott, 1978; Doyle & Widhalm, 1979). Corbett and Burst (1976) compared adolescents cared for by midwives and by physician residents in the adolescent clinic (N = 270) and concluded that the nurse-midwife's care was comparable to that of the physician, although the midwife tended to overdiagnose. However, 83% of the teenagers in the midwifery group ended pregnancy without anemia compared to 53% in the physician group.

A special antepartum clinic in the school resulted in more prenatal visits, fewer obstetrical complications, fewer low-birth-weight infants, and fewer complicated deliveries, when compared with subjects randomly matched for race and receiving care in a nonschool clinic (Berg, Taylor, Edwards, & Hakanson, 1979). A school clinic well may be more accessible and attractive to the teenager.

Crawford (1980, 1982) observed that social-emotional support accounted for 46% of the variance in pregnancy complications among 50 white, pregnant teenagers, all of whom were single. This finding may explain in part why special clinics directed by nurses who focus on the special needs of the teenager have favorable results.

In a comparison of 14- to 16-year-olds enrolled in a special clinic run by obstetricians and fellows in adolescent medicine (n = 135), with teenagers who received care at neighborhood clinics (n = 100), and 19- to 24-year-olds who were the next case delivered after a teenage subject (n = 100), few differences were found between the two teenage groups (Perkins, Nakashima, Mullin, Dubansky, & Chin, 1978). The risks of the teenagers were no greater than those of the older, more socially stable women. Fewer of the teenagers in the special clinic were seen during the first trimester; 12% were seen after 34 weeks.

In a Canadian study, 14- to 16-year-olds (n = 11) were compared with 25- to 38-year-olds (n = 11) by Hendry and Shea (1980). The teenagers had fewer antepartum visits, more antepartum problems and hospitalizations, with no differences in labor and delivery outcome, but a lower hemoglobin one week postpartum. Although the number of the well-baby visits the first 18 months was the same, the older women took the infants for well-baby care, and the teens went for episodic, special problems. All of the teens had been enrolled in high school, but dropped out during pregnancy.

Summary. Nurse scientists have played an important role in several areas of antepartum care for the adolescent. Nurses pioneered in implementing programs for students who had been expelled from school during the 1960s (Day, 1965; Knight, 1965). Careful work was done to identify the emotional needs of the pregnant adolescent, as well as her informational needs (Burton & Holter, 1966; Copeland, 1979; Dickerson & Ovellette, 1982; Frye & Barham, 1975; Iungerich, 1967; Knight, 1965; Schroeder, 1975).

Innovative antepartum clinics were developed for adolescents in which outcome variables such as anemia, infants with low birth weight, and obstetrical complications were more favorable when care was given by nurse-midwives (Abbott, 1978; Corbett & Burst, 1976; Doyle & Widhalm, 1979) or an interdisciplinary team in a school clinic (Berg et al., 1979). Improved health care with more optimal outcomes for the adolescent and her child has been facilitated greatly by the findings of nursing research.

If a consistent format could be adopted for reporting case studies as suggested by K. Barnard (1983), secondary analysis of several case studies could produce common themes and variables for testing. With some important descriptive work accomplished, quasi-experimental research could be undertaken to test some of the observations. Importantly, cost-effectiveness of different types of antepartum clinics should be measured systematically.

Another question to be addressed is whether antepartum and postpartum students should be separated for teaching purposes as indicated by Iungerich (1967). Usually this is not done in school health education programs.

Intrapartum, Postpartum

Eight of the studies (10.4%) related more to intrapartum, postpartum outcome. Four were case studies with investigators reporting different responses and support measures by nurses (Faril, 1968; Kuhn, 1982; Labrenz, 1976; Mercer, 1979a). Four were ex post facto designs.

In a comparison of 11- to 17-year-olds receiving care by nurse-midwives from 1968 to 1975 (n = 884) with the rest of the obstetric population delivering in 1973 at the same hospital (Chanis, O'Donohue, & Stanford, 1979), no differences were found in prematurity rates. Perinatal mortality was 4.56 per 1,000 among the teenagers compared to 17.6 per 1,000 in older women. Teenagers had higher occurrences of uterine dysfunction, contracted pelvis, toxemia, and anemia. These data showing no differences in prematurity rates and lower perinatal mortality rates among teenagers were in contrast to nonnursing studies (Alan Guttmacher Institute, 1981), which showed high prematurity and mortality rates and further supported the value of nurse-directed antepartum care.

Neeson, Patterson, Mercer, and May (1982a, 1982b) compared pregnancy outcome for three groups: teenagers attending a registered nurse-operated clinic (n = 261), teenagers attending the regular university clinic (n = 318), and 20- to 25-year-olds also attending the regular university clinic (n = 2,655). Teenagers attending the nurse-operated clinic had higher hematocrits on admission to labor and delivery, more spontaneous vaginal births, longer first stage of labor, and fewer cesarean births than the other two groups. They also had more average-size infants than the other two groups, and fewer small-for-gestational-age infants than the teens attending the regular clinic. Among the group managed antepartally by the nurses, fewer infants were admitted to the intensive care neonatal nursery, and infants had higher one- and five-minute Apgar scores compared to the teenage group cared for in the regular clinic. The differences were explained by the low provider-to-patient ratio, highly individualized physical and psychosocial care, and close attention directed to nutritional status during pregnancy.

Teenagers attending a special clinic run by an interdisciplinary team not only made more antepartum and postpartum visits than those attending the usual neighborhood clinics, but they also more often used contraceptives one year postpartum (McAnarney et al., 1978). There were no other differences between groups.

In a retrospective record review of 105 teenagers who were 17 years of age or younger, and who had delivered over a one-year period, 14 (13.3%) of the young women had threatened, attempted, or actually committed suicide (Gabrielson, Klerman, Currie, Tyler, & Jekel, 1970). Emotional illness, marital discord, and physical illnesses were associated with suicide attempts. The suicide attempt and the pregnancy were thought possibly to stem from a common process.

Summary. The absence of research beyond the case study stage in the nursing care of the adolescent during the intrapartum and postpartum leaves a void in evaluating nursing care. Since two researchers reported that adolescents have great concern about labor and delivery during the antepartum period, much more attention should be directed to what happens during this period, and how the adolescent responds to, and is affected by, the process of childbirth.

There was additional support that antepartum care delivered by nurse care providers leads to better postpartum outcomes. Why this occurs has not been tested, although greater emotional and informational support have been implicated. Prospective data are needed to make further comparisons and conclusions about different modes of management and treatment, since retrospective data are lacking in control of independent variables and are vulnerable to inconsistencies in records.

Family Relationships

All 6 of the 77 reports (7.8%) dealing with changes in family relationships brought about by the teenage pregnancy were at the descriptive level. Five dealt with the impact on the teenager's mother and the grandmother's role, and one focused on the teenage father. One case study illustrated how to change existing relationships in the family to prevent recurring problems with the second child of the 18-year-old-mother (Aradine, Shapiro, & Fraiberg, 1978).

Two researchers described phases that the teenager's mother passes through as she adapts to the reality of her daughter's pregnancy. E. W. Smith (1971) identified seven phases: (a) informing process, (b) period of disequilibrium, (c) restoring normalcy, (d) taking on the grandmother role, (e) reality period, (f) a three-generation confusion period following birth, and (g) internalization of the grandmother role. Bryan-Loan and Dancy (1974) observed that the teenager's mother viewed her daughter's pregnancy as a sign of her own inadequacy, a reflection of her own past vulnerabilities, and a threat to her daughter's achievement of desired goals. The first of three phases reported was the silent phase, when the mother knew the daughter was pregnant, and the daughter said nothing about it. This was followed by the question–denial phase during which the daughter denied the pregnancy. The accepting phase was characterized by rationalization, and the grandmother-to-be's active negotiation toward resolution of the problem.

Through exploration of the problems faced by the mothers of adolescent mothers, Poole and Hoffman (1981) described three different situations: (a) the daughter accepts no responsibility for the infant, and the entire burden is placed on the grandmother; (b) the grandmother feels disgraced and, in return, places restrictions on the adolescent, preventing her maturation; and (c) the daughter accepts responsibility for the infant, and the grandmother is available for help and guidance. In later work, Poole, Smith, and Hoffman (1982) surveyed 44 mothers who had a daughter of junior or senior high school age with a child ranging in age from three months to three years. The addition of the infant did not appear detrimental to the mother–daughter relationship; 71% of the grandmothers did not feel that the daughter's infant had affected their plans for their lives, and 79% did not see the child as affecting time available. Time appears to diminish the grandmother's feeling of responsibility for the untimely pregnancy; only three (7%) believed that they were in some way responsible for the pregnancy, but six (14%) believed that others blamed them. Eighty percent of the adolescent mothers in this sample were major caretakers for their child, and 91% of the grandmothers believed that their daughters were doing better than they had anticipated. Only 23% reported that it was strange to be a grandmother, and 95% reported that they enjoyed taking care of the grandchild.

Elster and Panzarine (1980, 1981) studied 15- to 19-year-old fathers-to-be who were of lower SES and mixed ethnicity (N = 16); the research interviews were conducted during pregnancy. These young fathers stressed the isolation, anger, and concern that they were feeling, along with concern about the changes in their lives and having enough money. Half were proud and pleased with the girlfriend's pregnancy, and 25% had negative feelings about the pregnancy. Nine of the 16 were coping adequately with the pregnancy, but six were referred for counseling because they were clinically depressed. Over two thirds (69%) were interested in the birth, and 81% were interested in learning how to take care of the child. The findings indicated that the young father needed more emotional and informational support than usually was forthcoming from health care professionals. This study should be replicated with a larger sample.

Summary. Valuable insights were provided into the adolescent's mother's experiences in resolving the crisis of her daughter's pregnancy. These data are important to the nurse clinician, who needs to assess where the adolescent's mother is in this process, since the young woman's mother often is her major source of support.

Further research is warranted in all areas of family relationships. This is particularly critical, since family relationships were reported as an etiological factor in adolescent pregnancy, and parents may need assistance in order to be helpful to their child during this difficult period. Action research to develop programs for the grandmother and the father-to-be, such as were initiated in the 1960s and 1970s to improve care for the pregnant teenager, is badly needed.

Mothering

Twenty-two of the 77 studies (28.6%) focused on the teenager's mothering, with 9 at the descriptive level of research. Four of the reports were action and 4 were evaluation designs. Two were longitudinal designs, and 1 each was correlational, ex post facto, and experimental.

An action research program of postpartum ward meetings with teenage mothers and nurses was established to overcome the communication barriers between the two groups (Cochran & Yeaworth, 1967). In this program the teenagers preferred to discuss how they felt about their changing bodies and whether they could maintain their social activities, rather than talk about infants and their care. Lenocker and Doughterty (1976) also observed among a small sample of five black mothers, 14 to 16 years of age, that their needs and concerns related more to adolescent needs than to mothering. These findings reflected the egocentrism characteristic of early and middle adolescence.

Shaw (1974) designed a structured child-care program in school to teach teenagers the art of parenting. Initially, the mothers' discussions were focused on particular problems and child development. After a period of time, the group discussion turned to broader issues and personal concerns of the mothers, such as their sexuality or marital problems. Tankson (1976) also described the establishment of a school-based day-care center. Mothers fed their children at lunch hour and attended a class four days a week on child care. The mothers as a group became more relaxed and confident and behaved in a more accepting way toward their infants. Peer pressure to avoid hitting or yelling at the infants was observed.

Others developed a program for a group of 56 mothers of either high-risk or mentally retarded infants, who were under 20 when their infants were born (Levenson, Hale, Hollier, & Tirado, 1978; Levenson,

Hale, Tirado, & Hollier, 1979). Through this program, mothers were able to move away from egocentrism that prevented their focusing on their children's needs and to learn the skills needed to meet their children's needs. Importantly, the mothers learned to make and to act on health-related decisions for their children.

Abbott (1980) analyzed a parenting program for teenagers that failed. Like Iungerich (1967), Abbott noted that postpartum needs were different; postpartum mothers monopolized the time, leaving little time for the frightened pregnant teenagers. Other factors leading to the parenting group's demise were inconvenient location of the meeting room, clique formations, overidentification with the leaders, changing leaders, and a lack of planning and evaluation. These findings provided direction for those planning parenting programs and identifying variables for testing.

In a case study, a 16-year-old's work in taking on the mothering role was described in relation to her self, family, and social systems (Mercer, 1976). Four phases in maternal role attainment were identified for teenage mothers: (a) fairyland phase during the hospitalization period when motherhood is unreal, (b) reality shock phase that occurs the first month at home, (c) give-and-take phase that occurs around the third to fourth months when the young mother decides on pursuing a career and other options, and (d) internalization of the maternal role, which occurs from the sixth through the ninth months (Mercer, 1979b). In this longitudinal study of 14- to 19-year-olds (N = 12) over the first year of motherhood, substantial support from families was observed, but little from peers (Mercer, 1980). Poole (1976) found that the teenage mother who received greater support had greater coping abilities.

Mercer et al. (1982a, 1982b) observed that 15- to 19-year-olds (n = 66) had more unrealistic expectations of their infants at birth and had been much less likely to attend antepartum classes than women 20 to 29 years old or women 30 to 42 years old. The teenage mothers also had a significantly less positive self-concept than the older mothers. However, Arnold (1980) found no correlation between the self-concept and maternal self-confidence among 13- to 17-year-olds (N = 60). No correlation between the self-concept and perceived mothering skills was found for those with no previous mothering skills. There was a significant correlation between the self-concept and maternal confidence among those who had had previous mothering experience.

Three researchers studied initial mother–infant interactional behaviors. Bampton, Jones, and Mancini (1981) tested Rubin's (1963) maternal touch progression among 24 black, low-income 15- to 24-year-olds (all but four were teenagers). There was no progression of maternal touch from fingertip exploration to encompassing the newborn as described by

Rubin, but an immediate reaching out and encompassing behavior. This suggests different behavioral patterns for different cultures, more so than for age. Hardman (1975) observed that 16- to 17-year-olds had more positive and fewer negative responses to their infants and showed greater readiness for maternal behavior than did 13- to 15-year-olds. Since all subjects were black, age was the significant factor.

In an experimental design, Mozingo (1981) tested whether early contact would increase attachment behaviors and promote positive perceptions of the neonate, and whether these behaviors would be mediated by age. Data were collected on 13- to 19-year-olds ($N = 54$) on the second or third postpartum day and again at one month. Adaptive maternal behaviors were influenced by age, but the relationship of contact to age had an additive rather than an interactional effect as hypothesized. Age was significant for the adaptive interactional behaviors at one month.

In an evaluation of 117 teenage mothers attending the well-child clinic specifically designed for them, Brown (1978) concluded that very few problems were encountered by teenagers that were not encountered by older mothers. Teenagers had more support at home and resumed better hygiene and dress sooner. Overfeeding their infants at the advice of grandmothers and peers, as well as inconsistency in care, were commonly observed problems. The young mother under 16 years old had more social problems. Since the teenagers used an authoritarian method of parenting, Brown suggested much support was needed to avoid abuse and neglect. Singer's (1974) observations of child-care methods of 11- to 22-year-olds ($N = 200$) were in agreement with those of Brown. Jarrett (1982) also observed that half of the 15- to 21-year-old mothers ($N = 86$) felt that it was good for babies to cry it out. Controlling behaviors were more frequently reported by older mothers 18 to 21 than by the 15- to 18-year-olds, however. A third felt that praise spoiled a child and did not offer it. Others observed that the majority of the teenagers tended to use the same techniques that their parents used with them (Smith, Mumford, & Hamner, 1979).

Abrums (1979, 1980) observed that teenagers had poor self-concepts as persons, but good self-concepts as parents. The 41 teenagers, 15 to 19 years old, had positive child-rearing attitudes and positive ways of handling irritating child behaviors compared with older women. However, when ways of handling irritating behaviors were categorized by punitive and positive actions, adolescents were more likely to use punitive actions and less likely to use positive behavior than nonabusive adults. Abrums' study was a secondary analysis of data collected for another project (Disbrow, Doerr, & Caulfield, 1977) and represented the richness and potential benefits of working with a mentor.

The physical growth of children of 14- to 16-year-old mothers (n = 3,124) when compared with 20- to 30-year-old mothers who delivered the same year (n = 100) did not differ (Finkelstein, Finkelstein, Christie, Roden, & Shelton, 1982). All children were normal during the first two years of life. Ninety percent of the teenagers who had dropped out of school had no day care for their children; less than 15% were employed. Lack of day-care facilities hampers the teenage mother in either school or employment opportunities. Without these opportunities the cycle of poverty cannot be broken.

Summary. The developmental needs of the early and middle adolescent mother appeared to take priority over infant caretaking needs. Evaluation of programs that focus on the adolescent's egocentric needs prior to introducing infant needs might be fruitful. Nursing research to date has supported the idea that a readiness for early mothering appeared to be more prevalent in the older teenager; however, the older teenager appeared more controlling in the Jarrett (1982) study. Cultural differences in early mothering practices were operative among teenagers and must be considered in future research. Developmental studies are needed to investigate the adolescents' infants over a long term to determine the full impact of rigid, authoritarian mothering practices. Lacking are studies of the adolescent father and his role following the birth of the child.

CONCLUSIONS AND RECOMMENDATIONS FOR FUTURE RESEARCH

Nurse scientists have made important contributions in promoting the health care of the pregnant adolescent and her child, through action and evaluation research, and descriptive survey research. Many variables have been identified which need further testing. Prospective research designed to study the high school student who does not get pregnant, along with the one who does, has much to offer in determining the etiology of teenage pregnancy. Bowns' (1969) research in which she tested a total population before the event of pregnancy occurred permitted the later random selection of groups to compare those who did not become pregnant with those who did. This kind of research is essential if preventive measures are to be effective and if the research is to have an impact on social policy.

The adolescent is faced with complex decision making at the time she is just developing her decision-making skills; to date there is a serious gap in research in this area. Family planning programs have been available readily for several years, yet teenagers continue to have unplanned pregnancies.

Unplanned pregnancies appear to be a combined result of inaccurate knowledge, a tendency to avoid contraceptives when sexual activity is initiated, and a failure to continue to use contraceptives consistently after the decision is made to contracept. There is no information to suggest why this sequence of behavior occurs. Howe's (1980/1981) research merits replication to determine whether role-taking and communication skills are a predictor of contraceptive use in other populations. Even schools that denounce sex education could foster the development of role-taking and communication skills among their students. The poverty-stricken student who has dropped out of school presents a social issue for which further data are needed to effect social policy that would provide a program of activities for these teenagers to enhance both their self-esteem and their communication skills.

Prospective evaluation of programs in which nurses are providing antepartum care assumes much importance in austere times. When outcomes are documented carefully without the hazard of relying on old records, improved outcomes can be proven cost-effective in two ways. The astronomical savings in the prevention of premature and small-for-gestational-age births, with all of their adverse sequelae alone, can be convincing to health policymakers. Further, the cost of care delivered by nurses in extended roles, such as midwifery and practitioner roles, needs further documentation for third-party payment and for public awareness.

Research focused on adolescent pregnancy has been hampered by the lack of measures. Further testing of some of the measures reported is warranted, with more careful attention to establishing validity and reliability. Pretesting is essential since adolescents may rebel at the format or wording of items.

Adolescent developmental theory and psychological changes of pregnancy concepts provide natural frameworks from which to approach many of the problems of adolescent pregnancy. Other theoretical frameworks may prove fruitful; some of the researchers identified motivations for and attitudes toward adolescent pregnancy for future study. Researchers would profit by testing some of the variables in reproductive decision making from a motivational theory framework.

Adolescent pregnancy affects the entire family unit dramatically. Family relationships have been identified as an etiological factor, yet little research has been focused on this area to date. Research including family members other than the adolescent and her mother is badly needed. How are the grandfathers affected? The siblings? The male adolescent and his family are affected also, and there is need for more data from these perspectives if nurses are to have a positive impact on the community by ameliorating the problems of adolescent pregnancy.

REFERENCES

Abbott, M. I. (1978). Teens having babies. *Pediatric Nursing, 4*(3), 23–26.

Abbott, M. I. (1980). Parenting group for teen-agers fails. *Pediatric Nursing, 4*(5), 54–56.

Abrums, M. E. (1979). *Adolescent pregnancy and parenthood.* Unpublished master's thesis, University of Washington, Seattle.

Abrums, M. E. (1980). Adolescent pregnancy and parenthood [Abstract]. In *Communicating nursing research* (Vol. 13, pp. 42–43). Boulder, CO: Western Interstate Commission on Higher Education.

Adams, B. N., Brownstein, C. A., Rennalls, I. M., & Schmitt, M. H. (1976). The pregnant adolescent—A group approach. *Adolescence, 11,* 467– 485.

Adams, M. M., Oakley, G. P., Jr., & Marks, J. S. (1982). Maternal age and births in the 1980s. *Journal of American Medical Association, 247,* 493–494.

Alan Guttmacher Institute. (1981). *Teenage pregnancy: The problem that hasn't gone away.* New York: Author.

Anderson, C. (1976). The lengthening shadow: A case study in adolescent out-of-wedlock pregnancy. *Journal of Obstetric, Gynecologic, and Neonatal (JOGN) Nursing, 5,* 19–22.

Aradine, C., Shapiro, V., & Fraiberg, S. (1978). Collaborating to foster family attachment. *MCN, The American Journal of Maternal Child Nursing, 3,* 92–98.

Arnold, D. (1980). *The adolescent mother: A comparison of her self-concept and her perceived mothering skills.* Unpublished master's thesis, Texas Woman's University, Denton, TX.

Bampton, B., Jones, J., & Mancini, J. (1981). Initial mothering patterns of low-income black primiparas. *Journal of Obstetric, Gynecologic, and Neonatal (JOGN) Nursing, 10,* 174 –178.

Barnard, J. E. (1970). Peer group instruction for primigravid adolescents. *Nursing Outlook, 18,* 42–43.

Barnard, K. (1983). The case study method: A research tool. *MCN, The American Journal of Maternal Child Nursing, 8,* 36.

Berg, M., Taylor, B., Edwards, L. E., & Hakanson, E. Y. (1979). Prenatal care for pregnant adolescents in a public high school. *Journal of School Health, 49,* 32–35.

Bomar, P. J. (1975). The nursing process in the care of a hostile, pregnant adolescent. *Maternal-Child Nursing Journal, 4,* 95–100.

Bowns, B. H. (1969, March). Early adolescent pregnancy in relation to girls' reports of their mothers' behavior. In American Nurses' Association, *Fifth Nursing Research Conference* (pp. 20–34). Kansas City, MO: American Nurses' Association.

Broussard, E. R., & Hartner, M. S. S. (1971). Further considerations regarding maternal perception of the newborn. In J. Hellmuth (Ed.), *Exceptional infant: Vol. 2. Studies in abnormalities* (pp. 432–449). New York: Brunner/Mazel.

Brown, C. A. (1978). Teen-age mother's well-child clinic. *Pediatric Nursing, 4*(3), 27–31.

Bryan-Logan, B. N., & Dancy, B. L. (1974). Unwed pregnant adolescents: Their mothers' dilemma. In H. K. Grace & G. A. Traver (Eds.), *Nursing Clinics of North America, 9,* 57–68.

Burbach, C. A. (1980). Contraception and adolescent pregnancy. *Journal of Obstetric, Gynecologic, and Neonatal (JOGN) Nursing, 9,* 319–323.

Burton, M., & Holter, I. (1966). Health education classes for unwed mothers. *Nursing Outlook, 14,* 35–37.

Chanis, M., O'Donohue, N., & Stanford, A. (1979). Adolescent pregnancy. *Journal of Nurse-Midwifery, 24*(3), 18–22.

Clark, A. L. (1964). Maturational crisis and the unwed adolescent mother. *Nursing Science, 2,* 113–124.

Clark, A. L. (1967). The crisis of adolescent unwed motherhood. *American Journal of Nursing, 67,* 1465–1469.

Cochran, M. L., & Yeaworth, R. C. (1967). Ward meetings for teen-age mothers. *American Journal of Nursing, 67,* 1044–1047.

Coddington, R. D. (1979). Life events associated with adolescent pregnancies. *Journal of Clinical Psychiatry, 140,* 180 –185.

Connell, E. D., & Jacobson, L. (1971). Pregnancy, the teenager and sex education. *American Journal of Public Health,* 61, 1840 –1845.

Cooper, H. M. (1982). Scientific guidelines for conducting integrative research reviews. *Review of Educational Research, 52,* 291–302.

Copeland, D. Z. (1979). Unwed adolescent primigravidas identify subject matter for prenatal classes. *Journal of Obstetric, Gynecologic, and Neonatal (JOGN) Nursing, 8,* 248–253.

Corbett, M., & Burst, H. V. (1976). Nurse-midwives and adolescents: The South Carolina experience. *Journal of Nurse-Midwifery, 21*(4), 13–17.

Crawford, G. (1980). Teen social support patterns and the stress of pregnancy. *Dissertation Abstracts International, 41,* 893B–894B. (University Microfilms No. 80-19,335)

Crawford, G. (1982). The concept of pattern in nursing: Conceptual development and measurement. *Advances in Nursing Science, 5*(1), 1–6.

Cressy, M. K. (1976). Factors related to the use of family planning services by low-income teen-age mothers. *Dissertation Abstracts International, 36,* 6072B. (University Microfilms No. 76-13, 793)

Curtis, F. L. S. (1974). Observations of unwed pregnant adolescents. *American Journal of Nursing, 74,* 100 –102.

Danforth v. Planned Parenthocd of Central Missouri, 428 U.S. 52 (1976).

Day, G. A. (1965). A program for teenage mothers. *American Journal of Public Health, 55,* 978–981.

Devaney, S. W., & Lavery, S. F. (1980). Nursing care for the relinquishing mother. *Journal of Obstetric, Gynecologic, and Neonatal (JOGN) Nursing, 9,* 375–378.

Dickerson, P. S., & Ovellette, M. D. (1982). Prenatal education for adolescents in a delinquent youth facility. *Journal of Obstetric, Gynecologic, and Neonatal (JOGN) Nursing, 11,* 39–44.

Disbrow, M. A., Doerr, H., & Caulfield, C. (1977). Measuring the components of potential for child abuse and neglect. *The Journal of Child Abuse and Neglect: An International Journal, 1,* 279–296.

Doyle, M. B., & Widhalm, M. V. (1979). Midwifing the adolescents at Lincoln Hospital's teen-age clinics. *Journal of Nurse-Midwifery, 24*(4), 27–32.

Elder, R. G. (1976). Orientation of senior nursing students toward access to contraceptives. *Nursing Research, 25,* 338–345.

Elster, A. B., & Panzarine, S. (1980). Unwed teenage fathers. *Journal of Adolescent Health Care, 1,* 116–120.

Elster, A. B., & Panzarine, S. (1981). The adolescent father. *Seminars in Perinatology, 5,* 39–51.

Faril, M. S. (1968). Adolescent in labor. *American Journal of Nursing, 68,* 1952–1954.

Finkelstein, J. W., Finkelstein, J. A., Christie, M., Roden, M., & Shelton, C. (1982). Teenage pregnancy and parenthood: Outcomes for mother and child. *Journal of Adolescent Health Care, 3,* 1–7.

Fischman, S. H. (1975). The pregnancy-resolution decisions of unwed adolescents. In E. R. Sharp & E. J. Worthy (Eds.), *Nursing Clinics of North America, 10,* 217–227.

Fischman, S. H. (1977). Delivery or abortion in inner-city adolescents. *American Journal of Orthopsychiatry, 47,* 127–133.

Fischman, S. H., & Palley, H. A. (1978). Adolescent unwed motherhood: Implications for a national family policy. *Health and Social Work, 3*(1), 30–46.

Fitts, W. H. (1965). *Tennessee Self Concept Manual.* Nashville: Counselor Recordings and Tests.

Frye, B. A., & Barham, B. (1975). Reaching out to pregnant adolescents. *American Journal of Nursing, 75,* 1502–1504.

Gabrielson, I. W., Klerman, L. V., Currie, J. B., Tyler, N. C., & Jekel, J. F. (1970). Suicide attempts in a population pregnant as teenagers. *American Journal of Public Health, 60,* 2289–2301.

Gimpel, H. S. (1968). Group work with adolescent girls. *Nursing Outlook, 16,* 46 – 48.

Greenberger, E., Josselson, R., Knerr, C., & Knerr, B. (1975). The measurement and structure of psychosocial maturity. *Journal of Youth and Adolescence, 4,* 127–143.

Hardman, M. (1975). The younger vs. the older adolescent black mother taking on the nurturing-mothering role. In American Nurses' Association, *Clinical Conference Papers 1973* (pp. 133–141). Kansas City, MO: American Nurses' Association.

Hendry, J. M., & Shea, J. A. (1980). Pre and postnatal care sought by adolescent mothers. *Canadian Journal of Public Health, 71,* 112–115.

Howe, C. A. L. (1981). Psychosocial maturity and adolescent sexual behavior and attitudes (Doctoral dissertation, University of California San Francisco, 1980). *Dissertation Abstracts International, 46,* 4458B–4459B.

Inman, M. (1974). What teen-agers want in sex education. *American Journal of Nursing, 74,* 1866–1867.

Iungerich, A. (1967). High school for unwed mothers. *American Journal of Nursing, 67,* 92–94.

Isaac, S., & Michael, W. B. (1971). *Handbook in research and evaluation.* San Diego, CA: Robert R. Knapp.

Jarrett, G. E. (1982). Childrearing patterns of young mothers: Expectations, knowledge, and practices. *MCN, The American Journal of Maternal Child Nursing, 7,* 119–124.

Jekel, J. F., Tyler, N. C., & Klerman, L. V. (1977). Induced abortion and sterilization among women who became mothers as adolescents. *American Journal of Public Health, 67,* 621–625.

Knight, E. (1965). Conferences for pregnant, unwed teen-agers. *American Journal of Nursing, 65,* 123–127.

Kocinski, R. (1965). The adolescent nursing student and the adolescent unwed mother: A nurse educator's view. *Nursing Science, 3,* 172–177.

Kuhn, J. C. (1982). Stress factors preceding postpartum psychosis: A case study of an unwed adolescent. *Maternal-Child Nursing Journal, 11,* 95–108.

Labrenz, M. (1976). We can help the unwed teen-ager during labor. *Registered Nurse, 39,* 53–56.

Lenocker, J. M., & Dougherty, M. C. (1976). Adolescent mothers' social and health-related interests: Report of a project for rural, black mothers. *Journal of Obstetric, Gynecologic, and Neonatal (JOGN) Nursing, 5,* 9–15.

Leppink, M. A. (1979). Adolescent sexuality. *Maternal-Child Nursing Journal, 8,* 153–160.

Levenson, P., Hale, J., Hollier, M., & Tirado, C. (1978). Serving teenage mothers and their high-risk infants. *Children Today, 7*(4), 11–15, 36.

Levenson, P., Hale, J., Tirado, C., & Hollier, M. (1979). A comprehensive interactional model for health education delivery to teenage mothers. *Journal of School Health, 49,* 393–396.

Lindemann, C. (1974). *Birth control and unmarried young women.* New York: Springer Publishing Company.

Lindemann, C. (1975). Stages of birth control behavior in young, unmarried women. In M. V. Batey (Ed.), *Communicating Nursing Research,* (Vol. 7, pp. 249–258). Boulder, CO: Western Interstate Commission on Higher Education.

Malo-Juvero, D. (1970). What pregnant teenagers know about sex. *Nursing Outlook, 18,* 32–35.

McAnarney, E. R., Roghmann, K. J., Adams, B. N., Tatelbaum, R. C., Kash, C., Coulter, M., Plume, M., & Charney, E. (1978). Obstetric, neonatal, and psychosocial outcome of pregnant adolescents. *Pediatrics, 61,* 199–205.

Mercer, R. (1976). Becoming a mother at 16. *MCN, The American Journal of Maternal Child Nursing, 1,* 45–52.

Mercer, R. T. (1979a). The adolescent experience in labor, delivery, and early postpartum. In R. T. Mercer (Ed.), *Perspectives on Adolescent Health Care* (pp. 302–347). Philadelphia: Lippincott.

Mercer, R. T. (1979b) The adolescent parent. In R. T. Mercer (Ed.), *Perspectives on Adolescent Health Care* (pp. 348–383). Philadelphia: Lippincott.

Mercer, R. T. (1980). Teenage motherhood: The first year. Part I. The teenage mother's views and responses. Part II. How the infants fared. *Journal of Obstetric, Gynecologic, and Neonatal (JOGN) Nursing, 9,* 16–27.

Mercer, R. T., Hackley, K. C., & Bostrom, A. (1982a). Adolescent mothers: Their assets and deficits [Abstract]. In *Communicating Nursing Research* (Vol. 15, p. 59). Boulder, CO: Western Interstate Commission for Higher Education.

Mercer, R. T., Hackley, K. C., & Bostrom, A. (1982b). Adolescent mothers: Their assets and deficits. *Western Journal of Nursing Research, 4,* 59.

Mozingo, J. N. (1981). *Influence of early maternal-infant contact on attachment behaviors of teenage mothers*. Unpublished doctoral dissertation, Walden University, Naples, FL. (University Microfilms No. LD-00491)

National Center for Health Statistics. (1982). *Monthly Vital Statistics Report, 30*(13), 2.

Neeson, J., Patterson, K., Mercer, R., & May, K. (1982a). Pregnancy outcomes in a R.N. run prenatal clinic for teens [Abstract]. In *Communicating Nursing Research* (Vol. 15, p. 60). Boulder, CO: Western Interstate Commission for Higher Education.

Neeson, J., Patterson, K., Mercer, R., & May, K. (1982b). Pregnancy outcomes in a R.N. run prenatal clinic for teens. [Abstract]. In *Western Journal of Nursing Research, 4,* 60.

Offer, D., & Offer, J. B. (1972). The Offer Self-Image Questionnaire for Adolescents. *Archives General Psychiatry, 27,* 529–537.

Orem, D. (1971). *Nursing: Concepts of practice*. New York: McGraw-Hill.

Panzarine, S., Elster, A., & McAnarney, E. R. (1981). A systems approach to adolescent pregnancy. *Journal of Obstetric, Gynecologic, and Neonatal (JOGN) Nursing, 10,* 287–289.

Perkins, R. P., Nakashima, I. I., Mullin, M., Dubansky, L. S., & Chin, M. L. (1978). Intensive care in adolescent pregnancy. *Obstetrics and Gynecology, 52,* 179–188.

Poole, C. J. (1976). Adolescent mothers: Can they be helped? *Pediatric Nursing, 2*(2), 7–11.

Poole, C. J., & Hoffman, M. (1981). Mothers of adolescent mothers: How do they cope? *Pediatric Nursing, 7*(1), 28–31.

Poole, C. J., Smith, M. S., & Hoffman, M. A. (1982). Mothers of adolescent mothers. *Journal of Adolescent Health Care, 3,* 41–43.

Reichelt, P. A., & Werley, H. H. (1975a). Contraception, abortion, and venereal disease: Teenagers' knowledge and the effect of education. *Family Planning Perspectives, 7,* 83–88.

Reichelt, P. A., & Werley, H. H. (1975b). A sex information program for sexually active teenagers. *Journal of School Health, 45,* 100–107.

Robbie, M. O. (1978). Contraceptive counseling for the younger adolescent woman: A suggested solution to the problem. *Journal of Obstetric, Gynecologic, and Neonatal (JOGN) Nursing, 7,* 29–33.

Robbins, R. (1981). A study of the relationship between adolescent pregnancy and life-change events. *Issues in Mental Health Nursing, 3,* 219–236.

Roe v. Wade, Doe v. Bolton, 410 U.S. 113, 179 (1973).

Rosenberg, M. (1965). *Society and the adolescent self-image*. Princeton, NJ: Princeton University.

Rubin, R. (1963). Maternal touch. *Nursing Outlook, 11,* 828–831.

Russell, L. K. (1975). Sexual counseling: An approach to the integration of sexual counseling into the antepartal management of teenagers. *Journal of Nurse-Midwifery, 20*(1), 24–30.

Sapala, S., & Strokosch, G. (1981). Adolescent sexuality: Use of a questionnaire for health teaching and counseling. *Pediatric Nursing, 5*(6), 33–34, 52.

Schodt, C. M. (1982). Grief in adolescent mothers after an infant death. *Image, 14,* 20 –25.

Schroeder, E. (1975). The teenage unwed mother. In A. J. Kalafatich (Ed.),

Approaches to the care of adolescents (pp. 31–47). New York: Appleton-Century-Crofts.

Shaw, N. R. (1974). Teaching young mothers their role. *Nursing Outlook, 22,* 695–698.

Singer, A. (1974). Mothering practices and heroin addiction. *American Journal of Nursing, 74,* 77–82.

Smigielski, P. A., & Steinmann, M. J. (1981). Teaching sex education to multiply handicapped adolescents. *Journal of School Health,* 51, 238–241.

Smith, E. W. (1971). Transition to the role of grandmother as studied with mothers of pregnant adolescents. In *American Nurses' Association clinical sessions, 1970, Miami* (pp. 140–148). New York: Appleton-Century-Crofts.

Smith, P. B., Mumford, D. M., & Hamner, E. (1979). Child-rearing attitudes of single teenage mothers. *American Journal of Nursing, 79,* 2115–2116.

Speraw, S. (1982). *Adolescent motivation for pregnancy in three cultures.* Unpublished master's thesis, University of California, Los Angeles.

Steinman, M. E. (1979). Reaching and helping the adolescent who becomes pregnant. *MCN, The American Journal of Maternal Child Nursing, 4,* 35–37.

Tankson, E. A. (1976). The adolescent parent: One approach to teaching child care and giving support. *Journal of Obstetric, Gynecologic, and Neonatal (JOGN) Nursing, 5,* 9–15.

Townsend, J. (1967). The unmarried, pregnant adolescent's use of educational literature. *Nursing Outlook, 15,* 48–50.

Treece, E. W., & Treece, J. W., Jr. (1977). *Elements of research in nursing.* St. Louis: Mosby.

Welches, L. J. (1977). Factors influencing decisions regarding sexual behavior of adolescent girls (Doctoral dissertation, University of California, San Francisco, 1976). *Dissertation Abstracts International, 37,* 4991B. (University Microfilms No. 77-5277)

Welches, L. J. (1978). Sexual behavior of adolescent girls and perceived parental relationships. *Issues in Mental Health Nursing, 1,* 82–87.

Welches, L. J. (1979). Adolescent sexuality. In R. T. Mercer (Ed.), *Perspectives on adolescent health care* (pp. 29–41). Philadelphia: Lippincott.

CHAPTER 4

Cross-Cultural Nursing Research

TONI TRIPP-REIMER
COLLEGE OF NURSING
UNIVERSITY OF IOWA
AND
MOLLY C. DOUGHERTY
COLLEGE OF NURSING
UNIVERSITY OF FLORIDA

CONTENTS

The purpose of this chapter is to provide a critical review of published cross-cultural nursing research. In conducting the literature search to find materials for this review the authors used the following process. Comput-

The authors wish to acknowledge the technical assistance of Steven D. Warner in the preparation of this manuscript.

erized literature searches were conducted using MEDLINE and MEDLARS for works pairing nursing with culture or ethnicity. The references Sociology, Anthropology, and Psychology Abstracts were surveyed for the topic "nursing." Library card catalogs were surveyed to identify books in this area. After the articles and books had been collected, the references cited in these sources were checked for omission and subsequent retrieval.

The scope of the field was exceptionally wide and the authors identified that a number of content areas could not be addressed in the space available. Consequently, the following topics have been omitted from this review: (a) the nursing profession in other cultures (international nursing), (b) nursing education of minority students, (c) physiological differences of racial groups, and (d) the culture of nursing. In addition, the authors excluded literature not readily available to other investigators including unpublished papers presented at conferences, abstracts, dissertations, theses, and working papers. The authors also generally omitted preliminary reports, works that were not clearly research based, and purported research of insufficient caliber.

This chapter begins with a critical review of works that have contributed substantially to the field's theoretical and methodological underpinnings. Subsequently, six areas of research in the field are outlined to indicate the knowledge which has been generated. Attention is given to trends in strengths and weaknesses found in each area; additionally, particularly illustrative works in each area are highlighted. In the final section the current status of cross-cultural nursing research is reviewed and direction for future study is provided.

THE BASIS OF CROSS-CULTURAL NURSING RESEARCH

Theory

The underpinning of all research is theory which guides scientific inquiry and serves to produce explanatory and predictive statements about phenomena under study. Cross-cultural nursing research has been influenced strongly by theory borrowed from anthropology and other social sciences. A number of nurse researchers have contributed to theory in cross-cultural nursing.

Caring has been a major theoretical focus in cross-cultural nursing research. Utilizing her research on the Papago Indians, Aamodt (1978) developed the concept of care along four dimensions: (a) the fit in a cultural system of health and healing, (b) the applicability of a multicultural environment for care, (c) the power belief, and (d) changes in mechanisms of care during the life cycle of human beings. These dimensions of care provide a basis for cross-cultural investigations of care and variation in the cultural content of care behavior. Aamodt's conceptualization illustrated ways in which "taking care of" is a culturally relevant domain that organizes human experience.

The concept of care was elaborated by Leininger (1977b, 1978a, 1978b, 1978d, 1978e, 1980a, 1981), who saw care as the central focus of nursing behaviors, processes, and intervention modalities. Leininger's (1977b) three-phase model for transcultural nursing is one approach to cross-cultural nursing research. (Transcultural and cross-cultural are synonymous, but because of this author's preference, the term transcultural is used when referring to her work.) A number of studies that employ the Leininger model are available (Leininger, 1977a, 1977c, 1977d, 1979a, 1979b, 1980b, 1981). These reports contain research findings about ethnonursing from one or more cultures. A major weakness of the model is that the assumptions on which the model are based are not separated from the theoretical statements (Leininger, 1978c, pp. 35–36).

The concept of care has been a fruitful theoretical approach in transcultural nursing research, and when examined in a wider context this concept is seen as a guide to several theoretical contributions. Exploration of the fit of health and healing in a cultural system and the multicultural environment of caring (Aamodt, 1978) is seen in the work of Byerly, Molgaard, and Snow (1979) and Molgaard, Byerly, and Snow (1979). Their research concerned alternative healing systems in an Anglo-American subculture, the New Age healers, who were counterculture migrant farm workers. From this focus, theoretical statements emerged about healing systems that arise in opposition to Western medicine and that represent syncretic belief systems and culture change. This array of explanatory theory in caring reveals characteristics seen in emerging systems: flexibility and the ability to draw from several healing or caring traditions. Such emerging traditions survive on faith (Aamodt, 1978) rather than science or one integrated theory of health and disease, as is usually seen in Western medicine.

Folk systems of caring have been an important aspect of cross-cultural nursing research. Byerly et al. (1979) and Molgaard et al. (1979) concluded that New Age healing is a lay system of healing rather than a folk system, because it has a subcultural locus and numerous sources of healing beliefs.

Underlying explanatory theories of caring or healing systems have been important analytical contributions to transcultural nursing theory.

Muecke (1979) reported on research in northern Thailand where she studied the etiology, symptomatology, and treatment of "wind illness." Accounts of the illness were gathered from women, victims of the conditions were followed over time, and indigenous healers who treated clients with the illness were interviewed. This multifaceted approach of teasing out the cultural context of the illness was a profitable tactic. When the cultural reality of wind illness was correlated with biomedical terms used to describe it, a sociocultural explanation of wind illness was posited. Muecke concluded that wind illness is a residual category of illness; for the natives it explains symptoms that do not fit elsewhere in their explanatory model of disease. The disease category wind illness is sufficiently nonspecific to take on new symptoms when they arise in the population. Muecke followed a careful theoretical and methodological plan to come to a more complete understanding of a particular syndrome. One value of research in another culture on a residual illness category is that it can be used to point out inconsistencies in prevailing disease categories in Western medicine; a parallel example of a residual category in Western medical theory may be collagen diseases.

The interest in understanding the underlying differences between biomedical and client models of health and illness has promoted the use of ethnoscience theory in cross-cultural nursing research. In ethnoscience, emic–etic distinctions are derived from the differences between phonemics and phonetics made by anthropological linguists (Pike, 1954). Phonemics is the study of sound used in a particular language; phonetics generalizes from studies of single languages to universals common to all language. In ethnoscience, emic categories are culture specific while etic categories are applicable across cultures (Pike, 1954, 1966). The discovery of significant distinctions made by the members of a particular culture is the purpose of emic analysis. The discovery of behavior that does not require learning the viewpoint of those being studied occurs in etic analysis. Etic categories can be applied across cultures, may be seen as culture free, and are derived from the examination of several cultures (Pike, 1954; Sturtevant, 1964).

With this background it can be seen that ethnoscience in which emic–etic analysis is used may be usefully developed in cross-cultural nursing research. The elicitation of emic categories such as care, illness, and health are of interest; the study of etic (culturally universal) distinctions along the same lines would facilitate culturally appropriate nursing care. Assumptions underlying the ethnoscience method include the following: (a) language or word symbols are an accurate reflection of cognition; (b) language is an accurate representation of culture; (c) what is stated to be true by an informant is reflective of culture, even though culture may be largely perceptual and unconscious; and (d) categories reported by an informant are a reflection of cultural patterns. These assumptions suggest that there are weaknesses in ethnoscience as a theoretical approach because the validity of the assumptions cannot be substantiated fully. Other weaknesses in the methods which apply to any ethnoscience research are that: (a) the research addresses a narrow segment of culture; (b) executing the method is tedious and time consuming; (c) a small number of subjects are involved, usually 10 or less; and (d) the representativeness of the subjects is open to question, even though, theoretically, any native speaker of a language is considered to be representative of the group. An important point about ethnoscience research is that the investigator does not make predictions. The purpose is to elicit emic categories, and to allow the organization to arise from the data. Therefore, hypothesis testing is reserved for research for which sufficient previous ethnoscience research has been conducted so that all basic categories have been discovered. Cross-cultural ethnoscience nursing research has not advanced to the hypothesis-testing stage in any area to date. Studies based on ethnoscience theory are discussed later.

Theoretical contributions of cross-cultural nursing research include theory relating care givers to clients and the models of health and disease. Barbee (1977) examined the potential sources of cooperation and conflict between scientific and indigenous health care professionals in Botswana, Africa. In a preliminary report, she found that in rural areas nurses functioned as diagnosticians and healers, but when in hospitals they were assigned roles subordinate to physicians. The theoretical contribution of her work was in the way roles were shaped in a system in which indigenous care providers and Western-trained personnel interacted.

Theory derived from anthropology and other social sciences has been adapted to guide nursing research. Bauwens and Anderson (1978) examined factors associated with environmental stresses in hospital births. The concepts of environmental stresses and cognitive dissonance were used to explain factors influencing home birth. Prediction of factors that influence how client groups perceive and relate to health care institutions and care providers is an important theoretical tactic. Approaches that include comparisons are often more valuable than those testing theory in only one setting. Kayser-Jones (1979) compared the care of the institutionalized elderly in Scotland and the United States. Employing exchange theory as a model, she found that the health care system and social structure in Scotland allowed the aged to be more independent and to have resources with which to engage in balanced social relationships. Tripp-Reimer (1982a) studied how Appalachians and non-Appalachian health professionals viewed the behavior of Appalachians, employing theory on cultural relativism and ethnocentrism to frame the research and findings.

Both Bauwens and Anderson (1978) and Kayser-Jones (1979) provided too limited information on methods or data analysis, and Kayser-Jones considered too many variables to support the predictive value of exchange theory. These studies and that of Tripp-Reimer (1982a) reflected the use of well-established anthropological theory to guide the interpretation of findings. A weakness of these studies is that there was not further refinement of these theories for cross-cultural nursing research.

Ragucci (1981) incorporated several theoretical elements in her work on Italian-Americans. She addressed care as experienced by clients (Bauwens & Anderson, 1978; Kayser-Jones, 1979), indigenous models of illness (Muecke, 1979), and the relationships among care providers (Barbee, 1977). Additionally, she emphasized the theoretical importance of considering synchronic and diachronic approaches when examining ethnic health patterns.

Drawing from the observations of Colson and Selby (1974), Barbee (1977) stated that the field of medical anthropology was characterized by little theory and an absence of a cumulative trend in research. Similarly, research in cross-cultural nursing has resulted in limited theoretical contributions because rarely does an investigator build progressively on research in one or two cultures.

Similarly, Osborne (1977) observed that in anthropology a distinction is made between the anthropologist as an ethnographer (one who describes a people) and an ethnologist (one who develops theories of culture and society). He stated that all competent anthropologists must be both ethnographers and ethnologists and must understand when they are performing one or the other role. A review of cross-cultural nursing research indicates that these studies primarily fit the definition of ethnography and have neglected the comparative, theory-building aspect seen in ethnology. However, the contributions of Aamodt (1978) and Leininger (1977b) provided a basis on which to pursue the ethnography of transcultural nursing and to develop a body of knowledge on which theory can be built.

Methods

The explication and implementation of qualitative methods have been major strengths of cross-cultural nursing studies. Given the close link with anthropology, which is probably the leading discipline in qualitative research, this is natural. Descriptive methodology is best illustrated in cross-cultural nursing research through the use of ethnography, traditionally defined as the study of a culture. In ethnographic research the basic approach is to define a field for observation and systematically to observe the environment, the personnel interacting in it, and influences on the field of observation from the wider environment. Repeated observation and ongoing analysis of field notes result in the development of categories for analysis. Examples may be the interaction of high- and low-status persons, the reenactment of cultural norms through ritual, and normative behaviors of young and old or men and women. The focus of the researcher is to produce a descriptive study, organized around anthropological theory; little detail is given on methods because they are relatively standard. The reader is expected to accept that the investigator is an accurate observer, that the field has been appropriately delimited, and that the analytical framework has been selected appropriately for the study.

As a result of this heritage, ethnographic studies conducted by nurses contain similar strengths and weaknesses. When evaluated according to the criteria established in nursing research, certain weaknesses appear in nearly all ethnographic studies. Generally, limitations of the ethnographic method are not addressed, but the research contains rich description and analysis. While many of the studies do not reach the hypothesis-generation stage, the analyses do generate innovative conceptualizations of issues or questions. There is usually little attention to the sample size or the representativeness of the sample. It is accepted as a weakness of the method that certain members of a group will be key informants and that other segments of the group will be underrepresented. In ethnographic studies, the methods section is usually brief. While this characteristic may be viewed as a weakness, it should be emphasized that participant observation is the primary data-collection technique and has been the standard in ethnography. Closely related to ethnography as a method is grounded theory, which has sociology as its heritage. Grounded theory's similarity to ethnography in strengths and weaknesses were described in Stern (1980).

There are useful criteria for evaluation of qualitative methods (Bruyn 1966), and ethnographic nursing research would be strengthened if investigators employed standard criteria for the development and evaluation of qualitative nursing research. In this chapter, each study was evaluated according to Bruyn's criteria. Studies were included only if they were reasonably sound, and if they contained strengths which contributed to the body of nursing knowledge in cross-cultural research.

The ethnographic approach has been explicated well by nurse anthropologists through nursing and other health-related research. Byerly and Molgaard (1982) noted a high potential for ethnographic research to contribute to health care by:

> 1) assessing risk factors for disease which supplement age, sex, occupation, socioeconomic status, marital status and other traditional and relatively avail-

> able epidemiologic variables; and 2) providing information on the degree to which cultural milieu and cognitive frame may constrain health care planning, intervention, and prevention for social groups that operate with very different conceptions of the significance of biological events. (p. 402)

Aamodt (1972) described the ethnographic method as beginning with central empirical questions. The questions guide the choice of techniques to obtain the answers: When the question implies that culture is behavior, observation is employed. When the question implies that culture is knowledge, interviewing is used. Ethnographic research is time consuming because the data collection and analysis occur simultaneously, with refinement of the questions and data collection techniques occurring as the research progresses. Through ethnographic interview data, areas of commonality bearing significance to the culture under study (called culturally relevant domains) emerge (Aamodt, 1981). Domains are consistent with or contrast with other domains. The process of discovering and describing the domains and their contrasts results in an ordering of the ethnographic data that reveals the content of the culture as seen and experienced by members of the culture. For example, in a study of New Age Healers, Molgaard and Byerly (1981) initially focused on disease concepts as a domain. However, the domain was not relevant because the group did not consider disease concepts relevant to the pursuit of health. The analytical frame was refocused onto types of energy and the nature of energy flow, permitting an accurate representation of the group's health belief system.

Aamodt (1982) addressed the erroneous idea that ethnography is a simple research method and discussed seven veiled interpretations about ethnographic methodology which she called myths. While providing a valuable overview of ethnography as a method, attention is drawn to several pitfalls that investigators may encounter. In ethnographic research, categories are allowed to arise from the observations of the field under study. The organization that arises from the data is the basis for the analysis. The use of the ethnographic method where categories are not allowed to arise naturally from the data is illustrated by Germain's (1979, 1980) study of a cancer unit. The analysis was superficial because the focus was nurses' activities rather than how the activities were patterned by the ongoing culture of the unit (i.e., norms and values). Because Germain emphasized description and neglected process, her results reflected the pitfalls that can occur in ethnographic research.

Several investigators (Aamodt, 1981; Byerly, 1969; Byerly et al., 1979; Ragucci, 1972) emphasized the importance of the investigators' initial entry into the research setting and establishment of rapport with subjects (usually called "informants" in ethnographic research). In all ethnographic research the relationship between the investigator and the informants and the interaction with the research environment is important. Participant observation is a research method in which the interrelating factors are brought under ongoing examination and analysis. Participant observation has broad application in qualitative research because it serves as a data-collection technique and is a way to monitor the research process. Byerly (1969) addressed the issues and the dilemmas involved in participant observation: (a) Objectivity versus subjectivity. How does the investigator's presence influence the setting? (b) Scientific integrity versus protection of individual rights. How should information that is given in confidence be used without violating the confidence? (c) Intervention versus nonintervention. Should the investigator intervene when information is important to the welfare of the informant? Byerly's (1969) work is a classic contribution to qualitative methodology in cross-cultural nursing research. The principles explicated were employed and refined in Byerly et al. (1979).

In basic cross-cultural nursing research, investigators have employed the ethnographic method, including interviewing and participant observation. A number of investigators have extended, developed, and refined this basic approach. In studies of Italian-Americans, Ragucci (1972, 1977, 1981) developed a method and rationale for combining ethnographic methods with historical materials. She emphasized the importance of examining and analyzing cultural differences and persistence over three generations. This approach introduces a diachronic dimension to ethnographic research that is especially important in settings where culture change is a factor. Kay (1973, 1976, 1977a, 1977b, 1977c, 1979) studied Mexican-Americans extensively in Arizona. Initially employing ethnographic methodology, she moved to precise, extensive examination of language and history. Important findings were that folk medical culture was not stable and that change occurred in the labeling of disease, with the direction of change being toward the scientific classification system. The methodological contribution of Kay was the demonstration of how ethnographic findings could be extended diachronically through the use of library sources.

The combination of ethnographic methods with other approaches was demonstrated productively in a study by Tripp-Reimer (1982b), in which interviews and documentation of vital statistics were employed, and in another Tripp-Reimer study (1983), in which qualitative and quantitative methods were combined to provide a comprehensive analysis of the retention of folk healing practices among urban Greek immigrants in the United States.

A major difficulty in conducting cross-cultural nursing research has been the problems of precise definition and clear delineation of differences in such areas as ethnic identity, cultural differences, and caring behavior. However, Flaskerud (1979, 1980b) has made encouraging progress in these areas. She developed a methodology to establish the validity of an instrument and used vignettes to differentiate a minority group's normative behavior from the mainstream culture's deviant behavior. Subsequently, Flaskerud (1980a, 1980b) presented a tool for comparing the perceptions of problematic behavior for use by other researchers. Her research demonstrated that valid measures of ethnic differences could be developed. Although it was not stated by Flaskerud, it is clear that painstaking effort is necessary with *each* ethnic group of interest if valid, quantifiable differences are to be discovered.

The discovery and documentation of ethnic group differences was addressed by Clinton (1982), who described the results of a project to measure ethnicity and define the influence of ethnicity on health-seeking behaviors. An integrative, multivariate, computer-assisted approach proved successful in the measurement of European-origin ethnic identity, and was a useful heuristic device for partitioning the sample for the analysis of health data. The use of computers to select and refine components of ethnic identity and for other applications in cross-cultural nursing research is a promising new methodological approach.

Another refinement of the ethnographic method has been ethnoscience, where emic–etic distinctions were elicited and analyzed. Evaneshko and Kay (1982) described ethnoscience as a research methodology. Evaneshko and Bauwens (1976) demonstrated the elicitation of categories, card-sort technique, and data analysis, using medical emergencies as the topic and medical personnel and lay persons as informants. Bush, Ullom, and Osborne (1975), Byerly et al. (1979), and Molgaard et al. (1979) further explicated the ethnoscience method. The method is valuable for eliciting the underlying categories of knowledge of informant groups. Given the persistence of language codes, informants who speak the same language will show great similarities in the organizational structure of categories about major phenomena. To date, ethnoscience studies have contained emic analyses (i.e., generating categories used by one to four groups), but have not reached the level of etic analyses (generating categories applicable across cultures).

The cultural context of caring has been a fruitful theoretical frame for cross-cultural nursing research but has not been matched by methods that produce useful analyses of care practices in cultural context. Binn (1980) advanced understanding of the meaning of illness to individuals within cultural context. Employing the explanatory model developed by Kleinman, Eisenberg, and Good (1978) and a question guide based on the model, Binn described the beliefs, expectations, and behaviors of hypertensive adults. The question guide is transferable to various groups or illness contexts and represents a refinement of methodology to explore the meaning of health and illness and the needs and expectations for care. This method may be applied productively to inquiry delineating the concept of care (Leininger, 1981) within cultural context.

A review of methodological approaches to cross-cultural nursing research is not complete without mentioning the potential of anthropometric measurement (Kroska, 1977; A. S. Lewis, 1979) as a quantitative method, the importance of using comparative studies (Stern, 1981a) to derive cultural similarities and differences, or the value of case study (Sohier, 1976) to generate empirical questions. At this point, however, investigations using these methods in nursing are not sufficiently developed to represent major methodological contributions. The principle methodological advances in cross-cultural nursing research have been through the ethnographic method, which includes ethnographic interviewing, participant observation, and the ethnoscience method.

RESEARCH ON NURSING AND CULTURE

Descriptive Ethnographic Works

In a wide variety of studies ethnographic methods and case studies have been used to describe characteristics of minority cultures. Reports have included descriptions of various cultural aspects of the following groups: Paiute Indians (Brink, 1971a, 1971b), Salish Indians (Horn, 1977), rural black Americans (Dougherty, 1978), Appalachians (Tripp-Reimer, 1980; Tripp-Reimer & Friedl, 1977), and Mormons (Peay, 1977). Similarly, studies have been conducted on culture groups abroad by nurse anthropologists (Brink, 1982; Kendall, 1977; Leininger, 1967, 1977b; Sohier, 1976). These studies tend to be descriptions about specific culture groups and life-style patterns. They add to nursing knowledge by giving baseline information about general cultural characteristics of the people studied. In a few studies (Glittenberg, 1981; Mackenzie, 1977; Osborne, 1972), investigators looked more specifically at the relationship of health care behaviors to other aspects of the social structure. With a few exceptions, these studies have little direct applicability to nursing practice. But they do give information on the culture context, which is important for a holistic nursing approach.

Belief Systems

A number of investigators have focused on a client population's belief systems concerning health and illness. The majority of this research is solid descriptive accounts of the health beliefs of specific groups. Some studies concerned the orthodox and unorthodox beliefs and practices of a specific group (Byerly et al., 1979; Kay, 1973, 1977a, 1977b, 1979; Molgaard et al., 1979). Bauwens (1977) conducted an ethnographic study of low-income Anglos describing causes of illness, beliefs about ways to maintain good health, the definition of good health, and what constituted deviations from good health. Bauwens' study was extended by Hautman and Harrison (1982) to a population of middle-income Anglos. In addition to providing baseline data on beliefs, these studies point out the important difference between the subjective perception of the client's health state and objective pathologies that may be evidenced. Hautman and Harrison found that a person may self-define a condition as "healthy" even in the presence of disease pathology. Similarly, in Ragucci's (1977) study of Italian-American women, she identified how social factors and activities of daily living were the most frequently mentioned indicators of health and well-being.

A few of the investigators focused specifically on folk health beliefs of a specific group (Tripp-Reimer, 1981) or on beliefs regarding specific conditions such as wind illness (Muecke, 1979), evil eye (Tripp-Reimer, 1983), hypertension (Ailinger, 1981, 1982; Binn, 1980), or vitamin use (Johnston & Sarty, 1978). Several important themes have emerged from these studies. In a sophisticated analytical study, Muecke (1979) explored the concept of wind illness. As previously described, this study provided the most complete example of the integration of emic and etic perspectives to come to a more complete understanding of a particular syndrome. A second theme has been the importance of considering diversity within cultures when describing traditional beliefs. A variety of factors (including age, sex, language fluency, education, and socioeconomic status) have been linked with retention of belief systems. Ragucci (1972) posited the importance of considering generational depth among immigrant populations. This was supported empirically by Tripp-Reimer (1983) in a study of Greek-Americans.

A number of investigators have stressed the syncretic nature of beliefs held by members of a culture group. In this regard, the works of Byerly and associates (Byerly et al., 1979; Molgaard et al., 1979), Ragucci (1977, 1981), and Kay (1976, 1977a, 1977b, 1979) are particularly informative. Refinements of the definition of folk health belief have resulted from the emphasis on syncretism. These refinements originated from Redfield's (1947) typology of great and little traditions, Ackerknecht's (1942) distinction between primitive and folk medicine, as well as Coe's (1970) and Freidson's (1961) differentiation of modern medical and layman's knowledge. For example, for the Italian-Americans Ragucci (1981) differentiated three types of lay traditions: (a) archaic (what was, but is no longer), (b) traditional (beliefs and actions derived from "little" and past "great" traditions of medicine), and (c) contemporary (popular medicine) beliefs and practices that have filtered down from the present "great" tradition of medicine as reinterpreted by laymen.

In a similar vein, Kay (1976, 1977a) looked for the origins of health beliefs of Mexican-American women. She posited convincingly that there was a dominant and common source for what is currently considered "indigenous" medicine in the Southwest. The 18th century work the *Florilegio Medicinal* was written by a Jesuit lay brother (Esteyneffer), who combined herbal lore of American Indians with the materia medica and disease categories of European physicians. Kay suggested that this book's descriptions of illnesses and therapies served to standardize them throughout the greater Southwest. Kay (1977b) clearly illustrated that what is currently categorized under the rubric of "folk" may have in the past been considered "scientific." Even the hot–cold folk system of Hispanics can be seen as a survival of a period when these notions were prevalent in orthodox medicine.

Some research has been conducted on the child's acquisition of traditional belief systems. An early effort by Aamodt (1972) focused on a Papago Indian community. She investigated how the content of health and healing systems are transmitted to a child. She indicated the mechanism and timing of the enculturative process by which health concepts were acquired as the child was socialized by family and community. This was an important early investigation of the way traditional health beliefs are learned. However, there is a marked need for further investigations in this area.

Kay (1979) traced linguistic use of disease names using the methods of ethnoscience. She pointed out that the lexicon (vocabulary) of illness terms used by Mexican-American women is affected by the practice of speaking both Spanish and English and by the coexistence of several health systems. Thus, she demonstrated that the illness terms are particularly dynamic, evidencing lexemic change and semantic shift. Further, she found that the direction of the semantic shift is in the direction of correspondence with concepts of scientific medicine.

Cognitive Nonsharing

Several studies have been conducted on an area that has been termed "cognitive nonsharing" by Molgaard and Byerly (1981). Investigators identified a topical area (definition of medical emergencies, mental health, and problematic or common behavior) and then studied the perceptions of this topic as held by members of two or more groups. The groups most often investigated were health care practitioners and lay persons (sometimes culturally specified). In a pioneering ethnoscience study, Bush et al. (1975) investigated cognitive differences in the meaning of mental health held by mental health specialists and inner-city clients. In another ethnoscience investigation, Evaneshko and Kay (1982) studied the cognitive maps of nurses and laypersons for the taxonomic category "medical emergencies." Their findings indicated that professional nurses operated with a much more complex taxonomy than did lay persons. Evaneshko and Kay (1982) suggested that these differences may lead the groups to define "medical emergencies" differently, resulting in over- or underusage by clients and friction in the emergency room. These investigators pointed out incongruities in perceptual and cognitive sets of practitioners and recipients of health care.

Flaskerud (1980a, 1980b) has been a pioneer in the development of the use of vignettes to identify ethnic differences in illness assessment and management. She investigated whether Appalachians, mental health professionals, and lay non-Appalachians differed in the way they labeled and managed sets of behaviors. Data indicated that the differences between Appalachians and each of the other groups were significant. The Appalachians and the other two groups demonstrated different explanations for client behavior and a different system for managing behavior.

In a complementary study of Appalachian and non-Appalachian health professionals, Tripp-Reimer (1982a) investigated whether the ethnic background of the health professionals was associated with their perceptions of client behavior. Like Flaskerud, she found that the interpretation of client behaviors was closely linked to the subject's ethnic background.

Health Behaviors

The syncretism that was documented for health beliefs is also evident in health behaviors. A number of investigators presented baseline descriptive data on ways orthodox (scientific) and unorthodox (indigenous) health practices coexisted in several populations (Aamodt, 1976; Bauwens, 1977; Ford, 1973; Hautman & Harrison, 1982; Powers 1982). These investigators pointed out that during illness episodes, individuals selected from a variety of practitioners and self-care options and used them concurrently or consecutively. For example, in an interesting case study of a black woman treated for hypertension and obesity, Powers (1982) found that the client used both the scientific health clinic and a "root doctor"; the client relied on the root doctor for the "cure" but used the health clinic staff's evaluation to gauge the efficacy of the root doctor.

Other investigators focused on decision making in pluralistic societies (Ailinger, 1977; Brink, 1977; McKenna, 1979). These investigations addressed factors that influence how people make decisions to seek health care. Brink, for example, demonstrated that much decision making about health care and illness was accomplished prior to the patient entering a health care system. Ailinger (1977) conducted an important study of illness referral in a Hispanic-American community. She used daily family-health histories with 19 Latin-American immigrant families. She found that family members did not necessarily pass through the steps of the illness referral process as conceptualized by medical sociologists. She found that in most cases when a person perceived him- or herself to be ill, the person self-treated, combining home and herbal remedies, nonprescription, and on-hand prescription medications. Only a relatively few cases (10%) sought recommendations for treatment from others in their social network. However, an important next step in this area that Ailinger did not address was to ascertain how decisions were made about home treatments or professional consultation.

Other aspects of health behaviors have been investigated. Elms, Kevany, Thomson, and Webb (1979) studied differences in presenting complaints and subsequent treatment of clients in psychiatric outpatient clinics in Ireland and California. They found important differences in clients' presenting complaints, referral process, expectations, and subsequent treatment plans. In a pioneering effort, Clinton (1982) used an integrative, multivariate approach to measure ethnic identity and posited its usefulness for health-seeking behaviors. Studying a variety of ethnic groups of European descent in Detroit, Clinton (1982) found significant differences among the European groups concerning a variety of health behaviors including exercise, medical checkups, and diet. This approach holds promise for future research on health data from an ethnic perspective.

Two investigators indicated that social class may be an overriding factor of importance in health behaviors. Milio (1967) documented that socioeconomic variables were most influential in predicting patterns of maternity activities. She also illustrated that what has been considered "ideal" maternity activities contained some features that were nonessential for the health of the infant. Some of these ideal behaviors may be considered more reflective of the dominant culture notions than of physiologically based requirements. Similarly, O'Brien (1982) studied the health behaviors of Mexican-American migrant laborers. Using grounded theory methodology, she found that the migrants' pattern of health behavior could be characterized as "pragmatic survivalism" in that they were selective in choosing those behaviors that would allow health maintenance or illness recovery in the most practical manner possible for the continuance of their productive life.

A related area concerns the social functions that are served by the health behaviors of lay health agents. Using ethnoscience, in a study of a New Age group in Washington, Byerly et al. (1979) identified a self-help emphasis. They suggested that the New Age therapies seemed to serve, not so much as rebellion against society, but as a vehicle for gaining self-respect and maintaining the social identity of the group. Other studies have identified that lay health agents (Dougherty, 1976; Muecke, 1976) and self-help groups (Lipson, 1980; Lipson & Tilden, 1980) may serve as socializing agents. Together, these studies indicated that in pluralistic societies, nonscientific practitioners may serve as instruments of social change and education.

Care as a Theoretical or Empirical Domain

A promising concept that has emerged for culture and health studies is the domain of care and caring behaviors. While literature concerning this construct has been predominantly theoretical, a number of empirical studies have been reported. Leininger (1978c, 1980a, 1981) wrote most extensively on this concept. In the proceedings of the first three National Caring Conferences, Leininger (1981) defined care or caring in a generic sense as "those assistive, supportive, or facilitative acts toward or for another individual or group with evident or anticipated needs to ameliorate or improve a human condition or lifeway" (p. 9). Based on several years of formulations, Leininger identified assumptions about the phenomenon of caring and devised 10 hypotheses concerning the construct. She identified 28 major taxonomic caring constructs and devised a model to study transcultural and ethnocaring constructs. Previously, Leininger (1977a) conducted an early ethnographic study of the Gadsup of New Guinea. In this study she identified dominant caring behaviors evidenced by the Gadsup. A limitation of this study was that these caring behaviors (surveillance, stimulation, nuturance, etc.) were etic categories; hence, it was unclear how the Gadsup themselves identified that they performed "caring."

Aamodt (1972, 1977, 1981) also explored the domain of care. In this series of studies, Aamodt built on her own field work with Papago Indians and Norwegian-Americans. In her earlier work, Aamodt (1972, 1977) identified themes among the Papago which were important for understanding care as a culturally relevant domain. Recently, Aamodt (1981) identified that an important domain of care among Norwegian-American women is the construct of "neighboring" and that being present was a major theme in neighboring. Aamodt's Norwegian-American work brings in the notion of support networks, which had not been explored previously as such in cross-cultural nursing research.

In a conceptually related study, Tripp-Reimer and Schrock (1982) investigated care preferences for the ethnic aged of European descent. Studying groups of Old Order Amish, Czechs, and Greeks in Iowa, they found that the groups differed from each other in residential care preferences given specified life conditions. These investigators documented that even in supportive groups with high degrees of ethnic retention, the elderly did not necessarily prefer to be "cared for" in the home of a relative.

Interrelationship of Culture and Biology

A few investigators focused on the interrelationship between cultural and biological variables. In particular, the influence of cultural patterns on fertility was addressed (Glittenberg, 1977; Tripp-Reimer, 1981, 1982b; Urdaneta, 1975; Wang, 1979). Similarly, investigators focused on the relationship of culture and disease transmission (Byerly & Molgaard, 1982), blood pressure (Segall, 1965), and postsurgical convalescence (Williams, 1972). In a particularly good study, Williams (1972) compared length of convalescence after hysterectomy in two groups: Anglo and Mexican-American women. Through this study Williams made important contributions to investigating stress levels and identifying the relative importance of lay versus professional advice. Research combining social and biological variables has high potential; it combines the holistic approach of both anthropology and nursing and it can contribute to a more complete understanding of the total health picture of the individual.

CURRENT STATUS AND NEW RESEARCH DIRECTIONS

Critique

In this review the careful, precise work necessary to demonstrate distinctions between ethnic groups was mentioned. The literature in cross-cultural nursing research contains many examples of empirical or inaccurate use of concepts and terms. An important example is the use of the term *culture*. Culture is usually defined as the integrated system of learned behavior patterns that are characteristic of a population living as a distinct entity, and that are not the result of biological inheritance (Hoebel, 1966). The use of the term culture or subculture to describe the elderly (Sullivan, 1977; Uhl, 1981) is an inappropriate use of the culture concept. More importantly, it sets a precedent in the literature which may be followed by others. Just as shared characteristics of the elderly such as retirement or declining physical vigor do not justify the application of the term culture or subculture, shared economic circumstances do not identify a culture. Milio (1967) inappropriately used the phrase "lower-class subculture," but it is recognized that this notion (culture of poverty) has been used widely in the social sciences, originating with O. Lewis (1966).

The inappropriate or inaccurate use of terms, concepts, and methods originating in anthropology creates imprecision and confusion in cross-cultural nursing research. Theory and research in all disciplines is a building process, each cycle of theory and research building squarely on earlier literature; additions, modifications, and adaptations must be specified clearly and justified. When one discipline borrows and adapts the terms, concepts, and methods of another, it is especially important to impart to fellow scholars the process involved. This is not evident in the literature reviewed and is especially problematic in the use of grounded theory (Stern, 1981a, 1981b) and in several ethnoscience studies.

In much of the literature reviewed, culture is characterized as a veneer, as if it could be removed for examination in isolation. Culture pervades the entire being of individuals and populations; it is the sum total of learned behavior. In a related way, cultures customarily are studied only once by an investigator. Lack of follow-up studies results in a static view of culture. Cultures are dynamic and incorporate change continually. The use of methods (Kay, 1979; Ragucci, 1972, 1977, 1981; Tripp-Reimer, 1983) by which the diachronic perspective is revealed are an encouraging development.

Too frequently research questions derive from intuition rather than a firm grounding in theory. For example, O'Brien (1982) followed a complex procedure to derive the construct of pragmatic survivalism as a determining factor in the health behavior of migrant laborers. But the observation that low-income groups attend only to severe problems is a straightforward notion dating from research by Koos (1954).

Similarly, there is too little attention to determinations of reliability and validity of measures and/or methods. Questions of accuracy must be addressed more thoroughly in qualitative studies; otherwise, the reports remain at an impressionistic level. Bruyn (1966) and others outlined excellent criteria for judging the accuracy of ethnographic research. It has been noted here that nursing has borrowed from anthropology. In the area of cross-cultural nursing research, investigators can borrow and employ techniques for the verification of reliability and validity from nursing and other sciences.

In an emerging science such as nursing, there is a great need for research. In the cross-cultural area, priorities are for more comparative studies, replications of studies, and research-based frameworks to provide direction to the area. Since these efforts are underrepresented in the available literature, it is not possible to ascertain whether reported findings represent only "the local village"; it is too early to generalize from available research.

Knowledge gained from cross-cultural research in nursing has been developed horizontally, that is, one culture is described, then another, and then another. The area will become theoretically substantial, however, when knowledge can be linked vertically with ethnographic accounts serving as the basis for general theory. To date, ethnographic studies have not resulted in models that could guide research to explain health behaviors in cross-cultural perspective.

Theory building is needed in this area. In scientific disciplines there is a reciprocal relationship between theory and research. Descriptive studies serve to generate hypotheses that are tested in research. In cross-cultural nursing research this occurs infrequently. The probable reason for lack of follow-through is that nurse investigators conducting ethnographic research are not expert in quantitative methods. The development of cross-cultural nurse investigators who are skilled in a range of qualitative and quantitative methods, or who collaborate with nurse investigators who are, will improve the quality of research and theory.

Most available cross-cultural nursing research does not derive from a clear theoretical base. When concepts are presented, they tend to come from anthropological rather than nursing theory. If research were based on models from nursing (Orem, 1980; Roy & Roberts, 1981) results would be more applicable for refining nursing theory and guiding cross-cultural research in nursing.

The limited applicability of cross-cultural nursing research to nursing practice is readily apparent. Cross-cultural nurse researchers who affiliate with anthropology (to the exclusion of nursing) diminish their contribution to advancing knowledge important to nursing. Rarely was it made clear how cross-cultural nursing research findings could be articulated with the function of assessment, diagnosis, or intervention. It is no longer sufficient for investigators to state that the nurse should be sensitive to the culture of the client. Research findings that identify the effectiveness of differing intervention strategies with culturally specific client groups is a clear need. In available research, individual variation within each culture group is generally not easily identified; findings represent dominant patterns. Nurses, however, provide care for individual clients. There is little attention by nurse researchers to the application of cross-cultural findings to the nursing needs of specific clients or client groups.

Nursing is intervention oriented; anthropology is oriented to recognizing and maintaining the integrity and stability of identifiable cultural groups (nonintervention). Both disciplines agree that understanding clients' values, beliefs, and customs is important. The assumption that these patterns are static and unchangeable may be patronizing. Incorporating folk beliefs and practices into biomedical care settings may be neither what clients desire nor health promoting. At times, "natives" are presented as if they wished to remain unassimilated; limited consideration is given to the preferences "natives" hold. To deny choice promotes subjugation. These issues represent a major research initiative needed in cross-cultural nursing research.

General Contributions of This Field

The most important contribution of this field is the descriptive data that have emerged concerning health beliefs and behaviors. Most of this critical review attests to the richness of research findings. A recent emerging focus of research is the popular, or general, American culture (vs. ethnic groups). The documentation of lay, or nonscientific, beliefs and practices that pervade the popular culture is receiving increasing attention. Generalization of the concept of culture from the study of discrete minority groups to the wider popular American culture and to that of the health professional holds promise for the wider application of cross-cultural nursing research in the future.

Human behavior and health are two constructs that are basic to nursing theory; research in this area may stimulate nursing theory development. The holistic focus of anthropology fits well with the holistic perspective of nursing and may contribute to more generalized models and theories of nursing.

Finally, emerging research gives importance to clients' social and physical experience with illness and health. No other field of research so clearly illustrates the subjective meaning of clients' health experiences and the dissonance of these subjective meanings with those of health professionals. Scotch's (1963) observations on the field of medical anthropology can be applied to the area of cross-cultural nursing research. He stated that there was a great deal of criticism of the poor quality of the literature, and truly, the quality of literature in this area was not always impressive. It has not, however, yet been documented that cross-cultural nursing differs in this respect from other substantive areas in nursing. Is all other nursing research uniformly rigorous, profound, and stimulating? Even accepting the assumption that the proportion of high-level research is smaller in cross-cultural nursing than in other areas should not be reason for rejection. Specific instances of unworthy research should be discounted, but not the whole area. It is the authors' contention that this area can be studied rigorously, be used to test hypotheses of a general nature, produce concepts and theory, develop systematic methodologies, and produce substantive data.

REFERENCES

Aamodt, A. M. (1972). The child view of health and healing. In M. Batey (Ed.), *Communicating nursing research: Vol. 5. The many sources of nursing knowledge* (pp. 38–54). Boulder, CO: Western Interstate Commission for Higher Education.

Aamodt, A. M. (1976). Observations of a health and healing system in a Papago community. In M. Leininger (Ed.), *Health care dimensions: Vol. 3. Transcultural health care issues and conditions* (pp. 23–36). Philadelphia: F. A. Davis.

Aamodt, A. M. (1977). The social-cultural dimensions of caring in the world of the Papago child and adolescent. In M. Leininger (Ed.), *Transcultural nursing care of infants and children: Proceedings from the First Transcultural Nursing Conference* (pp. 40–50). Salt Lake City: University of Utah College of Nursing.

Aamodt, A. M. (1978). The care component in a health and healing system. In E. Bauwens (Ed.), *The anthropology of health* (pp. 37–45). St. Louis: Mosby.

Aamodt, A. M. (1981). Neighboring: Discovering support systems among Norwegian American women. In D. Messerschmidt (Ed.), *Anthropologists at home in America: Methods and issues in the study of one's own culture* (pp. 133–149). Cambridge, MA: Cambridge University Press.

Aamodt, A. M. (1982). Examining ethnography for nurse researchers. *Western Journal of Nursing Research, 4,* 209–221.

Ackerknecht, E. H. (1942). Problems of primitive medicine. *Bulletin of the History of Medicine, 11,* 503–521.

Ailinger, R. L. (1977). A study of illness referral in a Spanish-speaking community. *Nursing Research, 26,* 53–56.

Ailinger, R. L. (1981). Cultural factors in hypertension of Spanish-speakers. *Virginia Nurse, 49*(3), 14–17.

Ailinger, R. L. (1982). Hypertension knowledge in a Hispanic community. *Nursing Research, 31,* 207–210.

Barbee, E. L. (1977). Health action and conflict between the professional health actors in Botswana. In M. Batey (Ed.), *Communicating nursing research: Vol. 10. Optimizing environments for health: Nursing's unique perspective* (pp. 265–277). Boulder, CO: Western Interstate Commission for Higher Education.

Bauwens, E. E. (1977). Medical beliefs and practices among lower-income Anglos. In E. Spicer (Ed.), *Ethnic medicine in the Southwest* (pp. 241–270). Tucson: The University of Arizona Press.

Bauwens, E. E., & Anderson, S. V. (1978). Home births: A reaction to hospital environmental stressors. In E. Bauwens (Ed.), *The anthropology of health* (pp. 56–60). St. Louis: Mosby.

Binn, M. (1980). Using the explanatory model to understand ethnomedical perceptions of hypertension and the resultant behaviors. In M. Leininger (Ed.), *Transcultural nursing care: Teaching, practice and research. Proceedings from the Fifth National Transcultural Nursing Conference* (pp. 60–76). Salt Lake City: University of Utah College of Nursing.

Brink, P. J. (1971a). Paviotso child training: Notes. *The Indian Historian, 4*(1), 47–50.

Brink, P. J. (1971b). Some aspects of change in northern Paiute childrearing practices. In C. Aikens (Ed.), *Great Basin Anthropological Conference, 1970: Selected Papers.* University of Oregon Anthropological Papers, Number *1,* 167–175.

Brink, P. J. (1977). Decision making of the health care consumer: A Nigerian example. In M. Batey (Ed.), *Communicating nursing research: Vol. 9. Nursing research in the bicentennial year* (pp. 351–362). Boulder, CO: Western Interstate Commission for Higher Education.

Brink, P. J. (1982). Traditional birth attendants among the Annang of Nigeria: Current practices and proposed programs. *Social Science and Medicine, 16,* 1883–1892.

Bruyn, S. (1966). *The human perspective in sociology: The methodology of participant observation*. Englewood Cliffs, NJ: Prentice-Hall.

Bush, M. T., Ullom, J. A., & Osborne, O. H. (1975). The meaning of mental health: A report of two ethnoscientific studies. *Nursing Research, 24,* 130–138.

Byerly, E. L. (1969). The nurse-researcher as participant-observer in a nursing setting. *Nursing Research, 18,* 230–236.

Byerly, E. L., & Molgaard, C. A. (1982). Social institutions and disease transmission. In N. Chrisman & T. Maretzki (Eds.), *Clinically applied anthropology: Anthropologists in health science settings* (pp. 395–409). Boston: Reidel.

Byerly, E. L., Molgaard, C. A., & Snow, C. T. (1979). Dissonance in the dessert: What to do with the golden seal? In M. Leininger (Ed.), *Transcultural nursing care: Culture change, ethics and nursing care implications. Proceedings from the Fourth National Transcultural Nursing Conference* (pp. 114–133). Salt Lake City: University of Utah College of Nursing.

Clinton, J. H. (1982). Ethnicity: The development of an empirical construct for cross-cultural health research. *Western Journal of Nursing Research, 4,* 281–300.

Coe, R. (1970). *Sociology of medicine*. New York: McGraw-Hill.

Colson, A. C., & Selby, K. E. (1974). Medical anthropology. *Annual Review of Anthropology, 3,* 245–262.

Dougherty, M. C. (1976). Health agents in a rural Black community. *Journal of Afro-American Issues, 4,* 61–69.

Dougherty, M. C. (1978). *Becoming a woman in rural black culture*. New York: Holt, Rinehart and Winston.

Elms, R., Kevany, J., Thomson, C., & Webb, M. (1979). Cross-cultural study of initial visits to psychiatric outpatient clinics. *Nursing Research, 28,* 81–84.

Evaneshko, V., & Bauwens, E. E. (1976). Cognitive analysis and decision-making in medical emergencies. In M. Leininger, (Ed.), *Health care dimensions: Vol. 3. Transcultural health care issues and conditions* (pp. 83–102). Philadelphia: F. A. Davis.

Evaneshko, V., & Kay, M. A. (1982). The ethnoscience research technique. *Western Journal of Nursing Research, 4,* 49–64.

Flaskerud, J. H. (1979). Use of vignettes to elicit responses toward broad concepts. *Nursing Research, 28,* 210 –212.

Flaskerud, J. H. (1980a). Perceptions of problematic behavior by Appalachians, mental health professionals, and lay non-Appalachians. *Nursing Research, 29,* 140 –149.

Flaskerud, J. H. (1980b). Tool for comparing the perceptions of problematic behavior by psychiatric professionals and minority groups. *Nursing Research, 29,* 4–9.

Ford, V. (1973). Cultural criteria and determinants of modern medicine among the Teton Dakota, Rosebud Indian Reservation, South Dakota. In M. Batey (Ed.), *Communicating nursing research: Vol. 6. Collaboration and competition* (pp. 41–62). Boulder, CO: Western Interstate Commission for Higher Education.

Freidson, E. (1961). *Patients' views of medical practice*. New York: Russell Sage.

Germain, C. (1979). *The cancer unit: An ethnography*. Wakefield, MA: Nursing Resources.

Germain, C. (1980). Where it's at: An ethnography of a cancer unit. In M. Leininger (Ed.), *Transcultural nursing care: Teaching, practice and research. Proceedings from the Fifth National Transcultural Nursing Conference* (pp. 19–32). Salt Lake City: University of Utah College of Nursing.

Glittenberg, J. E. (1977). Fertility patterns and child-rearing of the Ladinos and Indians of Guatemala. In M. Leininger (Ed.), *Transcultural nursing care of infants and children: Proceedings from the First Transcultural Nursing Conference* (pp. 140–155). Salt Lake City: University of Utah College of Nursing.

Glittenberg, J. E. (1981). Variations in stress and coping in three migrant settlements—Guatemala City. *Image, 13,* 43–46.

Hautman, M. A., & Harrison, J. (1982). Health beliefs and practices in a middle-income Anglo-American neighborhood. *Advances in Nursing Science, 4*(3), 49–64.

Hoebel, E. A. (1966). *Anthropology: The study of man*. New York: McGraw-Hill.

Horn, B. M. (1977). Transcultural nursing and child rearing of the Muckleshoot people. In M. Leininger (Ed.), *Transcultural nursing care of infants and children: Proceedings from the First Transcultural Nursing Conference* (pp. 51–67). Salt Lake City: University of Utah College of Nursing.

Johnston, M., & Sarty, M. E. (1978). Maternal beliefs about vitamin efficacy in four U.S. subcultures. *Journal of Cross-cultural Psychology, 9,* 327–337.

Kay, M. A. (1973). Disease concepts in the barrio today. In M. Batey (Ed.), *Communicating nursing research: Vol. 6. Collaboration and competition* (pp. 185–194). Boulder, CO: Western Interstate Commission for Higher Education.

Kay, M. A. (1976). The fusion of Utoaztecan and European ethnogynecology in the Florilegio medicinal. *Proceedings of the XLI International Congress of Americanists, 3,* 323–330.

Kay, M. A. (1977a). The Florilegio medicinal: Source of southwest ethnomedicine. *Ethnohistory, 24,* 251–259.

Kay, M. A. (1977b). Health and illness in a Mexican American barrio. In E. Spicer (Ed.), *Ethnic medicine in the Southwest* (pp. 99–166). Tucson: The University of Arizona Press.

Kay, M. A. (1977c). Mexican-American fertility regulation. In M. Batey (Ed.), *Communicating nursing research: Vol. 10. Optimizing environments for health: Nursing's unique perspective* (pp. 279–294). Boulder, CO: Western Interstate Commission for Higher Education.

Kay, M. A. (1979). Lexemic change and semantic shift in disease names. *Culture, Medicine and Psychiatry, 3,* 73–94.

Kayser-Jones, J. S. (1979). Care of the institutionalized aged in Scotland and the United States: A comparative study. *Western Journal of Nursing Research, 1,* 190 –200.

Kendall, K. (1977). Maternal and child nursing in an Iranian village. In M. Leininger (Ed.), *Transcultural nursing care of infants and children: Proceedings from the First Transcultural Nursing Conference* (pp. 19–33). Salt Lake City: University of Utah College of Nursing.

Kleinman, A. M., Eisenberg, L., & Good, B. J. (1978). Culture, illness and care: Clinical lessons from anthropologic and cross-cultural research. *Annals of Internal Medicine, 99,* 25–58.

Koos, E. (1954). *The health of Regionville: What the people thought and did about it*. New York: Columbia University Press.

Kroska, R. (1977). Physical appraisal of Minnesota Ojibwa and White school children. In M. Leininger (Ed.), *Transcultural nursing care of infants and children: Proceedings from the First Transcultural Nursing Conference* (pp. 102–112). Salt Lake City: University of Utah College of Nursing.

Leininger, M. (1967). The culture concept and its relevance to nursing. *Journal of Nursing Education, 6*(2), 27–37.

Leininger, M. (1977a). The Gadsup of New Guinea and early child-caring behaviors with nursing care implications. In M. Leininger (Ed.), *Transcultural nursing care of infants and children: Proceedings from the First Transcultural Nursing Conference* (pp. 201–219). Salt Lake City: University of Utah College of Nursing.

Leininger, M. (1977b). Transcultural nursing and a proposed conceptual framework. In M. Leininger (Ed.), *Transcultural nursing care of infants and children: Proceedings from the First Transcultural Nursing Conference* (pp. 1–18). Salt Lake City: University of Utah College of Nursing.

Leininger, M. (Ed.). (1977c). *Transcultural nursing care of infants and children: Proceedings from the First National Transcultural Nursing Conference*. Salt Lake City: University of Utah College of Nursing.

Leininger, M. (Ed.). (1977d). *Transcultural nursing care of the elderly: Proceedings from the Second Transcultural Nursing Conference*. Salt Lake City: University of Utah College of Nursing.

Leininger, M. (1978a). Changing foci in American nursing education: Primary and transcultural nursing care. *Journal of Advanced Nursing, 3*, 155–166.

Leininger, M. (1978b). Culturalogical assessment domains for nursing practices. In M. Leininger (Ed.), *Transcultural nursing: Concepts, theories and practices* (pp. 85–106). New York: Wiley.

Leininger, M. (Ed.). (1978c). *Transcultural nursing: Concepts, theories and practices*. New York: Wiley.

Leininger, M. (1978d). Transcultural nursing: A new and scientific subfield of study in nursing. In M. Leininger (Ed.), *Transcultural nursing: Concepts, theories and practices* (pp. 7–30). New York: Wiley.

Leininger, M. (1978e). Transcultural nursing: Theories and research approaches. In M. Leininger (Ed.), *Transcultural nursing: Concepts, theories and practices* (pp. 31–51). New York: Wiley.

Leininger, M. (Ed.). (1979a). *Transcultural nursing care: The adolescent and the middle years. Proceedings from the Third Transcultural Nursing Conference*. Salt Lake City: University of Utah College of Nursing.

Leininger, M. (Ed.). (1979b). *Transcultural nursing care: Culture change, ethics and nursing care implications. Proceedings from the Fourth Transcultural Nursing Conference*. Salt Lake City: University of Utah College of Nursing.

Leininger, M. (1980a). Caring: A central focus of nursing and health care services. *Nursing and Health Care, 1*(3), 135–143, 176.

Leininger, M. (Ed.). (1980b). Transcultural nursing care: Teaching, practice and research. *Proceedings from the Fifth Transcultural Nursing Conference*. Salt Lake City: University of Utah College of Nursing.

Leininger, M. (1981). The phenomenon of caring: Importance, research questions and theoretical considerations. In M. Leininger (Ed.), *Caring: An essential human need. Proceedings of the Three National Caring Conferences* (pp. 3–15). Thorofare, NJ: Charles B. Slack.

Lewis, A. S. (1979). Physical anthropology and transcultural nursing. In M. Leininger (Ed.), *Transcultural nursing care: The adolescent and middle years. Proceedings from the Third National Transcultural Nursing Conference* (pp. 12–39). Salt Lake City: University of Utah College of Nursing.

Lewis, O. (1966). The culture of poverty. *Scientific American,* 215, 19–25.

Lipson, J. G. (1980). Consumer activism in two women's self-help groups. *Western Journal of Nursing Research, 2,* 393–405.

Lipson, J. G., & Tilden, V. P. (1980). Psychological integration of the cesaerean birth experience. *American Journal of Orthopsychiatry, 50,* 598–609.

Mackenzie, M. (1977). Mana in Maori medicine—Rarotonga Oceania. In R. Fogelson & N. Adams (Eds.), *The anthropology of power* (pp. 45–56). New York: Academic Press.

McKenna, M. (1979). An ethnoscientific approach to selected aspects of illness behavior among an urban American Indian population. In M. Leininger (Ed.), *Transcultural nursing care: Culture change, ethics and nursing care implications. Proceedings from the Fourth National Transcultural Nursing Conference* (pp. 140–165). Salt Lake City: University of Utah College of Nursing.

Milio, N. (1967). Values, social class, and community health services. *Nursing Research, 16,* 26–31.

Molgaard, C. A., & Byerly, E. L. (1981). Applied ethnoscience in rural America: New Age health and healing. In D. Messerschmidt (Ed.), *Anthropologists at home in America: Methods and issues in the study of one's own culture* (pp. 153–166). Cambridge, MA: Cambridge University Press.

Molgaard, C. A., Byerly, E. L., & Snow, C. T. (1979). Bach's flower remedies: A New Age therapy. *Human Organization, 38*(1), 71–74.

Muecke, M. A. (1976). Health care systems as socializing agents: Childbearing the North Thai and western ways. *Social Science and Medicine, 10,* 377–383.

Muecke, M. A. (1979). An exploration of "wind illness" in northern Thailand. *Culture, Medicine and Psychiatry, 3,* 267–300.

O'Brien, M. E. (1982). Pragmatic survivalism: Behavior patterns affecting low-level wellness among minority group members. *Advances in Nursing Science, 4*(3), 13–26.

Orem, D. (1980). *Nursing: Concepts of practice.* New York: McGraw-Hill.

Osborne, O. H. (1972). Social structure and health care systems: A Yoruba example. *Rural Africana, 17,* 80–86.

Osborne, O. H. (1977). Emic-etic issues in nursing research: An analysis of three studies. In M. Batey (Ed.), *Communicating nursing research: Vol. 9. Nursing research in the bicentennial year* (pp. 373–380). Boulder, CO: Western Interstate Commission for Higher Education.

Peay, D. (1977). Some cultural values of Mormons and their implications for health care of the elderly. In M. Leininger (Ed.), *Transcultural nursing care of the elderly: Proceedings from the Second National Transcultural Nursing Conference* (pp. 105–121). Salt Lake City: University of Utah College of Nursing.

Pike, K. (1954). *Language in relation to a unified theory of the structure of human behavior.* Glendale, CA: Summer Institute of Linguistics.

Pike, K. (1966). *Language in relation to a unified theory of the structure of human behavior*. The Hague: Mouton.

Powers, B. A. (1982). The use of orthodox and Black American folk medicine. *Advances in Nursing Science, 4*(3), 35–47.

Ragucci, A. T. (1972). The ethnographic approach and nursing research. *Nursing Research, 21,* 485–490.

Ragucci, A. T. (1977). The urban context of health beliefs and caring practices of the elderly women in an Italian-American enclave. In M. Leininger (Ed.), *Transcultural nursing care of the elderly: Proceedings from the Second National Transcultural Nursing Conference* (pp. 33–51). Salt Lake City: University of Utah College of Nursing.

Ragucci, A. T. (1981). Italian Americans. In A. Harwood (Ed.), *Ethnicity and medical care* (pp. 211–263). Cambridge, MA: Harvard University Press.

Redfield, R. (1947). The folk society. *American Journal of Sociology, 52,* 293–308.

Roy, C., & Roberts, S. L. (1981). *Theory construction in nursing: An adaptation model*. Englewood Cliffs, NJ: Prentice-Hall.

Scotch, N. (1963). Medical anthropology. In B. Siegel (Ed.), *Biennial review of anthropology* (pp. 30–68). Hartford, CT: University Press.

Segall, M. E. (1965). Blood pressure and culture change. *Nursing Science, 3,* 373–382.

Sohier, R. (1976). Gaining awareness of cultural difference: A case example. In M. Leininger (Ed.), *Health care dimensions, Vol. 3: Transcultural health care issues and conditions* (pp. 67–81). Philadelphia: F. A. Davis.

Stern, P. N. (1980). Grounded theory methodology: Its uses and processes. *Image, 12,* 20–23.

Stern, P. N. (1981a). A comparison of culturally-approved behaviors and beliefs between Pilipina immigrant women, American-born, dominant culture women and Western female nurses. In P. Morley (Ed.), *Developing, teaching and practicing transcultural nursing. Proceedings of the Sixth Transcultural Nursing Conference* (pp. 85–95). Salt Lake City: University of Utah College of Nursing and the Transcultural Nursing Society.

Stern, P. N. (1981b). Solving problems of cross-cultural health teaching: The Filipino childbearing family. *Image, 13,* 47–50.

Sturtevant, W. C. (1964). Studies in ethnoscience. *American Anthropologist, 66,* 99–131.

Sullivan, R. (1977). Some values, beliefs and practices of elderly women in the United States: Implications for health and nursing care. In M. Leininger (Ed.), *Transcultural care of the elderly: Proceedings from the Second National Transcultural Nursing Conference* (pp. 13–26). Salt Lake City: University of Utah College of Nursing.

Tripp-Reimer, T. (1980). Appalachian health care: From research to practice. In M. Leininger (Ed.), *Transcultural nursing care: Teaching, practice and research. Proceedings from the Fifth National Transcultural Nursing Conference* (pp. 48–59). Salt Lake City: University of Utah College of Nursing.

Tripp-Reimer, T. (1981). Ethnomedical beliefs and practices among Greek immigrants: Implications for nursing intervention. In P. Morley (Ed.), *Developing, teaching and practicing transcultural nursing: Proceedings of the Sixth Trans-*

cultural Nursing Conference (pp. 129–140). Salt Lake City: University of Utah College of Nursing and the Transcultural Nursing Society.

Tripp-Reimer, T. (1982a). Barriers to health care: Perceptual variations of Appalachian clients by Appalachian and non-Appalachian health care professionals. *Western Journal of Nursing Research, 4,* 179–191.

Tripp-Reimer, T. (1982b). Cultural influences on the potential for natural selection. *Central Issues in Anthropology, 4,* 49–57.

Tripp-Reimer, T. (1983). Retention of a folk healing practice (matiasma) among four generations of urban Greek immigrants. *Nursing Research, 32,* 97–101.

Tripp-Reimer, T., & Friedl, M. (1977). Appalachians: A neglected minority. *Nursing Clinics of North America, 12,* 41–54.

Tripp-Reimer, T., & Schrock, M. M. (1982). Residential patterns and preferences of ethnic aged: Implications for transcultural nursing. In C. Uhl & J. Uhl (Eds.), *Focus on transcultural nursing: Arching the domains of practice. Proceedings of the Seventh Transcultural Nursing Conference* (pp. 144–157). Salt Lake City: The Transcultural Nursing Society.

Uhl, J. (1981). Caring as the focus of a multidisciplinary health center for the elderly. In M. Leininger (Ed.), *Caring: An essential human need* (pp. 115–125). Thorofare, NJ: Charles B. Slack.

Urdaneta, M. L. (1975). Fertility and the "pill" in a Texas barrio. In S. Ingman & A. Thomas (Eds.), *Topias and utopias in health: Policy studies* (pp. 69–83). The Hague: Mouton.

Wang, J. (1979). A cross-cultural study of educational level and family planning among Chinese in Pittsburgh, Pennsylvania, and in Taipei, Taiwan. In M. Leininger (Ed.), *Transcultural nursing care: The adolescent and middle years. Proceedings from the Third National Transcultural Nursing Conference* (pp. 96–124). Salt Lake City: University of Utah College of Nursing.

Williams, M. A. (1972). A comparative study of post-surgical convalescence among women of two ethnic groups: Anglo and Mexican American. In M. Batey (Ed.), *Communicating nursing research: Vol. 5. The many sources of nursing knowledge* (pp. 59–73). Boulder, CO: Western Interstate Commission for Higher Education.

PART II

Research on Nursing Care Delivery

CHAPTER 5

Nurse Practitioners and Primary Care Research: Promises and Pitfalls

SHERRY L. SHAMANSKY
SCHOOL OF NURSING
YALE UNIVERSITY

CONTENTS

This chapter includes discussion of research on primary care provided by nurse practitioners working in ambulatory settings. The studies included here are those in which nurses were the principal investigators or where nurses were members of the research team. The health care literature is replete with data about the characteristics of nurse practitioners (Jelinek, 1978; Pesznecker & Draye, 1978; Ward, 1979), the demographic characteristics of their clients (Pesznecker & Draye, 1978), their practice settings (Sullivan, Dachelet, Sultz, & Henry, 1978), their educational preparation (Sultz, Henry, Kinyon, Buck, & Bullough, 1983a, 1983b), and their economic advantage (Fagin, 1982; Prescott & Sorenson, 1978). Therefore, inclusions in this chapter are limited to those in which the impact on the care, on the health care system, and on the acceptance of nurse practitioners was examined. The studies are limited to those done in the United States since 1975; excluded was the nurse midwifery literature. Research examples cited in this chapter were identified through MEDLARS, the National Technical Information Service (NTIS), and the U.S. Department of Health, Education and Welfare Division of Nursing (1978) publication entitled *Nurse Planning Information Series: Nurse Practitioners and the Expanded Role of the Nurse: A Bibliography*. Readers are referred to several review articles, including one by a physician, Sox (Abdellah, 1982; Diers & Molde, 1979; Dunn & Chard, 1980; Edmunds, 1978; Fagin, 1982; Sox, 1979; C. A. Williams, 1975; Yankauer & Sullivan, 1982) that provide a broad, historical examination of the primary health care literature and its concomitant issues.

HISTORICAL PERSPECTIVE AND DEFINITIONAL DILEMMAS

The nurse practitioner movement began in 1965 (Ford, Seacat, & Silver, 1966; Ford & Silver, 1967; Lewis & Resnick, 1967; Silver, Ford, & Stearly, 1967) and gained momentum in the troubled 1960s and 1970s. It was against this backdrop that nurse practitioners were educated and introduced into the health care scene because of a perceived shortage of primary care physicians. For those who needed medical care and were not able to get it, the physician shortage was real. The right of access to health care for all, one goal of primary health care, was thus part of many larger social issues present at that time. The introduction of this new breed of health care provider could be understood as an attempt by the government to solve the health care crisis.

From 1968 through 1972 there was an explosion of studies, symposia, commission reports, comments, and diatribes about nurse practitioners and other new health professionals. Systems analysts and researchers had a field day with the plethora of information; they "catalogued, costed, and timed the maneuvers that constitute a medical work-up . . . [they] probed the subtleties of professional identities and dominance and of patient-provider, nurse-physician, and male-female relationships" (Yankauer & Sullivan, 1982, p. 252).

Part of the difficulty in conducting research about primary care was the lack of a clear definition of this care, which, in the early days, was read as medical care. David Rogers (1977), President of the Robert Wood Johnson Foundation, defined primary care:

> First, it is care of a continuing, longitudinal nature. It also implies continuing medical responsibility for groups of people, and not just for individuals who seek a physician. It has integrationist qualities in that it must combine concern for social and psychological factors which contribute to illness with concern for factors that are physiologic and disease-oriented. (pp. 10–11)

According to the U.S. Department of Health, Education and Welfare (USDHEW) (1976), primary health care means:

> care which may be initiated by the client or provider in a variety of settings and which consists of a broad range of personal health care services including (a) promotion and maintenance of health, (b) prevention of illness and disability, (c) basic care during acute and chronic phases of illness, (d) guidance and counseling of individuals and families, and (e) referral to other health care providers and community resources when appropriate. (p. 3555)

Similarly, nurse practitioners have had difficulty in reaching consensus on the definition of nurse practitioner. The USDHEW (1976) provided the following definition:

> a registered nurse who has successfully completed a formal program of study designed to prepare registered nurses to deliver primary health care including the ability to: (a) assess the health status of individuals and families through health and medical history taking, physical examination, and defining of health and developmental problems; (b) institute and provide continuity of health care to clients; . . . (c) provide instruction and counseling to individuals, families and groups; . . . (d) work in collaboration with our other health care providers and agencies. (pp. 3552–3556)

These confusing and often cumbersome definitions pervaded the primary health care literature and contributed to conceptual difficulties apparent in the research.

CONCEPTUAL AND METHODOLOGICAL PROBLEMS

Whether nurse practitioners take their rightful place in the health care system is in part contingent upon well-documented, quantitative evidence essential to increase both the supply and the demand for their services. The introduction of nurse practitioners has been examined in terms of changes in cost, accessibility, quality, and productivity. In fact, the quality of services delivered by nurse practitioners has received far more attention than the quality of services ever provided by physicians.

Edmunds (1978) analyzed 471 books and journal articles about the work of nurse practitioners. She concluded that patients fully accepted nurse practitioners, and nurse practitioners were competent in the delivery of high-quality care. Sox (1979) examined 21 studies of nurse practitioners who provided primary care and compared their efforts to those of physicians; he found no differences in care provision between the two types of providers. As the costs of care began to escalate, possible cost savings were examined. Fagin (1982) analyzed nursing research on the efficacy of care over the last 20 years. She found convincing evidence that nurses provided competent and efficacious health care, resulting in great savings of health care dollars.

From the early days, however, two disparate views were expressed about the role of nurse practitioners in primary health care—they either extended or replaced physician services or they functioned within a uniquely nursing role. Irrespective of the view, if the patient is the focus in any research, then the quality of care must be adequate and acceptable, regardless of who provides it (Bailit, Lewis, Hochheiser, & Bush, 1975).

After nearly two decades of experience, the nurse practitioner movement suffers from a dearth of research conducted by nurses. In part, nurse practitioners have been so engrossed in legitimizing their practice that they have had little time, energy, or support to conduct well-executed studies. Although the literature is replete with studies about nurse practitioners and their work in primary health care dating back to the early 1960s, most of the research has been done by physicians, sociologists, or program evaluators. It is difficult to determine whether those investigators understood the research needs of the nursing profession.

The conceptual and methodological problems outlined here were not unique to the studies done by nurse researchers; these same problems were evident in the preponderance of studies carried out by non-nurses. Edmunds (1978) alleged that when nurse practitioners and physicians found themselves in practice together, they suddenly had the need to write about this new phenomenon. Pressure to describe the new role and lack of research expertise undoubtedly contributed to the many difficulties in the early research. All of the studies were designed after the innovation was introduced; the designs were fraught with the problems of retrospective analysis, missing data, and difficulties in data retrieval. Most investigators employed descriptive designs concerned with one practitioner and one practice setting. Too often methodological problems were not reported, nor was the instrumentation included. Generally, the psychometric properties of the instruments were not established. Questionnaires and chart reviews were the most common means of data collection, although charting may have been incomplete, varied from provider to provider, and did not include nursing activities. The studies suffered from inadequate pretesting of instruments, small samples, and inappropriate statistical analyses. Absent were longitudinal studies that might account for changes in standards of practice over time. Inadequate attention was paid to thorough descriptions of the providers when nurse practitioners and physicians were compared. Issues such as number of years in practice, amount of time per week spent in practice, specialty preparation and preference, and other factors were seldom addressed (Diers & Molde, 1979).

One of the most significant problems in the primary care literature was the lack of conceptualization. Donaldson and Crowley (1978) noted that this is a familiar problem. Nurse researchers often seemed to function primarily with tacit rather than explicit awareness of broad nursing concepts. This lack of conceptualization also was evident in the work of investigators from other disciplines.

Diers and Molde (1979) contended that conceptual problems, including definition of both the independent and dependent variables, together with lack of theory about nurse practitioner practice, permeated nurse practitioner research. In most of this research, investigators construed the practitioner as the independent variable, when a more appropriate conceptual understanding would be the practice, or system of care. Nurse practitioner care is more than technical medical care. Nurse practitioner care includes counseling, health education, advocacy—the art-of-care elements. When only medical diagnostic categories or protocols were used to describe and define nurse practitioner practice, many other patient care needs were left without classification according to these definitions.

If primary care is to be seen as the independent variable, then a search for conceptual clarity must continue. Such a definition would be far more complex than what is already known as traditional medicine. When a circumscribed set of operational definitions is used, threats to validity can be introduced. Researchers often use limited conceptual and operational definitions to achieve consensus about the meaning of a concept. However, in behavioral research, multiple explanations of concepts are desirable; very narrow definitions offer little information about whether findings are applicable in a variety of situations (Cooper, 1982).

If primary care is to become the independent variable, then explicit criteria should guide the definition of an adequate index of quality, assuming that such an index will elicit differences in quality. A conceptual definition of primary care should reflect a broader range of conditions than do most of the existing indices of outcome. Little of the nurse practitioner's work is concerned with life-threatening events, and given that about half of the patients have more than one diagnosis, the customary indices, that is, morbidity and mortality, are of limited relevance. Nurses must develop reliable and valid measures that account for both medical criteria and also the client's ability to function normally. In addition to the medical diagnosis, a person's subjective reaction to the condition that gives rise to the medical problem and underlies the motives for seeking care must be considered. And the client must play an important role in judging the improvement (Kalinowski, 1978).

The evaluation of ambulatory care and its providers is appealing. Because an outcome approach involves a direct measure of health, it has inherent validity. It follows that since nurse practitioner care was seen as a subset of medical care, then patient outcomes were defined in the traditional ways. However, outcome appraisal has its own difficulties, not the least of which is that one's health is affected by many factors outside the purview of established medicine, and these confounding and intervening variables are difficult to control in establishing outcome measures. The more traditional measures (morbidity and mortality) can be insensitive in the short term (Mushlin, Appel, & Barr, 1978). Morbidity measures are also difficult to interpret because many of the health problems treated by primary care providers are self-limiting and eventually would resolve without medical or nursing intervention. Measurement of the disability or impairment caused by the illnesses would give a more valid indication of outcomes from short-term contacts with primary care providers (Kane et al., 1976). Epidemiological methods that account for both physiological and behavioral variables at the aggregate level would be useful in giving primary care providers the data with which to identify high-risk clients and their appropriate treatments (Yankauer & Sullivan, 1982).

It is well known that nurse practitioners tend to care for patients who either are essentially well, for example, well children, or have chronic illnesses. The measurement of outcomes in clients with chronic illnesses is, according to Diers and Molde (1979), a conceptually difficult task. Chronic illnesses are often multifactorial in nature. One cannot assume that the presenting problem is the only problem the client has. Therefore, it is almost impossible to develop measures of the effect of any kind of practitioner care that are valid, practical, or account for the other illnesses and treatments affecting the presenting condition. Moreover, according to Diers and Molde (1979) because the presenting problem is likely to be compounded by social or environmental problems, researchers frequently developed outcome measures that did not necessarily fit the target population.

There is one other reason why morbidity and mortality indicators are worrisome in nurse practitioner research. For patients with chronic illnesses, stability (rather than recovery) is usually the desired outcome. Similarly, for clients who are essentially well, stability is also the goal, since healthy people do not generally become more healthy. In these examples, the traditional indices again are unsuited to the population.

Several investigators (Diers & Molde, 1979; Edmunds, 1978; Prescott, Jacox, Collar, & Goodwin, 1981) held that much of the nurse practitioner research is atheoretical, as evaluation research tends to be. In defining the dependent variable and developing standards for care, evaluation strategies must be precise and sensitive enough to reflect the process of clinical judgment. Diers and Molde (1979) recommended that prescriptive theory (Dickoff & James, 1968) might be useful in defining nurse practitioner work as a system of care.

Other methodological problems precluded the conduct of true experiments through which investigators could examine the relationships between processes and outcomes (Prescott et al., 1981). Yet it is incumbent upon nurse researchers to begin to examine the process of care itself and to link the process components with outcomes. Nurses must begin to examine those elements of the nurse practitioner role and those interactions between nurse practitioner and client that account for positive changes (Sullivan, 1982).

C. A. Williams (1975) posed several considerations when evaluating the quality of decision making among nurse practitioners. Without accounting for the input of physicians who contributed to the protocols or, in some cases, conjointly managed the patients, it was difficult to evaluate the medical decisions made by nurse practitioners. Investigators also must attend to the arrangements between nurse practitioners and physicians for managing patients. Yankauer and Sullivan (1982) stated that according to empirical findings, role overlap was more apparent than role differentiation in primary care, and that it might be counterproductive to seek role clarity among primary health care providers. The purpose of primary care is to monitor the management of patients over time. Usually this involves several encounters; some of these are managed by the nurse practitioner and others by the physician. Therefore, it may be more appropriate to examine the care provided by the nurse practitioner–physician team.

RESEARCH EXAMPLES

Acceptance Studies

The attitudinal studies about nurse practitioners tended to fall into three categories: acceptance by patients and parents of patients, acceptance by physicians, and acceptance by other health professionals and agencies.

Connelly and Connelly (1979) surveyed 40 residents and interns in a primary care medical clinic to determine whether these physicians' behavior patterns in the referral of clients to nurse practitioners correlated with their attitudes. Data were obtained from patient data sheets and self-administered questionnaires. Although the physicians displayed positive attitudes about nurse practitioners and their potential impact on the health care delivery system, they referred patients to nurse practitioners at low rates. This study lacked both conceptual and methodological rigor. What the residents' and interns' backgrounds and past experiences with nurse practitioners had been, information about the nurse practitioner, and the effect of chronically ill patients on the health care providers were issues never discussed.

Levine, Orr, Sheatsley, Lohr, and Brodie (1978) undertook a comprehensive study of nurse practitioners to determine their responsibilities and effectiveness in various practice settings. Findings suggested that physicians tended to be satisfied with the performance of nurse practitioners, and patient attitudes indicated satisfaction with treatment by nurse practitioners. By including various settings, this study was a response to the problem of earlier data generated from only one practice setting. Although the researchers pretested the five instruments, they did not establish reliability and validity. The investigators did include the teaching and counseling activities of the nurse practitioner, but they did not link these functions to any conceptual understanding of nurse practitioner practice. It was assumed, then, that for these investigators the standard for practice was medical care.

In an interesting replication of the Lewis and Resnick (1967) Kansas Nurse Clinic Study, Lewis and Cheyovich (1976) examined the impact of two different styles of care provided by nurse practitioners on the patients and on physicians with whom they worked. Patients appropriate for the clinical trial were grouped according to referring physicians and primary diagnosis and then randomly allocated to the control or experimental group. Once assigned to the experimental group, they were further assigned at random to one of the two nurse practitioners who were matched in terms of educational preparation and experience. Patients in the control group continued to receive care from the physicians. Encounter sheets were used to describe the various process components of care. A one-year follow-up was done using the same questionnaire. One of the practitioners saw her patients more frequently, spent more time with them, ordered more medications, and used physician consultation less often. The other nurse practitioner tended to depend upon the physician for validation of her care. The physicians did not differentiate between the functioning of the two nurse practitioners in terms of their care. However, patients cared for by the more independent nurse practitioner saw nurses as a common source of information about illness and demonstrated more shifts in preference for care provided by nurse practitioners than by physicians.

This study was exciting in several ways: It was well-designed, both conceptually and methodologically. These researchers offered a conceptual approach to the roles of health care providers; these roles were defined as instrumental or expressive. The clinical trial was executed carefully. Perhaps most significantly, this study provided information on one of the central questions about nurse practitioner care. It was the rare study in which the investigator recognized the significance of individual style differences as relevant factors in evaluating the effectiveness of nurse practitioners. These data were critical in teasing out the special contributions that nurse practitioners make in primary health care. The researchers were also cognizant that the process components of care might have contributed to a different set of outcomes. The logical next step, then, would be to link processes with outcomes.

More recently, researchers opened promising lines of inquiry in the analysis of attitudes and acceptance. Derived from theories of the diffusion of innovations (E. Rogers, 1962), marketing concepts offered an exciting link between attitudes and acceptance and consumer demands and needs. Brands (1983) surveyed 331 people in a Southwestern urban community to determine whether selected demographic, experiential, or attitudinal characteristics were associated with retired people's acceptance of the nurse practitioner for performing traditional, transitional, and nontraditional primary care functions. Discriminant analysis differentiated the characteristics of people who chose the nurse or who had no preference for either nurse or physician from those who preferred the physician. Those retired persons who preferred the nurse were primarily English-speaking, younger than age 70, having at least seven years of formal education, and having a family income of $10,000 or more. These respondents agreed with the statement that nurses can do the same things that physicians can do. The findings suggested a likely relationship between the selection of the nurse and the knowledge of the independent activities of the nurse. This study corroborated the findings of Pender and Pender (1980), who determined that education beyond high school was one of the best predictors of intention to use nurse-provided services. These data reconfirmed E. Rogers' (1962) premise that people who are innovators have more education than those who are most traditional.

Similar results to those of Brands (1983) were found by Smith and Shamansky (1983). Using a stratified random sample of 239 people listed in the Seattle, Washington, telephone directory, a survey provided data about the relationships between consumer values and their intentions to use family nurse practitioner (FNP) services. Using the theory of diffusion of innovations as a conceptual base, these researchers hypothesized that consumers would be likely to purchase new health care options in the same way that they purchased new products. Discriminant analysis suggested that the best predictors of intention to use innovative services, such as FNP care, were age, family size, compatibility of such services with individual and family norms, prior knowledge of FNP care, and the value attached to health education. The profile of users included women, relatively more affluent, better educated, and younger than the general population. Data accumulated from these more rigorous studies (Brands, 1983; Smith & Shamansky, 1983) extended the available literature on attitudes and acceptance and provided much-needed theoretical approaches for the design of marketing strategies to reach particular target groups, while meeting the needs of both consumers and providers of care.

The data from the studies cited in this section demonstrated marked variability in attitudes and acceptance, depending upon the specific practice setting and the sample. The extent to which the role of the nurse practitioner was validated by physicians, the severity of the illness, and the experiences with nurse practitioners over time were important variables that contributed to acceptance among clients. Many of the findings must be viewed with caution, because many of the opinion surveys were limited by small, nonprobability samples or samples from single medical specialities. Regardless of the conceptual and methodological pitfalls, however, these studies provided evidence that nurse practitioners were accepted as primary care providers by clients.

Impact Studies

Impact studies were grouped into two broad categories: the impact of nurse practitioners on the quality and type of care delivered, and the impact of nurse practitioners on the practice setting itself. These studies can be divided further into those with (a) impact on physician activities, and (b) impact on the economics of the practice. For most studies in these categories investigators used comparative designs; comparisons almost always were made between nurse practitioners, or nurse practitioner–physician teams, and physicians. The methods most frequently used were observation, interview, questionnaire, or chart audit.

Chen, Barkauskas, Ohlson, and Chen (1977, 1978) systematically documented student–patient encounter data in order to classify and analyze health problems identified by the students. Because medical diagnostic categories derived from the International Classification of Diseases Adapted for Use in the United States (ICDA) were used, the categories were most applicable in classifying health problems when there was some pathophysiology present. The researchers concluded that the findings justified the need to develop problem classification systems that fit primary health care in its broadest sense and confirmed the need to examine carefully the unique contributions of nurse practitioners to a system of care. In a later study, Chen, Barkauskas, Ohlson, and Chen (1982) again construed the independent variable as the practitioner rather than the practice. Conceptualization of care, therefore, was quite narrow.

In a well-designed study that included evaluation of telephone management of five common conditions, Goodman and Perrin (1978) and Perrin and Goodman (1978) found that pediatric nurse practitioners scored significantly higher ($p < .001$) in terms of interview skills when compared with private pediatricians and pediatric residents. Nurse practitioners also scored higher on the content evaluation of history taking and referral. During well-child visits, nurse practitioners elicited more information on child development and behavior, were more direct in providing information to the parent, and offered more opportunities for parents to share information and ask questions. This study was an excellent sample of conceptual clarity about the expressive and instrumental process components of care.

Heagarty, Grossi, and O'Brien (1977) evaluated 29 pediatric nurse associates and 15 nurse associate trainees working in the child health care system of a large city health department. The comparative data on the productivity of dissimilar health workers were culled from system-wide information used for managerial rather than research purposes. This was another example of an atheoretical evaluation scheme in which productivity was defined in terms of medical tasks.

Komaroff, Sawayer, Flatley, and Browne (1976) examined patients with signs and symptoms of acute, minor illnesses. Using protocols, a nurse practitioner managed one group of patients, while a physician managed the other group. Safety, effectiveness, efficiency, and cost of care for minor, acute illnesses in both modes (nurse practitioner versus physician) were compared. No serious illnesses were missed by the nurse practitioners or physicians. Patients in the nurse practitioner group scored higher with regard to relief of symptoms. Patients in both groups reported equivalent satisfaction with care, and personnel costs were equal in both groups. However, costs for medications and laboratory tests were 27% less in the nurse protocol mode. Although protocols are an attempt to standardize care and an indirect effort to increase reliability and validity, they further restrict the conceptualization of care.

McLaughlin et al. (1978a, 1978b, 1978c, 1979a, 1979b) compared the clinical judgment of nurse practitioners to physicians in the management of essential hypertension and chronic obstructive pulmonary disease.

In these simulations the nurse group emphasized patient education approaches, compliance strategies, and reduction of risk factors to a greater extent than did the physicians. The family practice physicians tended to have the lowest scores on the use of the psychosocial nursing model in all applicable categories.

Diers and Molde (1979) argued that comparisons of nurse practitioners and physicians are problematic. It is assumed that health care providers define their ideas for practice according to the entrenched boundaries of their respective professional disciplines. Nevertheless, both physicians and nurse practitioners cross these boundaries; for example, physicians counsel and teach patients, and nurse practitioners make diagnosis and management decisions about their patients. Given the absence of precise and sensitive criteria to examine nurse practitioner practice, comparative studies of this nature are extremely difficult to execute.

Using the concept of hidden agendas, Molde and Baker (1983) examined the reasons that motivate people to request visits to a clinic staffed by nurse practitioners. Approximately 30% of the 128 patients sampled had hidden agendas that could not have been predicted without careful probing. For example, although someone presented with a headache, the patient really wanted to discuss concerns about a partner. Despite its methodological problems, this study added to the conceptual understanding of nurse practitioner practice. Findings from this study underscored the therapeutic and diagnostic significance of learning why patients seek care.

Cognizant of the fact that most nurse practitioner research included reliance upon instruments with unknown psychometric properties, Prescott et al. (1981) and Goodwin, Prescott, Jacox, and Collar (1981) developed an instrument to account for nurse practitioner practice when the role combined medical and nursing functions along a continuum of care/cure activities. Extensive reliability studies were conducted on this instrument over a two-year period; these were reported in detail by the authors. Some evidence existed for the validity of the observation form, especially in teaching activity categories. As one of the first efforts to establish the reliability and validity of instruments to be used in nurse practitioner research, this methodological work is indeed promising. However, its practicality will have to be weighed against its complexity.

FUTURE RESEARCH DIRECTIONS

The extensive literature available in the United States on nurse practitioners in primary health care seems to parallel the concern about physician work load, supply, and the escalation in health care expenditures. However, future directions must include rigorous scrutiny of the work of nurse practitioners, and these studies must be based upon nursing concepts reflecting both the art and the science of care.

If a conceptual definition of primary care is to include the humanistic and nontraditional approaches to health, then in future research investigators must consider individual health perceptions, beliefs about current and previous health status, susceptibility to illness, and anxiety about health. Researchers have demonstrated that personal health perceptions are significant in the demand for primary care services (Hamermesh & Hamermesh, 1983).

A fundamental concern about health care research is whether the presumed benefits of such research can be qualified, that is, can people discuss the degree to which they value health? Values about health are always relative to other personal, social, or national goals. These other goals may be significant motivating or intervening factors in the demand for health care, compliance with prescribed therapeutic regimens, and other health behaviors. Little research has been done on the issue of whether consumers and professionals understand the implications of their value choices. For example, is it believed that health care dollars spent on specialist care are health care dollars unavailable for primary care services? Although these relationships are not well understood at the moment, they are certain to have implications for nurse practitioner practice and research in the future (Williams & Brook, 1978).

Years of efforts directed toward quality assurance has led to recognition that quality of health care is an elusive notion. Much work examining process components separately from outcomes of health care has occurred; more recently researchers are attempting to relate process and outcome measures. Increasing numbers of instruments and methods are being developed and refined, and recently efforts have been directed toward measuring patient outcomes that are more consistent with nursing's goals and activities.

The basic activities of health care can be understood and monitored, but the precise deficiencies, especially in nurse practitioner practice, are not as well understood. One future direction for nurse researchers interested in primary care might be to examine the process of care for explanations when outcomes are deficient or absent. For example, deficient outcomes might be defined as the occurrence of preventable illnesses or conditions; then the process of care could be examined if these events occurred. Outcome strategies useful for common conditions require measures that are sensitive to the objectives of primary care, that is, measures that reflect the goals not only of treating and curing illnesses, but also of alleviating discomfort, disability, and distress (Mushlin et al., 1978).

Sullivan (1982) offered two suggestions for future studies:

> First, the "soft" process variables—such as communication factors, client participation in treatment, and continuity of provider—must be studied in combination with the "hard" clinical variables, such as serum chemistries, drug dosages, and diet and exercise regimens. In turn, outcome measures need to represent a combination of adherence/health promoting behaviors adopted by the client, together with the effect of the right processes and treatment combinations that lead to improved clinical outcomes. (p. 9)

Much work remains to be done on nurse practitioners' contributions to increasing the self-care capabilities of clients. It is expected that such research endeavors will promote a better understanding of the political issues today labeled as the supplemental or substitutive functions of nurse practitioners.

Although the quality of health care has been studied off and on for over a century, much conceptual and empirical work is yet to be done, especially in the primary care arena. It is essential that such issues as the extent to which patient outcomes can be related to the type of delivery in light of the predicted oversupply of physicians in the next decades be investigated. The impact on medical costs of nurse practitioner services must be evaluated, and explicit attempts must be initiated to examine the costs of achieving better quality care and to determine whether these efforts are balanced by eventual improvements in health.

Perhaps primary care needed little explicit definition until the societal changes extant in the last decades precipitated a search for the specific functional and qualitative attributes that differentiate primary care from the rest of the health–illness spectrum. Therefore, the following researchable questions must be considered in the next decade:

1. What are the benchmarks of primary care? Do family nurse practitioners make a difference in treating families? Are individuals and the family constellation improved because of family nurse practitioner intervention?
2. To what extent will a health orientation become a part of primary care? Will activities such as biofeedback, stress management, natural therapies, and other treatments still not definable in scientific terminology be incorporated into nurse practitioner practice models?
3. What are nurse practitioners in primary care doing about new illnesses and new epidemiology, for example, acquired immune deficiency syndrome (AIDS)? Are the chief problems with which clients present themselves in the primary care setting those which

nurse practitioners can resolve? Is there evidence that primary care prevents, anticipates, or corrects incipient illnesses?

4. Will responsibility for the health care of the individual extend to client groups and go beyond client-initiated contact? To what extent will interventions other than personal health care services be employed? Can the risk of illness in populations defined by enrollment or geography be decreased by nurse practitioners?
5. Can practice models be conceptualized in creative ways? Or are ill-conceived, restrictive practices ones which consumers will come to expect and demand to be delivered, without the realization that little good is done?
6. To what extent are teams, including primary care physicians and nurse practitioners, models that are reasonably cost effective and suitable for patients? Will those teams give way to the pressures of separate reimbursement, so that patients will have to negotiate yet another kind of fragmentation?

Answers to these questions will be contingent upon increased conceptual and methodological rigor in nurse practitioner research. Diers and Molde (1979) concluded that more careful attention should be paid to sampling, developing measures better suited to chronically ill and well populations, defining comparison groups and initiating longitudinal studies, considering new sources of data, examining charting practices, and establishing more relevant standards of care. Nurse researchers must select an appropriate paradigm for use in nurse practitioner research. Such a model might be based on clinical judgment, including gathering data, processing information, making decisions, and evaluating care.

There are several other issues germane to the discussion of future directions in nurse practitioner research. Individual studies must be related and elaborated, thereby creating a larger context for reference. This problem confronts all nurse researchers, but it becomes particularly important in primary health care research, the need for which grew out of an already fragmented system of health care. It is encouraging to observe that those nurse researchers interested in the work of nurse practitioners have begun to replicate earlier studies and elaborate the growing body of literature. It is also heartening to note that the primary health care research conducted by nurses, scant though it is, is appearing not only in refereed nursing journals, but also in other journals such as *Medical Care, New England Journal of Medicine, American Journal of Public Health, Evaluation and the Health Professions, Annual Review of Public Health,* and *Journal of Community Health,* among others.

When the volume of studies conducted by physicians and/or program evaluators is compared to the numbers conducted by nurse researchers, it is strikingly apparent that nurse researchers have received minimal financial support for work of this kind. Large-scale research on nurse practitioner practice, with nurse practitioners as principal investigators, must be developed and funded. The work of nurse practitioners is patient care; yet incentives and opportunities for them to initiate and participate in clinical research must be created. Fagin (1982) contended that additional funding will be forthcoming if the findings of nursing research are disseminated to those who influence decisions in the social and political spheres. Journal articles that include discussion of the impact of nurse practitioner practice could be abstracted and sent to decision makers and other nurse researchers. In this way access to and use of the data might be improved significantly. Finally, the large body of literature that is not research must not be ignored. Many of these "think pieces" present well-reasoned, stimulating, and challenging ideas that might evolve into future researchable issues.

REFERENCES

Abdellah, F. G. (1982). The nurse practitioner 17 years later: Present and emerging issues. *Inquiry, 19,* 105–116.

Bailit, H., Lewis, J., Hochheiser, L., & Bush, N. (1975). Assessing the quality of care. *Nursing Outlook, 23,* 153–159.

Brands, R. (1983). Acceptance of nurses as primary-care providers by retired people. *Advances in Nursing Science, 5*(3), 37–49.

Chen, S. C., Barkauskas, V. H., Ohlson, V. M., & Chen, E. H. (1977). Documented clinical experiences of primary care RN students: A preliminary report. *Nursing Research, 26,* 342–348.

Chen, S. C., Barkauskas, V. H., Ohlson, V. M., & Chen, E. H. (1978). Patient encounters by primary care nurse students. *Research in Nursing and Health, 1,* 18–28.

Chen, S. C., Barkauskas, V. H., Ohlson, V. M., & Chen, E. H. (1982). Health problems encountered by nurse practitioners and physicians. *Nursing Research, 31,* 163–169.

Connelly, S. V., & Connelly, P. A. (1979). Physicians' patient referrals to a nurse practitioner in a primary care medical clinic. *American Journal of Public Health, 69,* 73–75.

Cooper, H. M. (1982). Scientific guidelines for conducting integrative research reviews. *Reviews of Educational Research, 52,* 291–302.

Dickoff, J., & James, P. (1968). Theory of theories: A position paper. *Nursing Research, 17,* 197–203.

Diers, D., & Molde, S. (1979). Some conceptual and methodological issues in nurse practitioner research. *Research in Nursing and Health, 2,* 73–84.

Donaldson, S. K., & Crowley, D. M. (1978). The discipline of nursing. *Nursing Outlook, 26,* 113–120.

Dunn, B. H., & Chard, M. A. (Eds.). (1980). *Nurse Practitioners: A review of the literature 1965–1979* (ANA Publication No. NP-62 2M 10/80). Kansas City, MO: American Nurses' Association.

Edmunds, M. W. (1978). Evaluation of nurse practitioner effectiveness: An overview of the literature. *Evaluation and the Health Professions, 1,* 69–82.

Fagin, C. M. (1982). Nursing as an alternative to high-cost care. *American Journal of Nursing, 82,* 56–60.

Ford, L. C., Seacat, M. S., & Silver, G. G. (1966). Broadening roles of public health nurse and physician in prenatal and infant supervision. *American Journal of Public Health, 56,* 1097–1103.

Ford, L. C., & Silver, H. K. (1967). The expanded role of the nurse in child care. *Nursing Outlook, 15,* 43–45.

Goodman, H. C., & Perrin, E. C. (1978). Evening telephone call management by nurse practitioners and physicians. *Nursing Research, 27,* 233–237.

Goodwin, L., Prescott, P., Jacox, A., & Collar, M. (1981). The nurse practitioner rating form. Part II: Methodological development. *Nursing Research, 30,* 270–276.

Hamermesh, D. S., & Hamermesh, F. W. (1983). Does perception of life expectancy reflect health knowledge? *American Journal of Public Health, 73,* 911–914.

Heagarty, M. C., Grossi, M. T., & O'Brien, M. (1977). Pediatric nurse associates in a large official health agency: Their education, training, productivity, and cost. *American Journal of Public Health, 67,* 855–858.

Jelinek, D. (1978). The longitudinal study of nurse practitioners: Report of phase I. *Nurse Practitioner, 3*(1), 17–19.

Kalinowski, R. H. (1978). Primary care training: Some random thoughts. *Mount Sinai Journal of Medicine, 45,* 612–619.

Kane, R. L., Woolley, F. R., Gardner, H. J., Snell, G. F., Leight, E. H., & Castle, C. H. (1976). Measuring outcomes of care in an ambulatory primary care population. *Journal of Community Health, 1,* 233–240.

Komaroff, A. L., Sawayer, K., Flatley, M., & Browne, C. (1976). Nurse practitioner management of common respiratory and genitourinary infections, using protocols. *Nursing Research, 25,* 84–89.

Levine, J. L., Orr, S. T., Sheatsley, D. W., Lohr, J. A., & Brodie, B. M. (1978). The nurse practitioner: Role, physician utilization, patient acceptance. *Nursing Research, 27,* 245–254.

Lewis, C. E., & Cheyovich, T. K. (1976). Who is a nurse practitioner? Processes of care and patients' and physicians' perceptions. *Medical Care, 14,* 365–371.

Lewis, C. E., & Resnick, B. A. (1967). Nurse clinics in ambulatory care. *New England Journal of Medicine, 277,* 1236–1241.

McLaughlin, F. E., Cesa, T. A., Johnson, H. G., Lemons, M. M., Anderson, S. J., Larson, P. J., & Gibson, J. R. (1978a). *Primary care judgments of nurses and physicians: Vol. 1. Report of the research.* Springfield, VA: U.S. Department of Commerce, National Technical Information Service (NTIS No. HRP 0900605).

McLaughlin, F. E., Cesa, T. A., Johnson, H. G., Lemons, M. M., Anderson, S. J., Larson, P. J., & Gibson, J. R. (1978b). *Primary care judgments of nurses and physicians: Vol. 2. Clinical simulation test for hypertension*. Springfield, VA: U.S. Department of Commerce, National Technical Information Service (NTIS No. HRP 0900606).

McLaughlin, F. E., Cesa, T. A., Johnson, H. G., Lemons, M. M., Anderson, S. J., Larson, P. J., & Gibson, J. R. (1978c). *Primary care judgments of nurses and physicians: Vol. 3. Clinical simulation test for COPD*. Springfield, VA: U.S. Department of Commerce, National Technical Information Service (NTIS No. HRP 0900607).

McLaughlin, F. E., Cesa, T. A., Johnson, H. G., Lemons, M. M., Anderson, S. J., Larson, P. J., & Gibson, J. R. (1979a). Nurses' and physicians' performance on clinical simulation tests: Hypertension. *Research in Nursing and Health, 2,* 61–72.

McLaughlin, F. E., Cesa, T. A., Johnson, H. G., Lemons, M. M., Anderson, S. J., Larson, P. J., & Gibson, J. R. (1979b). Nurse practitioners', public health nurses' and physicians' performance on clinical simulation: COPD. *Western Journal of Nursing Research, 1,* 273–295.

Molde, S., & Baker, D. (1983, June). *Explaining primary care visits*. Paper presented at the meeting of the Fourth Annual Nurse Practitioner Symposium, Baltimore, MD.

Mushlin, A. I., Appel, F. A., & Barr, D. M. (1978). Quality assurance in primary care: A strategy based on outcome assessment. *Journal of Community Health, 3,* 292–305.

Pender, N. J., & Pender, A. R. (1980). Illness prevention and health promotion services provided by nurse practitioners: Predicting potential consumers. *American Journal of Public Health, 70,* 798–803.

Perrin, E. C., & Goodman, H. C. (1978). Telephone management of acute pediatric illness. *New England Journal of Medicine, 298,* 130–135.

Pesznecker, B. L., & Draye, M. A. (1978). Family nurse practitioners in primary care: A study of practice and patients. *American Journal of Public Health, 68,* 977–980.

Prescott, P. A., Jacox, A., Collar, M., & Goodwin, L. (1981). The nurse practitioner rating form, Part I: Conceptual development and potential uses. *Nursing Research, 30,* 223–228.

Prescott, P., & Sorenson, J. (1978). Cost-effectiveness analysis: An approach to evaluating nursing programs. *Nursing Administration Quarterly, 3*(1), 17–40.

Rogers, D. E. (1977). Primary care: Some issues. *Bulletin of the New York Academy of Medicine, 53,* 10–17.

Rogers, E. (1962). *Diffusion of innovations*. New York: Free Press.

Silver, H. K., Ford, L. C., & Stearly, S. G. (1967). A program to increase health care for children: The pediatric nurse practitioner program. *Pediatrics, 39,* 756–760.

Smith, D. W., & Shamansky, S. L. (1983). Determining the market for family nurse practitioner services: The Seattle experience. *Nursing Research, 32,* 301–305.

Sox, H. C. (1979). Quality of patient care by nurse practitioners and physician's assistants: A ten-year perspective. *Annals of Internal Medicine, 91,* 459–468.

Sullivan, J. A. (1982). Research on nurse practitioners: Process behind the outcome? *American Journal of Public Health, 72,* 8–9.

Sullivan, J. A., Dachelet, C. Z., Sultz, H. A., & Henry, M. (1978). The rural nurse practitioner: A challenge and a response. *American Journal of Public Health, 68,* 972–976.

Sultz, H. A., Henry, O. M., Kinyon, L. J., Buck, G. M., & Bullough, B. (1983a). A decade of change for nurse practitioners. *Nursing Outlook, 31,* 137–141.

Sultz, H. A., Henry, O. M., Kinyon, L. J., Buck, G. M., & Bullough, B. (1983b). Nurse practitioners: A decade of change—Part II. *Nursing Outlook, 31,* 216–219.

U.S. Department of Health, Education and Welfare, Division of Nursing. (1978). Nurse Planning Information Series: *Nurse practitioners and the expanded role of the nurse: A bibliography* (DHEW Publication No. HRA 79–20). Hyattsville, MD: Author. (NTIS No. HRP 0500601)

U.S. Department of Health, Education and Welfare. (1976). Nurse practitioner training: Proposed grant program. *Federal Register, 41,* 3552–3556.

Ward, M. J. (1979). Family nurse practitioners: Perceived competencies and recommendations. *Nursing Research, 28,* 343–347.

Williams, C. A. (1975). Nurse practitioner research: Some neglected issues. *Nursing Outlook, 23,* 172–177.

Williams, K. N., & Brook, R. H. (1978). Research opportunities in primary care. *Mount Sinai Journal of Medicine, 45,* 663–672.

Yankauer, A., & Sullivan, J. (1982). The new health professionals: Three examples. *Annual Review of Public Health, 3,* 249–276.

CHAPTER 6

Nursing Diagnosis

MARJORY GORDON
SCHOOL OF NURSING
BOSTON COLLEGE

CONTENTS

The purpose of this chapter was to summarize and critique the major investigations related to identification and validation of nursing diagnoses. The review of research spanned the years 1950 to 1983. This period encompassed the first reference to nursing diagnosis in the literature (McManus, 1950), the initiation of systematic efforts to identify the phenomena of concern to nurses, and attempts to validate nursing diagnoses through clinical research. No attempt was made to review research pertaining to each of the 50 to 70 currently identified nursing diagnoses because of the extensive nature of such a review. Literature indexes, computer listings, hand searches of major nursing research journals, proceedings of conferences, and informal contacts with colleagues in the United States and Canada were used to identify research reports. Included in the review were studies with the stated purpose of identification or validation of diagnostic concepts within the domain of nursing practice and studies in which directions for future research were identified. Eight studies were accessed in this review, none of which was published in research journals. One explanation for the small number of studies was the fairly recent attention to independent diagnostic and therapeutic judgments in nursing and to nursing diagnosis (American Nurses' Association, 1973, 1980; Clark, 1978; Mundinger, 1980). Autonomy in an area of clinical judgment implied responsibility for research; yet it also was noted that no nursing journal or research textbook provided information on the application of quantitative or qualitative research models to this area. Gordon and Sweeney (1979) outlined some approaches, but not in sufficient detail to guide investigators. The studies reviewed represented an attempt on the part of investigators to identify phenomena of diagnostic and therapeutic concern and to create a language to describe these phenomena.

OVERVIEW AND DEFINITIONS

The current effort to identify, validate, and classify nursing diagnoses (Kim, McFarland, & McLean, 1984, pp. 472–477; Kim & Moritz, 1982, pp. 283–319) rests on assumptions that a distinct group of actual and potential health conditions exists which are amenable to nursing intervention. The conceptual domain of health conditions to be described by nursing diagnoses lacks consensus (Roy, 1984). Conceptual definitions of nursing diagnoses are as varied as the views of nursing itself. For example, diagnoses are viewed as patterns of unitary man (Roy, 1984), self-care agency deficits (Orem, 1980), ineffective adaptions (Roy & Roberts, 1981), behavioral systems dysfunctions (Johnson, 1980), conflicts in needs (Soares, 1978), alteration in meeting human needs (Yura & Walsh, 1982, 1983), and dysfunctional health patterns (Gordon, 1982a, 1982b). Leaders in the American Nurses' Association (1980) view human responses as the focus of diagnosis and treatment, although others specify unhealthful responses (Jones & Jakob, 1982; Mundinger & Jauron, 1975).

In the studies reviewed, investigators bypassed the conceptual diversity and defined nursing diagnoses as problems, states, or responses that were treated by nursing intervention. Diagnoses were identified by induction, based on the health conditions nurses said they treated. As noted by Kritek (1978), this empirical method was first-level theory development. The major effort in recent years has been focused on naming, defining, and testing the clinical validity of diagnostic concepts. This could lead to standardization of terms and definitions, thereby reducing the continuing semantic discrepancies and errors in communication, and increasing the reliability of clinical judgments (Bircher, 1975; Gebbie, 1976; Kritek, 1978; Roy, 1984).

Naming implies recognition of a class of health conditions that eventually will be grouped in a hierarchial classification system. For example, potential skin breakdown is a concept that could be an element within a classification of nursing diagnoses. Conceptualization of a health condition is communicated by using a concise word-label that replaces long, narrative descriptions. Diagnostic concepts are defined by observable referents. For example, referents for potential skin breakdown are red skin over a bony prominence, repeated incontinence, decreased periodic body movement, and so forth. It is the interrelated cluster of signs, symptoms, or both, that are named. Perceptible signs or symptoms that have the highest probability of occurring when the health problem occurs are *diagnostic criteria*. Clear, precise criteria permit discrimination among health problems (Jones & Jakob, 1981). Summary definitions for each label are used to capture the meaning of the concept. When developed, formal standardized definitions and precise criteria for diagnostic labeling will provide a common frame of reference for describing health problems. This will reduce communication errors among care providers and permit comparisons across studies.

The nature of the phenomena presented to the senses is captured through inductive generalization from multiple specific instances of a health problem. Concepts are formulated by abstracting common, intelligible features. In reality, concepts usually do not capture the nuances of any particular individual's health problem, thus the often used comment, the textbook picture. What is lost is the complex individuality of the particular instance of the phenomenon. What is gained is cognitive control over the unmanageable diversity of experience.

Diagnostic concepts have to be sufficiently inclusive of individual variation to be useful. Overinclusiveness produces broad concepts that cannot be used as a basis for applying therapeutic knowledge. To reduce complexity and facilitate the development and use of accumulated knowledge, a unique diagnosis cannot be constructed for every client. Diagnoses have to be detailed and vivid enough to describe individual manifestations, but sufficiently general for applicability to groups of clients (Gordon, 1982b, p. 11).

Definitive treatment, as opposed to palliative symptom relief, requires understanding of the probable cause, or etiology, of a health problem (Carpenito, 1983; Gordon, 1976, 1982b; Mundinger & Jauron, 1975). Concepts of this type are used to explain contributing factors rather than to describe a health problem. Similar to diagnostic concepts, etiological concepts require criteria and definitions. With multifactorial conceptions of causality (Rogers, 1982), each diagnostic class will have subclassifications of etiological factors.

CONCEPT IDENTIFICATION AND VALIDATION

Systematic classification of diagnostic concepts becomes a reality when sufficient elements have been isolated, defined, and validated clinically. Identification and validation of diagnostic concepts requires a large number of studies in which there is explicit definition of the construct (nursing diagnosis) being studied, sampling and description of clients and contexts, and clear reports of reliability and validity estimates. Attention is given to these factors in the summary, critique, and recommendations for further research in this chapter.

Retrospective Identification and Validation

Retrospective identification of nursing diagnoses employed nurses' recall of health conditions experienced in clinical practice (Gordon & Sweeney, 1979). This was the method used by the North American Nursing Diagnosis Association (NANDA), an organization of nurses from the United States and Canada which was formed in 1973 to identify, develop, and classify diagnostic concepts (Gebbie & Lavin, 1975). The early work of this group was used in six studies; thus, their methods and outcomes were of interest.

Gebbie and Lavin (1975) reported an alphabetical classification of 30 diagnostic categories and 100 subcategories that were identified, defined, and validated consensually by 150 nurse participants in 1973 at the First National Conference for Classification of Nursing Diagnoses sponsored by NANDA. No specific conceptual model of the client was used. Nursing diagnoses were defined as products of the assessment phase of the nursing process and described as "health problems or health states diagnosed by nurses and treated by means of nursing intervention" (Gebbie & Lavin, 1975, p. 1). The health problems or states identified and alphabetically classified were described by concept labels, such as impairment in skin integrity, anxiety, altered self-concept, impaired mobility, pain, and grieving. Subcategories represented distinct types of these health problems, including potential problems. An acuity and etiological typology provided further specification of subcategories (Gebbie & Lavin, 1975, pp. 62–112).

Following retrospective identification, a study was conducted through NANDA to test the clinical validity of the diagnostic concepts for describing clients health problems (Gebbie, 1976, pp. 19–21). A nonrandomized sample of nurse volunteers submitted 2,338 diagnostic labels and supporting data used in the care of 588 clients (newborn to 100 years) in 28 geographically distributed agencies. Analysis of data for congruence with the previously identified diagnoses by a panel of six nurses resulted in 19% being judged incongruent; these were medical diagnoses, interventions, and unclassified entities. Within the remaining 81%, diagnoses were similar (53%) or discrepant in label or defining characteristics (47%). Only general statements regarding frequently occurring diagnostic concepts were reported; these were pain, problems related to mobility, anxiety, and impaired skin integrity. Conclusions regarding validity of specific concepts were not reported.

Additions, deletions, and revisions at four national conferences (Gebbie, 1976; Kim et al., 1984, pp. 472–477; Kim & Moritz, 1982) between 1975 and 1982 resulted in an alphabetical listing of 50 diagnostic concepts, definitions, and defining characteristics accepted for clinical testing. Diagnostic labels are contained in Table 1; discussion will be deferred until the other studies are reviewed.

Retrospective identification of diagnostic concepts using nurses' recall of client conditions, consensual validation, and one clinical study were the procedures employed by NANDA (Gebbie, 1982). These methods provided a grounded, empirically based, set of diagnostic concepts representing phenomena of concern recalled by nurse participants. Involvement of large groups of nurses within the profession increased representativeness of opinion. Participation also may have stimulated interest in the use of nursing diagnosis, and thus provided a setting for research. What was lost with large group methods was the concentration of expertise found in highly selected, clinician panels, such as those used by other classifiers (American Psychiatric Association, 1980; World Health Organization, 1977). Retrospective identification can be used to sample the prevailing "folk taxonomy" and was a starting point for generating hypotheses about the concepts that direct nursing intervention. Systematic field trials of nursing diagnoses have been recommended repeatedly to reveal the adequacy of emerging concepts (Gebbie, 1976, 1982; Gebbie & Lavin, 1975; Gordon, 1976, 1982b; Kim & Moritz, 1982) but not carried out to the extent needed.

Identification and Clinical Validation of Phenomena

In addition to retrospective recall, diagnostic concepts can be identified by literature review and observations of practice. Once identified, concepts can be field tested. The knowledge gained could be used to discard or further refine the concepts. Studies using a clinical validation model

Table 1. Nursing Diagnoses Accepted for Clinical Testing by the North American Nursing Diagnosis Association (1982)

Nursing Diagnoses
Activity Intolerance
Airway Clearance Ineffective
[a]Anxiety
[a]Bowel Elimination, Alterations in: Constipation
[a]Bowel Elimination, Alterations in: Diarrhea
[a]Bowel Elimination, Alterations in: Incontinence
[a]Breathing Patterns, Ineffective
[a]Cardiac Output, Alterations in: Decreased
[a]Comfort, Alterations in: Pain
[a]Communication, Impaired Verbal
Coping, Ineffective Individual
Coping, Ineffective Family: Compromised
Coping, Ineffective Family: Disabling
Coping, Family: Potential for Growth
[a]Diversional Activity, Deficit
Family Process, Alteration in
[a]Fear
[a]Fluid Volume Deficit, Actual
[a]Fluid Volume, Alterations in: Excess
Fluid Volume Deficit, Potential
[a]Gas Exchange, Impaired
Grieving, Anticipatory
Grieving, Dysfunctional
Health Maintenance, Alterations in
[a]Home Maintenance Management, Impaired
[a]Injury, Potential for
[a]Knowledge Deficit (Specify)
Mobility, Impaired Physical
Noncompliance (Specify)
[a]Nutrition, Alterations in: Less Than Body Requirement
[a]Nutrition, Alterations in: More Than Body Requirements
Nutrition, Alterations in: Potential for More Than Body Requirements
Oral Mucous Membranes, Alterations in
Parenting, Alterations in: Actual
Parenting, Alterations in: Potential
Powerlessness
Rape-Trauma Syndrome
[a]Self-care Deficit (Specify Level) Feeding, Bathing/hygiene, Dressing/grooming, Toileting
[a]Self-concept, Disturbance in
[a]Sensory Perceptual Alterations
Sexual Dysfunction
[a]Skin Integrity, Impairment of: Actual
[a]Skin Integrity, Impairment of: Potential
[a]Sleep Pattern Disturbance
[a]Social Isolation
[a]Spiritual Distress (Distress of the Human Spirit)
Thought Processes, Alterations in
[a]Tissue Perfusion, Alteration in
[a]Urinary Elimination, Alteration in Patterns
[a]Violence, Potential for

[a]Nursing Diagnoses also listed by Jones and Jakob (1982)

NOTE: From Kim, M. J., & Moritz, D. A. (Eds.). (1982). *Classification of nursing diagnoses: Proceedings of the Third and Fourth National Conference* (pp. 281–319). New York: McGraw-Hill; Kim, M. J., McFarland, G., & McLean, A. (Eds.) (1984). *Classification of nursing diagnoses: Proceedings of the Fifth National Conference*. St. Louis: Mosby.

(Gordon & Sweeney, 1979) could provide information regarding whether the concepts represented realities of experience and could be applied consistently, and whether the set was sufficiently comprehensive.

From work begun in the early 1970s, Campbell (1978) identified and classified 721 diagnoses into categories of human responses or resource limitations. Using a broad conceptual focus, diagnostic terms were compiled from nursing literature, field tested by 233 junior and senior students in assessments of 550 patients with 344 different medical diagnoses. The total number of nursing diagnoses field tested was not reported. Instructors and a panel of clinical experts were used to review diagnoses for inclusion. Examination of the 721 diagnostic terms revealed extremely high specificity, compared to the NANDA listing included in Table 1 (Kim et al., 1984, pp. 472–477; Kim & Moritz, 1982, pp. 283–319). For example, whereas NANDA listed one diagnosis related to pain, Campbell (1978, pp. 1812–1813) listed 56. Pain was subcategorized using a typology: body systems, management, reactions, psychic, and nonspecific. Subcategories permitted finer discriminations, an important factor if interventions differed. Examination of interventions listed for each diagnosis revealed minimal differences; yet any difference made fine, diagnostic discriminations important. No further validation of diagnoses or interventions published by Campbell was found.

The use of professional nurses or specialists, as opposed to undergraduate students, would increase the credibility of findings. A major limitation of both Campbell's (1978) project and the study conducted by NANDA (Gebbie, 1976, pp. 19–21) was the absence of reliability estimates for each diagnosis. Reporting frequencies and results of interrater reliability would suggest which diagnoses required further refinement. For neither study did the investigators report training of data collectors nor means of assuring consistency of assessment relative to the conceptual model employed. Panel reviews were used, but estimates of reliability and validity were not reported.

Although not designed specifically as a study of nursing diagnosis, Halloran's (1980) study of nursing work load provided further support for the clinical validity of emerging diagnostic concepts. Nursing diagnosis was defined operationally as the labels and defining characteristics listed by NANDA in 1975 (Gebbie, 1976, pp. 19–21). In the Halloran study nurses documented diagnoses of 2,560 adults in a community hospital, 45% of whom had surgical procedures. Frequency of usage of the 37 diagnostic labels ranged from 53 (bowel impaction) to 2,181 (mild anxiety). This sampling of individual diagnoses provided support for many of the concepts as descriptors of the reality nurses perceived in this setting. Other diagnostic labels used in 900 or more cases were discomfort, altered ability to perform self-care activities, moderate anxiety, and less nutrition than required. Of the 2,560 clients, 80% had the diagnoses of anxiety and discomfort. The prior training of nurses, the relatively large sampling of individual diagnostic concepts, and the provision of defining characteristics for each concept were the bases for assumptions of accuracy and reliability of diagnostic judgments. Interobserver reliability measures were reported for a pilot study (Halloran, 1980).

Jones and Jakob (1982) reported a three-phase clinical study in Canada conducted between 1974 and 1981. This identification, validation, and refinement project involved 878 clients with 5,521 nursing diagnoses. The NANDA listing of diagnostic concepts (Gebbie, 1976, pp. 19–21) was incorporated into phase two, field trials (Jones, 1982). Similar to the NANDA (Gebbie, 1976, pp. 19–21) and Halloran (1980) studies, practicing nurses were employed as data collectors. The definition of nursing diagnosis used to guide data collectors and to review the submitted diagnoses was "responses to a situation or illness which are actually or potentially unhealthful and which nursing interventions can help to change in the direction of health" (Jones & Jakob, 1982, p. 3). Twenty-eight of the 71 diagnostic concepts contained in the Jones and Jakob listing also were listed by NANDA and are included in Table 1 (Kim et al., 1984, pp. 472–477; Kim & Moritz, 1982, pp. 283–319). Others were in the same conceptual area but were more specific, addressed different problems (lactation, avoidance coping, drug use, developmental delay), or had been deleted by NANDA (Kim & Moritz, 1982, pp. 283–319). In addition to the 64 diagnoses used in the final phase of the field testing, nurses generated seven other diagnoses.

Fifty percent of all health problems were described by 13 diagnostic labels. All but three (depression, potential for infection, discomfort) also were identified by NANDA and included in Table 1 (Kim et al., 1984, pp. 472–477; Kim & Moritz, 1982, pp. 283–319). Consistent with the findings of the NANDA study (Gebbie, 1976, pp. 19–21) and the Halloran study (1980), Jones and Jakob (1982) found pain, anxiety, mobility impairment, and impaired skin integrity to occur with high frequency. The high frequencies of discomfort and impaired hygiene self-care were consistent with Halloran's findings. Since nursing diagnoses can be expected to vary, to some extent, with medical conditions and acuity, these studies that were based on predominantly hospitalized adult populations cannot be generalized to other groups.

Strengths of the Jones and Jakob (1982) study were the large sample of diagnoses, multiple field trials, detailed reporting of analyses, and the attention to reliability of the diagnoses. Congruence of diagnostic labels and supporting clinical data were reported for 76% of the 2,772 diagnoses in the final field trial and for 95% in a second random sampling of 277 diagnoses. Congruence for the 13 highest frequency diagnoses ranged from 49% to 89%. Sampling of each of the 64 diagnoses in the final field trial was not controlled; frequencies ranged from 2 to 179 with an average of 43. Lack of control for reliability at the point of nurse–client encounter (assessment) was recognized. Threats to reliability of observations may have resulted in overdiagnosis, misdiagnosis, or underdiagnosis of conditions since procedures such as paired observations were not used.

Studies that were focused on a particular care setting or population of clients have yielded information about the specific applicability of diagnostic concepts. Simmons (1980) studied health problems in community health nursing to facilitate computerization of records. Essentially, the same methodology as the Jones and Jakob (1982) study was used, practicing nurse data collectors and an identify–test–retest model with repeated revisions. A set of 45 health problems were derived empirically from the home care practice of community health nurses. Nursing diagnosis was defined broadly as "an actual or potential deficit in the health status of an individual or family that is in need of primary, secondary, or tertiary methods of prevention" (Simmons, 1980, p. 57). Client data bases (N = 125) from agencies in four geographic areas were used to validate the occurrence of 45 health problems and their supporting signs and symptoms. Problems represented four domains: environmental, psychosocial, physiological, and health behaviors. Four refinements following field testing resulted in a final 73% to 90% average agreement between project and agency staff for the problems identified from data bases submitted by three agencies. Percentage of agreement for each diagnosis and the frequency of occurrence of diagnoses were not reported.

The 45 diagnostic labels (Simmons, 1980) did not include potential problems; these were created by adding a modifying term, but risk factors for these potential problems were not specified. Whereas NANDA as included in Table 1 (Kim et al., 1984, pp. 472–477; Kim & Moritz, 1982, pp. 283–319) and Jones and Jakob (1982) identified specific family-focused diagnoses, Simmons (1980) reported that each problem listed may have been referenced to a family or individual. This may be possible but could not have applied in the physiological domain. High-frequency diagnoses common to previous studies (Gebbie, 1976, pp. 19–21; Halloran, 1980; Jones & Jakob, 1982) were contained in Simmons' listing: pain, anxiety, impaired mobility (as impairment in neuromuscular skeletal function with the sign, gait, or ambulation disturbance), impairment of skin integrity (as integument: impairment), and personal hygiene deficit. Further comparisons were difficult. Is growth and development lag (Simmons, 1980) the same as developmental delay (Jones & Jakob, 1982)? Definitions indicated that they were different and that the differences were purely semantic. In future studies when two different labels are applied to the same cluster of signs and symptoms, justification of labeling should be reported.

Examination of concepts identified in the Simmons (1980) project revealed that the level of generality was higher than in the NANDA (Kim et al., 1984, pp. 472–477; Kim & Moritz, 1982, pp. 283–319), Jones and Jakob (1982), and Campbell (1978) lists. For example, impairment of respiration was one diagnosis in the Simmons (1980) list, but NANDA and Jones and Jakob listed three specific impairments. This makes comparisons difficult. General labels also may inflate the percentage of agreement attained between raters. For example, nurses may agree that assessment data points to a behavioral pattern impairment (Simmons, 1980, p. 22), but there may be less agreement when impairments are specified, such as body-image, self-esteem, personal identity, and role adaption disturbances.

The greater generality of the Simmons labeling system may be explained by the way in which terms such as problems, signs, and symptoms were used. Although defined in the traditional sense (Simmons, 1980), signs and symptoms were not always observations (signs) or reports (symptoms). For example, the signs of behavioral pattern impairment were (a) demonstrates inappropriate suspicion, (b) demonstrates inappropriate manipulation, (c) exhibits compulsive behavior, and (d) demonstrates passive-aggressive behavior (Simmons, 1980, p. 22). Many signs or symptoms were inferences and resembled problems, or diagnoses, in the NANDA (Kim et al., 1984, pp. 472–477; Kim & Moritz, 1982, pp. 283–319) and Jones and Jakob (1982) listings.

Large-scale clinical identification and validation studies have been costly. It was interesting to note that some investigators used retrospective record review, a less costly procedure. This method presupposed the implementation of nursing diagnosis and accurate, reliable diagnosticians. The validity of the 1973 NANDA listing of nursing diagnoses (Gebbie & Lavin, 1975) for long-term care was studied by Leslie (1981). Professional nursing staff's recordings of 1,521 diagnoses in 210 clients' charts comprised the study sample. Median age of clients was 85; predominant medical conditions were blood vessel disease (49%) and neurological conditions (22%). Nursing diagnosis was defined as the 1978 NANDA (Kim et al., 1984, pp. 472–477; Kim & Moritz, 1982, pp. 283–319) listing of diagnostic concepts.

One diagnostic concept, impairment of skin regulatory function, was not useful (Leslie, 1981). Consistent with others' findings (Jones & Jakob, 1982), nurses created concepts when the listing was incomplete. Three concepts were added: depression, impairment of circulation, and impaired sexual function. These concepts were listed by Jones and Jakob (1982) and the latter two were added to the NANDA (Kim & Moritz, 1982, pp. 283–319) list after 1973. In the Leslie (1981) study, the sample of 1,521 diagnoses contained 35 different concept labels. Ten labels described 66% of the total number of diagnoses recorded. Impaired mobility, self-care deficit, pain, anxiety, and impairment of skin integrity, reported with high frequency in previously reviewed studies (Gebbie, 1976, pp. 19–21; Halloran, 1980; Jones & Jacob, 1982; Simmons, 1980), were also among the 10 most frequently used diagnoses in the long-term care setting. The frequency of these 10 diagnoses on records ranged from 54 to 169. Other high-frequency diagnoses recorded also were contained in the Jones and Jakob (1982) and the NANDA (Table 1) listings (Kim et al., 1984, pp. 472–477; Kim & Moritz, 1982, pp. 283–319). Analysis of supporting data for diagnoses was not reported by Leslie (1981), leaving the question of whether phenomena were labeled consistently and accurately. Training procedures prior to the start of data collection also could have been used to increase credibility of the findings.

A second study employing hospital records was reported by Sweeney and Gordon (1983). They studied the use of nursing diagnoses identified by NANDA (Kim & Moritz, 1982, pp. 283–319) and the incidence of the problems described. Diagnoses ($N = 568$) were reviewed from discharge records (1975 to 1978) of 163 obstetrical and gynecological patients referred for continuing nursing care. The term nursing diagnosis was defined as an actual or potential health problem recorded by nurses on the referral record in a section labeled nursing diagnosis. Diagnoses were extracted verbatim and randomly checked for reliability of transcription. Thirty-one percent of the diagnoses were identical in wording to the NANDA listings between 1973 and 1978 (Gebbie, 1976, pp. 19–21; Gebbie & Lavin, 1975, pp. 62–112; Kim & Moritz, 1982, pp. 283–319).

Further analyses were done on the supporting clinical data for one high-frequency diagnosis, anticipatory observation for alteration in parenting (McKeehan & Gordon, 1982; Nicoletti, Reitz, & Gordon, 1982). The signs and symptoms recorded by nurses were congruent with the NANDA listing (Kim & Moritz, 1982, pp. 283–319), potential for alteration in parenting. This suggested that findings regarding use (as well as incidence) may have varied depending on whether labels, or labels and supporting data, were compared. Similar to other investigators (Jones & Jakob, 1982; Leslie, 1981; Simmons, 1980), Sweeney and Gordon (1983) concluded that the NANDA listings (Gebbie, 1976, pp. 19–21; Gebbie & Lavin, 1975, pp. 62–112; Kim & Moritz, 1982, pp. 283–319) of diagnostic concepts (1973 to 1978) described realities encountered, but that the listing of diagnostic concepts was incomplete. Also, similar to other investigators,

Sweeney and Gordon reported that nurses created new labels, such as loneliness and isolation, and added qualifications, such as potential, high-risk, and anticipatory observation for . . . (followed by a nursing diagnosis). Parenting problems (actual, potential, and anticipatory observation for . . .) were the most frequent diagnoses on the discharge referrals. This was explained by the high percentage of young, unmarried, postpartum clients.

Retrospective study of records has been used traditionally in epidemiological studies. Validity and reliability of diagnoses have been assumed (Kurland & Molgaard, 1981). Assumptions about the accuracy and consistency of diagnoses on referral records in the McKeehan (1979) study were based on (a) a hospital training program in diagnosis-based discharge planning, (b) provision of the 1973 to 1978 NANDA list of nursing diagnoses and their signs and symptoms (Gebbie, 1976; Gebbie & Lavin, 1975), (c) guidance on adding new diagnoses when needed, (d) consultation to nurses on each patient by an expert in nursing diagnosis, and (e) interdisciplinary team review of referrals by members of the interdisciplinary health team. To further strengthen this study, congruence of diagnostic labels and supporting clinical data should be evaluated. Lack of standardization of diagnostic terms and definitions increased the possibility of errors in labeling. Reporting the frequency of each diagnosis would have permitted comparisons across studies. In future research, it would be interesting to see whether discharge nursing diagnoses, such as parenting problems, would be confirmed during an immediate, postdischarge community nurse visit.

Gould (1983) reported a small study of the nursing diagnoses ($N = 68$) occurring in 15 clients with multiple sclerosis in nine acute settings and six ambulatory or home settings. The 1982 NANDA listing as reflected in Table 1 (Kim et al., 1984, pp. 472–477; Kim & Moritz, 1982, pp. 283–319), participant observation, and a grounded theory approach were used. Self-care deficit involving bathing, self-esteem disturbance, potential ineffective family coping (compromised), sleep pattern disturbance, and social isolation was diagnosed in five or more clients. Strengths of the study were specification of a framework for assessment, presentation, and discussion of data supporting each diagnostic concept, and comparisons of variations by care level. Findings were limited by the small sample and absence of interobserver reliability estimates. However, this study demonstrated the type of information that could be obtained with close attention to the structure of individual concepts and detailed reporting.

Small studies of a particular population of clients can be designed to control for accuracy and reliability of diagnoses. Kim et al. (1982) used both training and interobserver reliability in a clinical study of cardiovascular clients. Nurses were trained in diagnosis using videotapes, the NANDA

(Kim & Moritz, 1982, pp. 283–319) listing of diagnoses, assessment guidelines, and practice sessions. Twelve diagnoses were used most frequently. The strength of the study was in the design. Incomplete reporting and presentation of consensual validity analyses and the use of reliability estimates per patient, rather than by diagnosis, prohibited comparisons.

In contrast to other studies, Castles (1982) reported minimal agreement on diagnoses and on supporting data used in diagnoses among intensive care nurses. This may have been due to the lack of protocols for assessment and diagnoses and the time period. The study was done in 1975 when relatively little attention was given to the role of nurses as diagnosticians.

Only two investigators included etiological factors in their reports (Gould, 1983; Jones & Jakob, 1982). Yet, as Mundinger and Jauron (1975) clearly pointed out, definitive treatment (as opposed to palliative symptom relief) is not possible without understanding the probable cause of health problems. The data from the Jones and Jakob study indicated that 14 different categories of factors were specified as contributing to clients' nursing diagnoses. Interestingly, 49% of etiological factors specified were the same as the list of diagnostic concepts used in field testing. Similarly, approximately 50% of etiological factors reported by Gould (1983) were concepts listed by NANDA (Table 1) or adaptations of these (Kim et al., 1984, pp. 472–477; Kim & Moritz, 1982, pp. 283–319). This similarity suggested that the listings of diagnoses were used as a general diagnostic language, that is, as either descriptive or explanatory concepts. It may be that nurses used the diagnostic language terms available in a creative manner, individualizing their formulation of clients' diagnoses, and describing each situation in the way most useful for planning care. Underlying the nurses' specification of etiological factors in the Jones and Jakob study (1982) was a theory of multiple rather than single causality. A mean of 1.9 (range of 1.2 to 2.7) contributing factors per diagnosis was identified. Additional studies that include the explanatory concepts used by nurses may clarify conceptions of causality. It will be important that validity and reliability for explanatory concepts should be determined. In addition, the reliability of the causal relationship should be specified for etiological data.

SUMMARY AND FUTURE RESEARCH DIRECTIONS

Accurate, cross-study, summarization of the nursing diagnoses identified or validated in clinical settings was limited by a number of factors. These included (a) lack of consistency in concept labels, definitions, and diagnostic criteria, and (b) variations in reliability and validity estimates in both analyses and reports. If assumptions are made that nurses used the definitions of the diagnostic concepts they were given and labeled their observations according to these definitions, then all the diagnoses studied were valid representations of health conditions encountered in the practice settings sampled. The degree to which general validity was supported depended upon sampling of each diagnosis. Support for the most frequent diagnoses (1,100 to 3,240 cases across studies) was strongest in acute care settings. These examples of diagnoses were impaired mobility, pain, anxiety, actual and potential impairment in skin integrity, and hygienic or self-care impairment (self-care deficit). The breadth of sampling in the studies was small. The number of settings generally was not specified, but was greater than four (Gebbie, 1976; Halloran, 1980; Jones & Jakob, 1982; Leslie, 1981) and the number of countries was two. Even given these limitations, these health conditions represented some of the traditional phenomena of concern to nurses.

The list of diagnoses in Table 1 published by an international group, the North American Nursing Diagnosis Association, in 1982, has not been validated in its present form. Many of the concepts, presented at earlier stages of development (Gebbie, 1976; Gebbie & Lavin, 1975; Kim & Moritz, 1982), were field tested within the studies reviewed. In general, investigators concluded that the listings were incomplete, they identified other concepts (Jones & Jakob, 1982; Leslie, 1981) or they generated a different listing with some conceptual relationship (Campbell, 1978; Simmons, 1980). It was interesting to note that the average number of nursing diagnoses per client ranged from 3.4 to 11.5 in long-term care. It has been speculated that acuity of disease is related inversely to problems described by nursing diagnoses (Gordon, 1982b). This may be an explanation for the number of nursing diagnoses in long-term care.

Clinical validation studies of the North American listing (Kim et al., 1984, pp. 472–477; Kim & Moritz, 1982, pp. 283–319) of diagnostic concepts have to be done in Canada and the United States, as well as in other countries. International studies are of interest from three perspectives. First, they contribute to general clinical validation of diagnostic concepts. Second, they test the international usefulness of concepts for describing the reality perceived. This is a prerequisite for developing an international nursing classification of health-related conditions. Third, international studies permit comparisons across nations and cultures.

The study of diagnostic concepts will occupy the careers of many researchers and theorists in this century and beyond. Identification, refinement, and validation of diagnostic concepts are difficult activities to prioritize. Each is critically important in specifying the elements for a classification system. Assuming that the prime focus of the profession is nursing care delivery, then refinement of diagnostic concepts, especially their diagnostic criteria, assumes first priority. As Gebbie (1982) remarked, nurses have thrust the emerging diagnostic concepts quickly into practice. Lack of clear definitions and criteria can lead to errors and influence quality of care delivered. Since the mid 1970s, suggestions for new conceptual areas of diagnosis have been few. This also suggests that the research pertaining to nursing diagnoses should be refinement of current concepts, rather than generation of new concepts. Refinement of concepts is also necessary prior to experimental studies of treatment modalities. A second priority for research is identification of predictor variables, such as age, sex, or medical diagnosis. Knowing the co-occurrence of nursing diagnoses and other variables increases diagnostic sensitivity (Gordon, 1982b). For example, if the findings of Gould (1983) are supported, nurses can be taught to observe for certain nursing diagnoses co-occurring with multiple sclerosis. Another set of variables possibly influencing the occurrence of certain nursing diagnoses are practice setting, specialty, and level of care. Brown (1974) argued for epidemiological studies of nursing diagnoses 10 years ago. Yet epidemiological, intervention, or outcome studies have to be based on operationally defined criteria for each diagnostic concept. Descriptive studies also are needed to reveal the etiological factors associated with health problems. Studies of different populations can be used to further validate associations between etiological factors and health problems (Ryan, 1983).

It is critically important to development and standardization of diagnostic labels, definitions, and diagnostic criteria that investigators relate their findings to previous studies. Similarities and differences should be reported. Reasons for differences in labeling similar concepts, or different definitions for similar labels, should be discussed. Reporting of interrater reliability and frequencies for each diagnosis is also important. This information would provide an estimate of validity and reliability.

Refinement of diagnostic concepts has to be based on research findings regarding clinical validity and reliability. Validity is determined by studying whether a concept represents practice realities, that is, the health problems encountered, attended to, and treated by nurses in one or more practice settings. Validity is influenced by the conceptual models employed by practitioners. The current debate over physiological diagnoses (Dracup, 1983; Gordon, 1982b; Guzzetta & Dossey, 1983; Kim, 1983), health diagnoses (Gleit & Tatro, 1981; Gottlieb, 1982), and certain diagnostic terms (Stanitis & Ryan, 1982) is centered on their validity. Conceptual models for viewing client behavior and personal concepts of nursing diagnosis influence which concepts are considered representative of practice realities.

Reliability of a diagnostic concept is determined by research that demonstrates (a) consistency of application to the same clinical data, across clients, by one diagnostician, and (b) agreement in application across diagnosticians exposed to the same clinical data. Low inference and concrete diagnostic criteria increase diagnosticians' reliability and interdiagnostician agreement. Errors by trained diagnosticians probably can be attributed to lack of precision of diagnostic categories. Refinement of diagnostic concepts is a continual process. The Jones criteria for rheumatic fever (American Heart Association, 1965; Feinstein, 1982) and psychiatric nomenclature (American Psychiatric Association, 1980) exemplify this. At present, criticisms have been directed at inconsistencies in level of abstraction of nursing diagnoses listed by NANDA (Gordon, 1982b; Roy, 1984) and complexity of the nomenclature system (Lunney, 1982; Shamansky & Yanni, 1983). Both conceptual analysis and data on nurses' responses regarding usefulness of each diagnosis (Jones & Jakob, 1982; Kim et al., 1982) will provide ideas for further refinement and testing.

Both qualitative and quantitative research designs are applicable to research on nursing diagnoses. Qualitative methods (Evaneshko & Kay, 1982; Oiler, 1982; Schatzman & Strauss, 1973), including taxonomic and comparative analyses, are useful for generating, refining, and validating concepts and diagnostic criteria. Studies can be done within and across populations, settings, or age-groups (Burgess & Holmstrom, 1974, 1978). Each diagnosis may be studied separately, or related clusters may be described and analyzed. For example, is there a difference in the experiences of pain and discomfort (Jones & Jakob, 1982)? What are the differentiating criteria? Are there subcategories of pain (Campbell, 1978) relevant to nursing? Is there a difference between a lag and a delay in development (Jones & Jakob, 1982; Simmons, 1980)? Would comparative analysis of ineffective coping patterns across age-groups or cultural groups suggest different diagnostic criteria? Also, nurses, as well as clients, could be studied to isolate the characteristics of a diagnostic entity.

When diagnoses are identified, quantitative methods can contribute to further refinement of concepts. Development of instruments for measuring criteria (Atwood, 1980) and correlational or factor analyses (Diers, 1979; Hudson, 1982) can contribute to identifying diagnostic criteria. Studies by

Avant (1979), Cranley (1981), Field (1979), and Guzzetta & Forsythe (1979), provide examples. The future may bring investigators and university departments known for their work on one diagnostic area, studies and the nursing literature indexed by nursing diagnoses, and comparative, international studies.

REFERENCES

American Heart Association. Ad hoc Committee to Revise the Jones Criteria of the Council on Rheumatic Fever and Congenital Heart Disease. (1965). Jones criteria (revised) for guidance in the diagnosis of rheumatic fever. *Circulation, 32,* 664.

American Nurses' Association. (1973). *Standards of nursing practice.* Kansas City, MO: Author.

American Nurses' Association. (1980). *Nursing: A social policy statement* (Publication No. NP-63 20M 9/82R). Kansas City, MO: Author.

American Psychiatric Association. (1980). *Diagnostic and statistical manual of mental disorders* (3rd ed.). Washington, DC: Author.

Atwood, J. R. (1980). Developing instruments for measurement of criteria. *Nursing Research, 29,* 104–108.

Avant, K. (1979). Nursing diagnosis: Maternal attachment. *Advances in Nursing Science, 2*(1), 45–55.

Bircher, A. U. (1975). On the development and classification of diagnoses. *Nursing Forum, 14,* 11–29

Brown, M. (1974). The epidemiologic approach to the study of clinical nursing diagnoses. *Nursing Forum, 13,* 346–359.

Burgess, A. W., & Holmstrom, L. L. (1974). Rape trauma syndrome. *American Journal of Psychiatry, 131,* 981–986.

Burgess, A. W., & Holmstrom, L. L. (1978). Recovery from rape and prior life stress. *Research in Nursing and Health, 1,* 165–174.

Campbell, C. (1978). *Nursing diagnosis and intervention in nursing practice.* New York: Wiley.

Carpenito, L. J. (1983). *Nursing diagnosis: Application to clinical practice.* New York: Lippincott.

Castles, M. R. (1982). Interrater agreement in the use of nursing diagnosis. In M. J. Kim & D. A. Moritz (Eds.), *Classification of Nursing Diagnoses: Proceedings of the Third and Fourth National Conferences* (pp. 153–158). New York: McGraw-Hill.

Clark, J. (1978). Should nurses diagnose and prescribe? *Journal of Advanced Nursing, 4,* 485–488.

Cranley, M. S. (1981). Development of a tool for measurement of maternal attachment during pregnancy. *Nursing Research, 30,* 281–284.

Diers, D. (1979). *Research in nursing practice.* Philadelphia: Lippincott.

Dracup, K. (1983). Nursing diagnosis: A rose by another name. [Editorial]. *Heart and Lung, 12,* 211.

Evaneshko, V., & Kay, M. A. (1982). Ethnoscience research technique. *Western Journal of Nursing Research, 4,* 49–64.

Feinstein, A. R. (1982). The Jones Criteria and the challenges of clinimetrics. *Circulation, 66,* 1–5.

Field, M. (1979). Causal inference in behavioral research. *Advances in Nursing Science, 2*(1), 81–93.

Gebbie, K. M. (Ed.). (1976). *Summary of the Second National Conference: Classification of nursing diagnoses.* St. Louis: Clearinghouse for Nursing Diagnoses, St. Louis University School of Nursing.

Gebbie, K. M. (1982). Toward the theory development of nursing diagnosis classification. In M. J. Kim & D. A. Moritz (Eds.), *Classification of Nursing Diagnoses: Proceedings of the Third and Fourth National Conferences* (pp. 8–12). New York: McGraw-Hill.

Gebbie, K. M., & Lavin, M. A. (Eds.). (1975). *Classification of Nursing Diagnoses: Proceedings of the First National Conference.* St. Louis: Mosby.

Gleit, C. J., & Tatro, S. (1981). Nursing diagnoses for healthy individuals. *Nursing and Health Care, 2,* 456–457.

Gordon, M. (1976). Nursing diagnosis and the diagnostic process. *American Journal of Nursing, 76,* 1298–1300.

Gordon, M. (1982a). *Manual of nursing diagnoses.* New York: McGraw-Hill.

Gordon, M. (1982b). *Nursing diagnosis: Process and application.* New York: McGraw-Hill.

Gordon, M., & Sweeney, M. A. (1979). Methodological problems and issues in identifying and standardizing nursing diagnoses. *Advances in Nursing Science, 2*(1), 1–15.

Gottlieb, L. N. (1982). Small steps toward the development of a health classification system for nursing. In M. J. Kim & D. A. Moritz (Eds.), *Classification of Nursing Diagnoses: Proceedings of the Third and Fourth National Conference* (pp. 203–213). New York: McGraw-Hill.

Gould, M. T. (1983). Nursing diagnoses concurrent with multiple sclerosis. *Journal of Neurosurgical Nursing, 15,* 339–345.

Guzzetta C. E., & Dossey, B. M. (1983). Nursing diagnosis: Framework, process, and problems. *Heart and Lung, 12,* 281–291.

Guzzetta, C. E., & Forsythe, G. L. (1979). Nursing diagnostic pilot study: Psychophysiological stress. *Advances in Nursing Science, 2*(1), 27– 44.

Halloran, E. J. (1980). Analysis of variation in nursing workload by patient medical and nursing condition (Doctoral Dissertation, University of Illinois, 1980). *Dissertation Abstracts International, 41,* 3385B.

Hudson, H. C. (1982). *Classifying social data.* San Francisco: Jossey-Bass.

Johnson, D. (1980). The behavioral systems model. In J. P. Riehl & C. Roy (Eds.), *Conceptual models for nursing practice* (pp. 207–216) (rev. ed.). Norwalk, CT: Appleton-Century-Crofts.

Jones, P. E., (1982). Developing terminology: A University of Toronto experience. In M. J. Kim & D. A. Moritz (Eds.), *Classification of Nursing Diagnoses: Proceedings of the Third and Fourth National Conference* (pp. 138–145). New York: McGraw-Hill.

Jones, P., & Jakob, D. (1981). Nursing diagnosis: Differentiating fear and anxiety. *Nursing Papers, 14,* 20–29.

Jones, P., & Jakob, D. (1982). *The definition of nursing diagnoses: Phase 3.* Unpublished manuscript. Toronto: University of Toronto, Faculty of Nursing.

Kim, M. J. (1983). Nursing diagnoses in critical care. *Dimensions of Critical Care Nursing, 2,* 5–6.

Kim, M. J., Amoroso, R., Gulanick, M., Moyer, K., Parsons, E., Scherubel, J., Stafford, M., Suhayda, R., & Yocum, C. (1982). Clinical use of nursing diagnoses in cardiovascular nursing. In M. J. Kim & D. A. Moritz (Eds.), *Classification of Nursing Diagnoses: Proceedings of the Third and Fourth National Conferences* (pp. 184 –190). New York: McGraw-Hill.

Kim, M. J., McFarland, G., & McLean, A. (Eds.). (1984). *Classification of Nursing Diagnoses: Proceedings of the Fifth National Conference,* St. Louis: Mosby.

Kim, M. J., & Moritz D. A. (Eds.). (1982). *Classification of Nursing Diagnoses: Proceedings of the Third and Fourth National Conferences* (pp. 281–319). New York: McGraw-Hill.

Kim, M. J. Suhayda, R., Waters, L., & Yocum, C. (1982). Effect of using nursing diagnosis in nursing care planning. In M. J. Kim & D. A. Moritz (Eds.), *Classification of Nursing Diagnoses: Proceedings of the Third and Fourth National Conferences* (pp. 158–165). New York: McGraw-Hill.

Kritek, P. B. (1978). Generation and classification of nursing diagnoses: Toward a theory of nursing. *Image, 10,* 33–40.

Kurland, L. T., & Molgaard, C. A. (1981). Patient record in epidemiology. *Scientific American, 245,* 54–63.

Leslie, F. M. (1981). Nursing diagnosis: Use in long-term care. *American Journal of Nursing, 81,* 1012–1014.

Lunney, M. (1982). Nursing diagnosis: Refining the system. *American Journal of Nursing, 82,* 456–459.

McKeehan, K. M. (1979). Use of nursing diagnoses in a continuing care program. *Nursing Clinics of North America, 14,* 517–524.

McKeehan, K. M., & Gordon, M. (1982). Utilization of accepted nursing diagnoses. In M. J. Kim & D. A. Moritz (Eds.), *Classification of Nursing Diagnoses: Proceedings of the Third and Fourth National Conferences,* (pp. 190–195). New York: McGraw-Hill.

McManus, L. (1950). Assumption of functions of nursing. In Teachers College, Division of Nursing Education. *Regional planning for nursing and nursing education.* New York: Teachers College Press.

Mundinger, M. O. (1980). *Autonomy in nursing.* Germantown, MD: Aspen.

Mundinger, M., & Jauron, G. (1975). Developing a nursing diagnosis. *Nursing Outlook, 23,* 94–98.

Nicoletti, A. M., Reitz, S. E., & Gordon, M. (1982). Descriptive study of the parenting diagnosis. In M. J. Kim & D. A. Moritz (Eds.), *Classification of Nursing Diagnoses: Proceedings of the Third and Fourth National Conferences* (pp. 176–183). New York: McGraw-Hill.

Oiler, C. (1982). Phenomenological approach in nursing research. *Nursing Research, 31,* 178–181.

Orem, D. E. (1980). *Nursing: Concepts of practice* (2nd ed.). New York: McGraw-Hill.

Rogers, M. E. (1982). Theoretical framework for classification of nursing diagnoses. In M. J. Kim & D. A. Moritz (Eds.), *Classification of Nursing Diagnoses: Proceedings of the Third and Fourth National Conferences* (pp. 221–224). New York: McGraw-Hill.

Roy, C. (1984). Framework for classification system development: Process and issues. In M. J. Kim, G. McFarland, & A. McLean (Eds.), *Classification of Nursing Diagnoses: Proceedings of the Fifth National Conference* (pp. 26–45). St. Louis: Mosby.

Roy, C., & Roberts, S. L. (1981). *Theory construction in nursing: An adaptation model*. Englewood Cliffs, NJ: Prentice-Hall.

Ryan, N. M. (1983). The epidemiological method of building causal inference. *Advances in Nursing Science, 2*(1), 73–81.

Schatzman, L., & Strauss, A. L. (1973). *Field research: Strategies for a natural sociology*. Englewood Cliffs, NJ: Prentice-Hall.

Shamansky, S. L., & Yanni, C. R. (1983). In opposition to nursing diagnosis: A minority opinion. *Image, 15*, 47–50.

Simmons, D. A. (1980). *Classification scheme for client problems in community health nursing* (DHHS Publication No. HRA 80-16). Washington, DC: U.S. Government Printing Office.

Soares, C. A. (1978). Nursing and medical diagnoses: Comparison of essential and variant features. In N. L. Chaska (Ed.), *The nursing profession: Views through the mist* (pp. 269–278). New York: McGraw-Hill.

Stanitis, M. A., & Ryan, J. (1982). Noncompliance, an unacceptable diagnosis? *American Journal of Nursing, 82*, 941–942.

Sweeney, M. A., & Gordon, M. (1983). Nursing diagnosis: Implementation and incidence in an obstetrical-gynecological population. In N. L. Chaska (Ed.), *The nursing profession: A time to speak* (pp. 294–305). New York: McGraw-Hill.

Yura, H., & Walsh, M. B. (Eds.). (1982). *Human needs 2 and the nursing process*. Norwalk, CT: Appleton-Century-Crofts.

Yura, H., & Walsh, M. B. (Eds.). (1983). *Human needs 3 and the nursing process*. Norwalk, CT: Appleton-Century-Crofts.

World Health Organization. (1977). *International classification of diseases*. Geneva: Author.

PART III

Research on Nursing Education

CHAPTER 7

Research on Continuing Education in Nursing

ALICE M. KURAMOTO
SCHOOL OF NURSING
UNIVERSITY OF WASHINGTON

CONTENTS

The field of continuing nursing education grew rapidly during the last decade when mandatory continuing education for relicensure became a much discussed topic. There was a proliferation of educational offerings and increased involvement by nursing organizations, schools, and hospitals in providing continuing education. The increase in continuing education offerings has made nurses more aware of their need for continued professional growth and lifelong learning.

Research on continuing education in nursing has been limited. This has been due primarily to the limited number of nurses prepared at the graduate level in the field of adult and continuing education. Also, prior to the 1970s there was not as much emphasis on studying the effects of continuing education on the learner or on patient care. Mandatory continuing education for relicensure raised many questions such as: Who participates in continuing nursing education? What courses are needed? Does continuing education improve patient care? What are effective methods of teaching continuing education? How do we evaluate a continuing education program?

Many continuing nursing education studies conducted in the 1960s were of a descriptive, exploratory design (Nakamoto & Verner, 1972). In over half of the studies the investigators described nurse manpower resources and the nurses' perceptions of their learning needs. Studies in the 1970s focused on the characteristics of the participants, educational achievement and competencies, the planning process, recruitment and retention of participants, instructional methods, and program and learner evaluations.

The majority of the studies in continuing nursing education were published in the *Journal of Continuing Education in Nursing,* which has been available since 1970. Research abstracts from dissertations on continuing nursing education were published in this particular journal. Other publications that included citations of continuing education studies were *Nurse Educator, Journal of Nursing Education, Occupational Health Nursing, Nursing Research, Journal of Advanced Nursing,* and *International Journal of Nursing Studies*.

DEFINITIONS

In this chapter research on continuing education in nursing is reviewed. In the broadest sense, continuing education in nursing includes all educational activities beyond the basic nursing program. Continuing education is often seen as being limited to noncredit courses, rather than courses leading toward a degree. The American Nurses' Association (1975) defined continuing education as "planned, organized learning experiences designed to augment the knowledge, skills and attitudes of registered nurses for the enhancement of nursing practice, education, administration and research, thus improving the health care to the public" (p. 2).

Inservice education is one aspect of continuing education, but the terms are not interchangeable. Inservice education is part of the learning that the employing agency offers to increase the employees' knowledge and skills in relation to the role expectations within the agency. The term staff development is larger in scope than inservice education and may include orientation, skills training, management training, and inservice education.

CRITERIA FOR SELECTION OF STUDIES

Reports selected for review included only those which have been published in nursing literature. Unpublished doctoral dissertations were eliminated. Studies on registered nurses enrolled in baccalaureate programs also were eliminated since definitions of continuing education usually refer to courses not leading toward a degree.

This review of research on continuing education in nursing did not include local staff development programs. The rationale for this was that these reports were not actual studies, but only descriptions of the staff development programs. This review included continuing education on a broader scope, which enhanced the professional knowledge base. Such areas of study included characteristics of nurse learners, learning needs, teachers and teaching methods, evaluation of continuing education courses, and mandatory continuing education.

CHARACTERISTICS OF NURSE LEARNERS

Nine studies were categorized into this group; in these, the investigators studied a number of characteristics for learning, such as motivation, barriers to participation, environmental factors, and demographic background of nurse learners. Only Bevis (1973) and A. B. O'Connor (1979) used measurement scales from previous research. These scales were the Corwin Scale (Corwin, 1961) and the Education Participation Scale (Boshier, 1971). Further psychometric evaluation should be done on both of these scales if they are to be used in future studies. The Corwin Scale measured role conception and role deprivation. It was applicable to nurses' roles in the 1950s, and needs revising for today's nurses. The Education Participation Scale is a self-report instrument that consists of 48 statements of possible reasons for participating in adult education courses. Learners in adult education courses are a different audience than professional nurses, who take courses for professional advancement.

Nurses' motivations for participating in continuing education were studied by A. B. O'Connor (1979). The sample included 843 nurses participating in university-sponsored continuing education programs from various geographical regions. Using the Education Participation Scale and a personal data sheet for demographic information, A. B. O'Connor found that for these nurses, the presence or threat of a mandatory continuing education law had little influence in motivating participation. Seven motivational orientations were identified: compliance with authority, improvement in social relations, improvement in social welfare skills, professional advancement, professional knowledge, relief from routine, and acquisition of credentials. The credentials orientation, which was not identified in previous research, may represent further clarification of either the professional advancement or compliance with authority orientations. On the basis of these findings, program administrators should base appeals to participants on professional responsibilities rather than on societal mandates. Furthermore, nurse researchers investigating program effectiveness should consider the various motivations of nurse participants when designing evaluation tools.

The A. B. O'Connor (1979) investigation contained a definite professional component not evident in the Clark and Dickinson (1976) study. Clark and Dickinson investigated 220 nurses' involvement in conventional forms of educational programs, as well as participation in self-planned and self-managed learning situations, such as reading and use of audiovisual resource materials. They found that all of the nurses participated in some form of continuing learning. The nurses engaged in self-directed learning activities more than in group-oriented programs that were planned and managed by an instructor. Scores on the attitude scale showed that the majority of respondents had a favorable attitude toward continuing nursing education.

Mathews and Schumacher (1979) studied the conceptions, needs, and participation factors of registered nurses in two different hospital settings in a Southern metropolitan area. An eight-item questionnaire was developed and revised three times with the assistance of two inservice education directors. Of the 150 practicing registered nurses who responded to the questionnaire, 89 were from a university hospital and 61 were from a community hospital. The nurses characterized continuing education activities as being of relatively short duration, on a specific topic, and resulting in a certificate of completion or credit toward a higher academic or professional degree. These nurses believed that continuing education activities were necessary to maintain professional competence and that annual credits should be required by state law. The most important participation factors included relatedness of the topic to the nurse's job, personal interest in a topic, perceived need, and the time of the activity.

Bevis (1973) explored the relationship between the role conception held by a nurse at the end of her first year of practice in a bureaucratic environment and her participation in continuing learning activities. The following conclusions about role conception were reached: (a) The service component was the primary influence on participation in continuing learning activities, (b) the professional and service components were complementary influences on participation in continuing learning activities, and (c) conflict between the bureaucratic and service components exerted a negative influence on participation in continuing learning activities. The chief limitations of the study concerned the Job Activity Survey (JAS) and the Corwin Scale (Corwin, 1961). The JAS is an instrument developed by Bevis (1973) to measure the educational participation of staff nurses, and the Corwin Scale measured role conception. Preliminary assessment of the validity of the JAS was reported by Bevis; both instruments need further psychometric evaluation before they are used in other studies.

The typical Indiana nurse attending a continuing education activity was young, single, employed full time, and a baccalaureate nurse. These characteristics were identified by Puetz (1979, 1980b) after surveying 1,423 Indiana nurses on their participation in continuing education. Most respondents indicated that the most important reason for attending continuing education courses was to keep abreast of changes and learn more in a specific field.

Schoen (1981) surveyed 395 Illinois nurses with results similar to those of Puetz (1979, 1980b). Nurses took classes to continue personal and professional development. Seventy-two percent took at least one continuing education course and 53% took 20 or more hours of continuing education per year.

There were more studies on why nurses participated in continuing education than on why nurses did not participate. Deterrents or barriers to participation in continuing education were identified by Puetz (1979, 1980b), Sorensen (1979), and Winters, Lum, and Faustino (1977). These reasons included inconvenient location, no release time, scheduling problems, cost, and family obligations.

Factors that may affect learning behavior and participation in continuing education were explored by Sorensen (1979). A model of learning included several important resources and/or barriers: previous education, type of job, promotional opportunities, existing relevant courses, family situation, and working conditions. An interesting feature was that the family could be both a supporting and a hindering factor for the same person. Motivation toward job-related education was probably dependent on general job satisfaction, although dissatisfaction with one's present job may be a motivating factor toward education. Factors such as the degree of tiredness after work also may be connected with the psychosocial stimuli of the job. Sorensen's findings suggested that continuing education should be organized as inservice education within normal working hours. The study took place in two general hospitals and a nursing home in Norway and involved structured interviews with 362 people. The results of this study cannot be generalized to the United States, where the role of female health workers is different.

LEARNING NEEDS

Participation in continuing education is related closely to the learner's interest in or need to know about a particular topic. A learning need often is defined as a discrepancy between what individuals know and can do and what they need to know and do to achieve a higher level of performance (Cooper, 1983). Learning needs are not fixed, but are constantly changing. Individuals have different learning needs. Specialty groups within the nursing profession also have different needs.

In 11 studies (Bernhardt, 1980; Binger, 1979; Brown & Brown, 1982; Craytor, Brown, & Morrow, 1978; Ferris & Pierce, 1982; Headricks, 1982; Parker, Wood, & Millsop, 1982; Pounds, 1976; Puetz, 1980a; Squires, 1979; Volinn, 1982) the investigators assessed learning needs of specific groups of nurses, such as school nurses, geriatric nurses, cancer nurses, and occupational health nurses. The data-collection tool for all these studies was a questionnaire to determine perceived needs for further continuing education.

The literature showed more needs assessment surveys done on occupational health nurses than on any other specialty group (Bernhardt, 1980; Brown & Brown, 1982; Parker, Wood, & Millsop, 1982). These investigators discovered the following: There was high interest in occupational health continuing education topics; one-day programs were the most popular length; the majority favored voluntary continuing education as opposed to mandatory continuing education; interest in occupational health certification and membership in the professional association correlated with planning to attend classes; the reason for attending continuing education courses was to update knowledge and skills; and nurses licensed the longest period of time showed the most interest in continuing education, but also were less likely to have attended continuing education in the past two years. Investigators need to explore factors that inhibit older nurses from participating in continuing education. Perhaps certification and professional membership offer motivation for participation in continuing education.

Pounds (1976) and Puetz (1980a) examined learning needs of operating room nurses. Puetz found continuing education attendance by operating room and recovery room nurses to be much higher than the rate of attendance of other specialty groups of nurses in Indiana. Nurses did not participate because of scheduling problems and family obligations. Nurses participated in continuing education because of a desire to learn more in their field and improve their nursing skills. Pounds surveyed 1,201 operating room nurses who attended the National Association of Operating Room Nurses Congress. The survey research approach was used to investigate the influence of education, experience, and professional rank on nurses' perceptions of their learning needs. The data-collection instrument was a self-report questionnaire consisting of demographic information and 24 behavioral learning needs; no assessment of reliability and validity was reported. Pounds identified learning needs in four categories of skills: technical operating room, research and evaluation, direct patient care, and personnel management. She recommended a formal continuing education program in operating room nursing with the format, scope, and content of the curriculum structured according to these needs. An adaptation of this model could be used in assessing the learning needs of other professional nursing groups.

Craytor et al. (1978) discovered that nurses with the fewest years of education and working in small agencies in rural areas felt a greater need for continuing education than nurses with more years of education and working experience in large agencies in urban areas. A series of three studies was carried out by these investigators to determine nurses' needs for continuing education in cancer nursing care. In the first study, a stratified sample of 187 nurses in a 10-county region in upstate New York answered a questionnaire on learning needs. In the second study, a random sample of 100 nurses working in direct patient care in an acute general hospital was surveyed. For the third study, a quasi-experimental design was used to test the nursing staff on one inpatient unit before and after a 13-week planned educational intervention. Groups in all three studies indicated a need to keep up with current therapy for cancer and the nursing measures necessary to help patients tolerate therapy. The findings of these studies were that increased knowledge and skills decreased feelings of helplessness, learning took place when learners were anxious because of the inability to meet perceived demands, and learners sought more knowledge and/or skills. The unique aspect of this project was the systematic process of coordinating these studies over a six-year period. Based on the defined needs, an educational intervention was planned and the usefulness of such a program was demonstrated. The process, or parts of it, may be appropriate for use in other health care settings.

The effects of anxiety can be a motivating stimulus for a nurse to learn. Carter and Mills (1982) determined the effect of cognitive learning on anxiety occurring in low and high test-anxious subjects. One experimental and two control groups were used. The teacher and instructional format remained the same for all three groups. The dependent variables were trait anxiety, test anxiety, state anxiety, objective test performance, and self-perception of learning. The independent variables were the expectation of an objective posttest and differential motivating instructions of continuing education units (CEU) contingent or noncontingent on evaluation. Cognitive learning was not affected when receipt of continuing education units was contingent upon test performance. When CEU receipt was not contingent upon test scores, the highly anxious subjects surpassed the low anxious ones on posttest performance. Nurses who expected an objective test of knowledge at the program conclusion more accurately evaluated their own learning. The major limitation of this study was that the subjects self-selected the groups, and thus there were uneven numbers of subjects within the groups as well as small sample sizes for the three groups (n = 13, n = 18, and n = 8).

Binger (1979) studied 123 nursing program directors and found that their learning needs related to their job tasks and functions and included writing grant proposals, systematic decision making, budgeting, and writing for publication. Most (99%) of the nurses in this sample had their learning needs met by attending professional workshops. Another means of learning was self-directed study, since a majority read at least four nursing journals and also interacted with their peers.

In previously cited studies investigators (Binger, 1979; Craytor et al., 1978; Pounds, 1976; Puetz, 1980a) assessed the learning needs of specific nursing populations. In a study that was broader in scope, Curran (1977) examined the relationship of employment factors to the learning needs and continuing education activities of registered nurses for a sample of staff nurses in six Chicago area hospitals. Courses on physical assessment, as well as on patient teaching, were rated very or somewhat important by 90% of the nurses in every clinical setting. Responses to a questionnaire showed that over 40% had not attended a workshop in a one-year time period, and 56% had read professional literature only one hour a week. These statistics are discouraging for proponents of voluntary participation in continuing education activities. Administrators and supervisors reported the greatest frequency of reading professional literature. Nurses employed full time consistently reported greater participation in continuing education activities. These data should stimulate employers to investigate the educational efforts of their part-time employees to determine how current their knowledge and skills are.

The most common method for assessing learning needs has been the distribution of questionnaires and surveys. The problems of using a questionnaire are poor returns, poorly designed questionnaires, and difficulty in analyzing open-ended questions. Beach (1982) took a different approach in assessing learning needs. The purpose of her study was to identify the learning needs of community health nurses as perceived by these nurses and their supervisors. The learning needs were placed into four categories: A shared need was one identified by both the nurses and the supervisors; a blind need was one identified by the supervisors but not by the nurses; a hidden need was identified by the nurses but not the supervisors; and an undiscovered need was one identified by the nurse or the supervisor as a priority less than 10% of the time. Beach found that nurses were more likely to be given time to attend programs that were either in the shared or blind categories. This framework for assessing learning needs could be a useful teaching and supervisory tool. For example, sharing the blind needs of a nurse with her might help her recognize more areas of growth and learning. Sharing the hidden needs with a supervisor might increase her data base, enabling her to assist in meeting the professional learning needs of her staff.

TEACHERS AND TEACHING METHODS

Research in instructional technology has been difficult to design. It is often difficult to control the various intervening variables, such as teacher and student characteristics. Huckabay, Cooper, and Neal (1977) studied the effects of four different teaching techniques on learning, transfer of learning, and affective behaviors of nurses in an inservice education setting. The subjects included a combination of 131 staff nurses, team leaders, and charge nurses from 15 hospitals who were enrolled in an inservice education class. The experimental group was taught by filmstrips and discussion, and the three control groups were taught by lectures alone, lectures with discussion, and filmstrips alone. Cognitive learning was measured in a pre- and posttest. Subjects' feelings about the program and the format were assessed by an affective measure. There were no significant overall differences in cognitive learning, transfer of learning, or affective behavior between the experimental group and the control group. Each of the four teaching strategies enabled learners to acquire knowledge, but nurses preferred a teaching strategy that facilitated two-way communication between themselves and the teacher. This study did not seem to have a clear research design as to the differences between the experimental and control group. A follow-up study could include designation of the experimental groups as teacher-directed and the control group as nonteacher-directed.

Instructional technology has expanded from teleconference via telephones and video satellite transmission to sophisticated computer systems. R. J. O'Connor (1980) used a posttest-only design on two experimental groups and one control group to determine the educational effectiveness of instructional television. The three groups consisted of: Group 1 experimental (view and response), Group 2 experimental (view only), and Group 3 control (no view). The view and response group made the fewest errors on the posttest. The view-only group was next. And the no-view group made the most errors. This study reaffirmed the need to conduct validation studies of media-based instructional material to determine its educational effectiveness. A pretest and posttest design would be stronger than the posttest-only control design for replication.

Teleconferencing is an instructional method of reaching a large audience over a broad geographical area. Rost, Barber, and Frank (1981) evaluated Maine's telelecture continuing education for nurses, assessing program financing and utilization. They found decreased utilization of the telelecture system during the second year. Interviews with hospital administrators and directors of nursing indicated that health facilities did not want to pay an annual enrollment fee when only 60% of the employed nurses were taking advantage of the program. A revised fee policy was established and new programming was planned. This study pointed out the importance of evaluation data when decisions are made about whether to try a different type of instructional delivery. The most frequently cited barrier to using an innovative teaching method was the cost. Yet it appeared cheaper to have faculty deliver their content via teleconferencing rather than traveling to every small town in the state. However, high fixed costs to maintain a telelecture system made this project too expensive to continue.

The latest technological delivery system is the computer. This form of delivery was not found in many continuing education programs, so there was only one study published about computer-assisted instruction in continuing education. Valish and Boyd (1975) used an experimental design, with posttest-only format. These investigators found no significant difference between nurses who participated in computer-assisted instruction programs and those who did not use computers. A factor that may have influenced performance was that the use of the computer was a new experience for all subjects, and, therefore, the concentration could have been focused on the physical manipulation of the machine rather than on the benefits derived from the course.

Moran (1977) and Hansell and Foster (1980) compared independent learning with conventional classroom teaching. Moran (1977) interviewed 30 staff nurses and found that these nurses spent more time (469 hours) on their independent efforts to learn than was spent in staff development attendance (22.4 hours) during a 12-month period. The younger staff nurses were more active in professional independent learning than older staff nurses. Moran found that staff nurses who have less education spend more time in professional learning. Staff nurses who were satisfied with their job had a higher rate of professional independent learning. Hansell and Foster (1980) tested 32 nurses using the programmed instructional module approach. With an experimental design Hansell and Foster used pretests and posttests, the Spielberger State Anxiety Test, and three-month job performance interviews. The programmed instruction method was nearly half the cost of the classroom teaching and was as effective a method for critical care orientation. Programmed instruction encouraged flexibility and individualized attention and, by self-pacing, allowed several nurses to begin practice in the critical care setting earlier than usual. The limitations of both of these studies were the small sample size, lack of randomization to control and experimental groups, and lack of attention to instrument assessment.

A different approach to evaluating the delivery method was to examine the characteristics and qualities of a good instructor. Floyd (1982) mailed questionnaires to 1,500 registered nurses in a 16-county area. Two pilot groups were used in developing the instrument. In each pilot study, participants were asked to list five qualities or characteristics they preferred in continuing education instructors. The final questionnaire contained 10 qualities or characteristics preferred in a continuing education instructor which the subjects ranked from 1 to 10. Respondents on 463 questionnaires preferred the following characteristics as important qualities of faculty in rank order: (a) knowledge, (b) ability to present knowledge, (c) openness to audience responses, and (d) evidence of ability to do clinical practice in the area discussed. The limitations of the study were that students may not have been able to identify qualities and characteristics preferred in continuing education instructors and that individual differences may have affected responses to specific qualities or characteristics in an instructor.

EVALUATION OF CONTINUING EDUCATION COURSES

Evaluations of continuing education courses often were not planned with enough sophistication in methodology. Systematic evaluation frequently was intended for continuing education courses but seldom was depicted in a formal process. Systematic evaluation of continuing education could help determine the effectiveness of teaching for the learner and ultimately improve patient care.

Patient improvement in relation to continuing education has been difficult to study. Examples of experimental approaches to assessing patient outcomes were reported by del Bueno (1977). These examples included the implementation of a cardiopulmonary resuscitation team with a program success rate increased to 54%, and a drop of 20% in urinary tract infection following a course on this topic. Lack of good studies relating continuing education to improved patient care was a major gap in present evaluation research. Forni and Overman (1974) found that the effect of continuing education on the practice of nursing could not be determined unequivocally in their study. The problems in obtaining definitive results were primarily methodological, concerning instrument construction, including the development of precise statements of course objectives in terms of changes to be expected in the practice of nursing, and the development of appropriate methods to determine whether such outcomes occurred.

It is sometimes assumed that continuing education makes a difference in practice without having enough documentation to justify this statement. And studies in which a difference was not found might not be published in the literature. Doran (1973) evaluated the therapeutic treatment delivered by nurses and aides in a drug-treatment unit. Observational techniques and questionnaires were used preworkshop and postworkshop on both an experimental and a control group. It would be expected that the group that participated in the educational program would perform better than the group that had not attended the program. However, the results showed no significant differences.

Derby (1982) attempted to relate the learners' goals and the educational processes used to improved patient care. Results showed that goal congruence occurred in relation to learners' intent to use content. A self-report questionnaire on health professionals' intent to use continuing education content in actual patient care was used immediately postcourse and then four weeks later. There was a decrease in the learners' stated use of course content four weeks postcourse. Derby's findings were influenced by poor follow-up returns. Also, it is questionable how valid the tool was with subjects self-assessing their use of content in patient care; no report was made of the reliability or validity of the questionnaire. A peer review or performance review by a supervisor would be a more objective means of verifying improvement in patient care due to a continuing education course.

Often continuing education courses are one- or two-day programs, and it is questionable whether a change in behavior can occur in so short a time. Ferris and Pierce (1982) evaluated change after a six-month program. These investigators, however, found that 87% of the practicing nurses indicated a need for a cardiovascular nurse specialty program, but only 12% could arrange to attend a six-month course. This demonstrated that the need for short-term programs was greater. The question of which preparation (long-term specialist type or short-term course) has the greatest impact on patient care has not been answered.

Another characteristic of evaluation studies done in continuing education is that a quasi-experimental, untreated control group design with pretest and posttest measures was not often conducted. Typically, in evaluation studies investigators used only immediate posttest measures on the conference participants. This could be due to too little time, too little money, and difficulty matching a control group. In four studies (Cox & Baker, 1981; Hamrin, 1982; Ingmire, 1973; Sessions & Van Sant, 1966) investigators used a quasi-experimental design. Cox and Baker (1981) did a longitudinal study involving 24 community health nurses to determine the impact of a two-week continuing education offering on their practice. The *t* test value produced on the pretest and posttest differences was 19.27, significant beyond the .001 level, thus confirming that the participants' knowledge base had been increased significantly when completing a continuing education course. An interesting finding was that nurses, regardless of age and experience, who received praise, support, and reinforcement from their immediate supervisor continued to adopt the new skills in their clinical settings. Nurses who did not receive reinforcement utilized their skills less consistently.

Ingmire (1973) conducted evaluation studies of a regional continuing education program for nurses in leadership positions. The leadership conference series was sponsored by the Western Interstate Commission for Higher Education (WICHE) and was held over a two-year period, 1962 to 1964. The conference group of 410 nurse leaders (experimental group) and another 450 nurses serving as control subjects took paper-and-pencil attitude tests and two performance tests. The outcomes indicated that the program had a definite impact on the participants' attitudes and beliefs concerning leadership roles and interpersonal relationships. The use of a combination of written tests and a simulated nursing situation in conjunction with on-the-job ratings may prove to be an excellent model for future evaluation studies.

Sessions and Van Sant (1966) also evaluated the leadership conference sponsored by WICHE and the University of Utah College of Nursing. The evaluation scale, called the WICHE Supervisor Rating Scale, was used preconference and postconference on 30 head nurses who completed the leadership course. In general, the conference participants (experimental group) improved, while nonconference nurses (control group) did not. The investigators reported problems with validity and reliability for this scale and recommended additional instrument evaluation.

The impact of continuing education may not be measurable immediately following a course. Changes in behavior may take more than three or six months. Most evaluation studies did not include measures of long-term outcomes. Hamrin (1982) found more improvement after six months than after three months. This is an important finding for follow-up evaluation techniques, since a three-month follow-up evaluation may not provide sufficient time for maximum change in behavior.

Job performance improvement has been an expectation of many inservice education programs. Skipper and King (1974) found that taking courses improved nurses' individual practice, but had little impact on the employing institution. The weakness of this study was that it was a self-report questionnaire and not an observation of actual performance.

Valencius (1980) stated the need for more objective means to follow up actual change in nursing practice. Her tool for evaluation of cancer nurses was a questionnaire, constructed for this study, which was used at three and six months following a course. The validity of using a self-report of one's own practice was a major limitation.

A more objective way to evaluate performance is to audit nursing charts and care plans. Hedman, Thatcher, Givner, and Erixon (1976) found improvement on nursing care plans in nursing homes following a continuing education course. Data were collected using pretests, posttests, observation, and a patient assessment questionnaire. In this instance, the patients were asked to rate their satisfaction with their care. Preconference and postconference chart audits also were done in the study by Cox and Baker (1981). Nursing audits are effective as follow-up evaluations, and also can indicate additional educational needs.

Most continuing education programs include evaluation of cognitive knowledge, since it is easy to administer a paper-and-pencil test. Five studies (Cox & Baker, 1981; Hedman et al., 1976; Kanto, Maples, Goldberg, & Miller, 1979; Plein, Plein, Kent, & Wallace, 1979; Westfall & Speedie, 1981) involved pretest and posttest measures. In all of these studies posttest scores of cognitive knowledge improved. Plein et al. (1979) and Westfall and Speedie (1981) did recall testing on drug knowledge in long-term care facilities and found that subjects had greater ability to make appropriate drug therapy decisions following an inservice education program.

Observation is a useful method of evaluation but can be time consuming and expensive. If a psychomotor skill is a component of the continuing education course, then it is appropriate to use skill checklists for recording observations. Many evaluation tools used in continuing education were self-report questionnaires that yielded subjective data. There was a lack of pilot testing and psychometric evaluation of instruments. This was a major weakness in studies on continuing education.

Another area that is difficult to evaluate is attitude change. Evaluations of most continuing education courses are conducted immediately following a workshop. A change in attitude may take several months. Therefore, evaluations administered three to six months following a continuing education course may measure change more accurately. Laube (1977) determined the effect of a two-day death and dying workshop on the death anxiety level of participating nurses. She tested levels of death anxiety at the beginning of the workshop, one month postworkshop, and three months following the workshop. Significant levels of reduction were not found three months following the workshop, but the death anxiety level did decrease over time. It is important to note that even three months postworkshop, the subject's level of death anxiety remained below the preworkshop level of anxiety.

Attitudes toward human sexuality were studied by Mims (1978). Pretests and posttests were administered to 93 health professional students. A two-day workshop on human sexuality led to change in their sexual knowledge, but basic attitudes, such as those measured on the abortion scale, did not change. This study design could be improved with comparison of a longer term course and by conducting a three- and six-month follow-up evaluation on sexual knowledge and attitude.

Holzemer, Barkauskas, and Ohlson (1980) conducted a study with a follow-up evaluation. Four separate workshops entitled Preparation in Primary Care for Nurse Faculty were held for 83 nurse faculty in 1975 to 1976. The evaluation activities were focused on the participants' cognitive and clinical learning, participants' attitudes toward the workshops, their views on the effectiveness of the workshops, preceptors' and participants' evaluations of the workshops, and a follow-up questionnaire mailed to the participants six months after completion of the workshop to examine the impact of the workshop. Overall, the participants evidenced satisfactory learning as measured by the cognitive and clinical examinations. The most important finding was that all of the participants were working with health assessment skills six months after the workshop in their own environments. This was a good study in attempting a workshop follow-up, although the evaluation method was a self-report questionnaire designed for the study.

A definite change in attitude and performance in the leadership role was measured by Ingmire (1973). She used several types of evaluation tools, including attitude and opinion scales, performance measures, and job rating forms to determine the degree of change resulting from participation in a six-week leadership course. She found that, given an opportunity, nurses in leadership positions can use the skills they learned in the training program to influence better relationships and improve techniques for patient care. A one-year follow-up questionnaire was completed by only 58 of the original 377 experimental subjects studied. This poor response raises questions as to the actual success of this project. More studies should be designed to assess the degree to which participants modify their behavior in the brief exposure to the activities of a training program.

There were few studies that dealt with cost analysis and the cost effectiveness of continuing education. Deets and Blume (1977) collected direct costs of continuing education programs, but did not report the indirect costs. The total costs of operating continuing education courses must include the administrative costs and other indirect fixed costs.

Kase and Swenson (1976) conducted a study to estimate the total national cost of orientation and inservice teaching in hospitals. Until this study was conducted, very little was known about hospital education costs. The national cost of hospital education was estimated at $226 million, of which 60% was for orientation and 40% for inservice education. Retrospective data were supplied by a stratified random sample of 998 hospitals from which 394 usable responses were received. A problem with the questionnaire was that hospital staff had difficulty answering some questions because accurate records were not kept and only cost estimates were given. Another problem was that the pretest was conducted within a single geographic region (New England), but the questionnaire was sent to a larger geographic area. Hospitals in other regions of the country collected different data than those in New England. This study should be replicated since most hospitals now have better record-keeping systems and more accurate data can be obtained.

MANDATORY CONTINUING EDUCATION

Mandatory continuing education for relicensure became a controversial topic during the 1970s. As more states have mandatory continuing education requirements for relicensure, the question is raised whether nurses will be attending continuing education courses to meet those requirements rather than to meet an identified learning need.

Miller and Rea (1977) found the opposite opinion from nurses in northern Illinois. Seventy percent of the nurses surveyed favored mandatory continuing education, 23.3% opposed mandatory continuing education, and 6.7% were undecided. Diploma nurses and staff nurses were more reluctant to accept mandatory continuing education. A small sample size of 30 nurses was a major limitation of this study.

A larger sample of 395 Illinois nurses participated in an attitude survey conducted by Schoen (1982). An excellent return rate of 82% showed an almost evenly divided opinion on whether continuing education should be mandated for relicensure. Nurses in the study had positive attitudes toward continuing education as it enabled them to keep up with current knowledge. Those nurses who were members of a professional organization or who had received additional education were more likely to support requiring continuing education for relicensure. Age, initial nursing program, and current employment status were not related significantly to attitudes toward mandatory continuing education.

Several articles on the subject of mandatory continuing education concluded with a statement that research should be done on the effectiveness of mandatory continuing education and its impact on the profession (Cox & Baker, 1981; Forni & Overman, 1974; Gaston & Pucci, 1982; Miller & Rea, 1977). Evaluation studies of this nature had not been published in the literature at the time of this writing. Gaston and Pucci (1982) and Rizzuto (1982) described some of the positive and negative effects from mandating continuing education for relicensure. Limited funding for maintaining continuing education records, lack of computer services, lack of evaluation of the effect of continuing education upon practice, and lack of courses in rural areas were some of the problems cited. Rizzuto's (1982) conclusion was that mandatory continuing education is an expensive burden on nurses, employing institution, and society.

SUMMARY AND RESEARCH DIRECTIONS

There were several significant limitations to the majority of the studies reviewed on continuing nursing education. First, most of the investigators used small samples and measured outcomes of a workshop by means of a posttest. Some of these studies had no baseline testing or pretesting, so it is difficult to determine whether change occurred. Generalizability to other populations and settings is limited by poor research design.

Many studies conducted in the 1960s and early 1970s included descriptive, exploratory designs. A second limitation was the small number of experimental design studies. Many of the studies were focused on assessment of learning needs or analyses of nurses' participation in continuing education. Cooper (1983) stated that studies are needed to answer the following questions: Does continuing education have an impact on practice and on patient care? How can standards of practice be related to educational offerings? How can one determine individual learning styles in the clinical setting? Who is the continuing learner in nursing? What are the characteristics of effective teachers of adults? What is the cost of continuing education?

Another issue concerns nurses whose training is obsolete. The research literature contains little evidence that mandatory continuing education is the best solution to this problem. One cannot disagree that there are incompetent individuals in every occupation. Yet nowhere in the literature was the estimated degree of professional obsolescence stated. Tools for evaluating the level of competence in nursing practice need to be developed and tested for proper psychometric properties. Given adequate evaluation tools, those who currently are responsible for quality of nursing care could identify incompetent nurses or nurses with outdated education more readily. These nurses could then be sent to inservice education classes and be reevaluated.

Another deficiency of the studies reviewed was the high attrition rates with follow-up evaluations. Many of the investigators conducted paper-and-pencil testing immediately following a course. Attitudinal change or change in practice must be evaluated at a later time. The difficulty with follow-up paper-and-pencil evaluations is getting the participants to return the evaluations. Observational rating scales used in the work setting three to six months after a course would eliminate the problem of poor follow-up returns.

The major problems have been in the areas of research design and techniques. Investigators should control for intervening variables, but it was not always possible to obtain control and experimental groups with similar educational preparation, work experience, and reasons for attending a continuing education program. Evaluation techniques should be developed further and validated. Some of the techniques of peer review, record audit, and observations were excellent but were very time consuming and expensive. Pretest and posttest measurements were not always reliable or valid for testing specific course objectives. Problems in the use of these designs and techniques leave the field wide open for more sophisticated research.

The need for research on continuing education in nursing is urgent. Most of the research in continuing education has been done by graduate students in their master's theses and doctoral dissertations. Some of these studies have not appeared in the nursing literature since they have been completed relatively recently.

The quantity and quality of research in this area can be expanded in a supportive climate. Adult educators and nurses need to work together in critically evaluating and discussing scholarly work. Nurses can be encouraged strongly to publish their research in continuing education or research journals. Continuing education conferences and conventions should schedule program time for research in the field of continuing education.

The field of continuing education borrows and reformulates knowledge from other disciplines. Sociology, social psychology, psychology, history, and adult education are examples of some of these other disciplines. Research on the nature of adult development and learning only recently has provided a base for continuing nursing education. Research gaps in the field of continuing education include marketing, economics, quality assurance in the health field, cost-effectiveness, program efficiency, competency-based education, changes in nursing practice resulting from continuing education, evaluation of patient care outcomes in relation to a specific continuing education offering, and evaluation models.

The increase of research will occur in the future with a commitment for such investigation. This requires allocation of financial and human resources for the work. The number of continuing nursing education directors at the doctoral level must increase for future conduct and dissemination of research in the field. However, an increase in numbers alone is not the solution. These individuals have a responsibility to teach research methods to inservice educators and other nurses who may or may not be pursuing advanced degrees. Study clubs could be formed through local inservice educators for sharing research ideas and findings on a particular topic. A mentor role could be developed with persons who desire to learn more about research.

The increased demand for continuing nursing education offerings in the 1980s will increase the number of continuing education providers and consumers. It is imperative for both providers and consumers of the future to be informed better about conducting and receiving continuing education based on past and current research. The purpose of both nursing research and continuing education is the improvement of care, and continuing education provides an appropriate means for the dissemination of research results.

REFERENCES

American Nurses' Association. (1975). Standards for nursing education (Publication Code NE-1 10M 6/75). Kansas City, MO: Author.

Beach, E. K. (1982). Johari's window as a framework for needs assessment. *Journal of Continuing Education in Nursing, 13*(3), 28–32.

Bernhardt, J. H. (1980). Survey of interest in continuing education for occupational health nurses in Wisconsin. *Occupational Health Nursing, 28*(11), 35–38.

Bevis, M. (1973). Role conception and the continuing learning activities of neophyte collegiate nurses. *Nursing Research, 22*, 207–216.

Binger, J. L. (1979). Perceived learning needs and resources of undergraduate and diploma program directors. *Journal of Nursing Education, 18*(6), 3–7.

Boshier, R. W. (1971). Motivational orientations of adult education participants: A factor analytic exploration of Houle's typology. *Adult Education, 21*, 3–26.

Brown, V. A., & Brown, K. C. (1982). Continuing education needs of occupational health nurses. *Occupational Health Nursing, 30*(4), 22–26.

Carter, L. B., & Mills, G. C. (1982). Cognitive learning and anxiety in registered nurses in CEU—contingent and noncontingent continuing education courses. *Journal of Continuing Education in Nursing, 13*(3), 19–27.

Clark, K. M., & Dickinson, G. (1976). Self-directed and other-directed continuing education: A study of nurses' participation. *Journal of Continuing Education in Nursing, 7*(4), 16.

Cooper, S. S. (1983). *The practice of continuing education in nursing*. Rockville, MD: Aspen.

Corwin, R. G. (1961). Role conception and career aspirations: A study of identity in nursing. *American Journal of Sociology, 66,* 604–615.

Cox, C. L., & Baker, M. G. (1981). Evaluation: The key to accountability in continuing education. *Journal of Continuing Education in Nursing, 12*(1), 11–19.

Craytor, J. K., Brown, J. K., & Morrow, G. R. (1978). Assessing learning needs of nurses who care for persons with cancer. *Cancer Nursing, 1,* 211–220.

Curran, C. L. (1977). What kind of continuing education? *Supervisor Nurse, 8*(7), 72–75.

Deets, C., & Blume, D. (1977). Evaluating the effectiveness of selected continuing education offerings. *Journal of Continuing Education in Nursing, 8*(3), 63–71.

del Bueno, D. J. (1977). Evaluation on a continuing education workshop for inservice educators. *Journal of Continuing Education in Nursing, 8*(2), 13–16.

Derby, V. L. (1982). Learners and course goal congruence: Impact on learning outcomes. *Journal of Continuing Education in Nursing, 13*(4), 16–25.

Doran, M. O. (1973). A nursing approach to the treatment of drug addicts: Evaluation of an educational programme. *International Journal of Nursing Studies, 10,* 217–228.

Ferris, L., & Pierce, S. (1982). Evaluation for change. *Journal of Continuing Education in Nursing, 13*(1), 14 –20.

Floyd, G. J. (1982). Qualities/characteristics preferred in continuing education instructors. *Journal of Continuing Education in Nursing, 13*(3), 5–14.

Forni, P. R., & Overman, R. (1974). Does continuing education have an effect on the practice of nursing? *Journal of Continuing Education in Nursing, 5*(4), 44–51.

Gaston, S., & Pucci, J. (1982). Mandatory continuing education in Kansas—three years later. *Journal of Continuing Education in Nursing, 13*(2), 15–17.

Hamrin, E. (1982). Attitudes of nursing staff in general medical wards towards activation of stroke patients. *Journal of Advanced Nursing, 7,* 33–42.

Hansell, H. N., & Foster, S. B. (1980). Critical care nursing orientation: A comparison of teaching methods. *Heart and Lung, 9,* 1066–1072.

Headricks, M. M. (1982). Determining the learning needs of nursing personnel in nursing homes. *Journal of Continuing Education in Nursing, 13*(2), 18–22.

Hedman, L. L., Thatcher, R. M., Givner, N., & Erixon, J. E. (1976). Assessing continuing education course outcomes in gerontological nursing. *Journal of Gerontological Nursing, 2,* 10–14.

Holzemer, W. L., Barkauskas, V. H., & Ohlson, V. M. (1980). A program evaluation of four workshops designed to prepare nurse faculty in health assessment. *Journal of Nursing Education, 19*(4), 7–18.

Huckabay, L. M., Cooper, P. G., & Neal, M. (1977). Effects of specific teaching techniques on cognitive learning, transfer of learning, and affective behavior of nurses in an inservice education setting. *Nursing Research, 26,* 380–385.

Ingmire, A. E. (1973). The effectiveness of a leadership program in nursing. *International Journal of Nursing Studies, 10,* 3–19.

Kanto, W. P., Maples, J. C., Goldberg, G. H., & Miller, M. D. (1979). Evaluation and need of education programs for community hospital nurses providing neonatal care. *Journal of Obstetric, Gynecologic, and Neonatal (JOGN) Nursing, 8,* 98–103.

Kase, S. H., & Swenson, B. (1976). Costs of hospital-sponsored orientation and inservice education for registered nurses (DHEW Publication No. HRA 77-25). Washington, DC: U.S. Government Printing Office.

Laube, J. (1977). Death and dying workshop for nurses. *International Journal of Nursing Studies, 14,* 111–120.

Mathews, A. E., & Schumacher, S. (1979). A survey of registered nurse conceptions of participation factors in professional continuing education. *Journal of Continuing Education in Nursing, 10*(1), 21–27.

Miller, J., & Rea, D. (1977). How nurses perceive mandatory continuing education. *Journal of Continuing Education in Nursing, 8*(1), 8–15.

Mims, F. H. (1978). Human sexuality workshop: A continuing education program. *Journal of Continuing Education in Nursing, 9*(6), 29–36.

Moran, V. (1977). Study of comparison of independent learning activities vs. attendance at staff development by staff nurses. *Journal of Continuing Education in Nursing, 8*(3), 14–21.

Nakamoto, J., & Verner, C. (1972). *Continuing education in nursing: A review of the North American literature*. Vancouver: Adult Education Research Centre, University of British Columbia.

O'Connor, A. B. (1979). Reasons nurses participate in continuing education. *Nursing Research, 28,* 354–359.

O'Connor, R. J. (1980). Evaluation of an interactive instructional television program in Hansen's disease. *Journal of Continuing Education in Nursing, 11*(2), 47–49.

Parker, J. E., Wood, J., & Millsop, M. (1982). Illinois occupational health nurses express continuing education needs. *Occupational Health Nursing, 30*(4), 27–32.

Plein, J. B., Plein, E. M., Kent, S., & Wallace, D. L. (1979). Drug therapy update for the long-term care nurse assessment of needs and evaluation of method. *American Journal of Hospital Pharmacy, 35,* 44 – 49.

Pounds, E. (1976). Assessing learning needs of OR nurses. *Association of Operating Room Nurses Journal, 24,* 433–436.

Puetz, B. E. (1979). Continuing education participation of occupational health nurses in Indiana. *Occupational Health Nursing, 27*(10), 24–28.

Puetz, B. E. (1980a). Continuing education and OR and RR nurses. *Association of Operating Room Nurses Journal, 31* 652–662.

Puetz, B. E. (1980b). Differences between Indiana registered nurse attenders and nonattenders in continuing education in nursing activities. *Journal of Continuing Education in Nursing, 11*(2), 19–26.

Rizzuto, C. (1982). Mandatory continuing education: Cost versus benefit. *Journal of Continuing Education in Nursing, 13*(3), 37–43.

Rost, M. A., Barber, G. M., & Frank, T. (1981). Evaluation of Maine's telelecture continuing education program. *Journal of Continuing Education in Nursing, 12*(3), 23–30.

Schoen, D. C. (1981). Who takes CE and why? *Nurse Careers, 2*(1), 16–21.

Schoen, D. C. (1982). The views of Illinois nurses toward requiring continuing education for relicensure. *Journal of Continuing Education in Nursing, 13*(1), 28–37.

Sessions, F. Q., & Van Sant, G. (1966). Evaluation of regional continuing education conferences. *Nursing Research, 15,* 75–79.

Skipper, J. K., & King, J. A. (1974). Continuing education feedback from the grass roots. *Nursing Outlook, 22,* 252–253.

Sorensen, K. H. (1979). The learning needs of female health-workers and their consequences for the planning of continuing education programmes. *Social Science and Medicine, 13A,* 797–805.

Squires, R. L. (1979). Assessing the continuing education needs of school nurses. *Journal of School Health, 49,* 493–495.

Valencius, J. (1980). Impact of a continuing education program in cancer nursing. Part I: Results affecting patient care. *Journal of Continuing Education in Nursing, 11*(2), 14–18.

Valish, A. U., & Boyd, N. J. (1975). The role of computer assisted instruction in continuing education of registered nurses: An experimental study. *Journal of Continuing Education in Nursing, 6*(1), 13–32.

Volinn, I. J. (1982). Geriatric nurses assess their educational needs. *Geriatric Nursing, 3,* 106–107.

Westfall, L. K., & Speedie, S. (1981). The effect of inservice education provided by consultant pharmacists in the behavior of nurses in long-term care facilities. *Drug Intelligence and Clinical Pharmacy, 15,* 777–781.

Winters, B., Lum, J., & Faustino, S. (1977). Hawaii nurses express continuing education needs and preferences. *Journal of Continuing Education in Nursing, 8*(1), 30–36.

CHAPTER 8

Doctoral Education of Nurses: Historical Development, Programs, and Graduates

JUANITA F. MURPHY
COLLEGE OF NURSING
ARIZONA STATE UNIVERSITY

CONTENTS

Doctoral education of nurses is a relatively new phenomenon, and research on this phenomenon is even more recent. Only within the past decade has there been a systematic attempt to describe and evaluate the impact of doctoral education on the practice, education, and research of professional nurses in this country. Included in this review and critique of research are descriptive studies regarding the development of nursing doctoral programs, evaluative studies of program quality, and descriptive studies of graduates.

A computerized literature search was conducted using the generic retrieval index of Doctoral Education of Nurses and the following subtopics: historical development of doctoral education of nurses; nursing doctoral education programs, courses, dissertations, socialization processes, and conceptual frameworks; and sociodemographic and other relevant descriptors of nurses with earned doctoral degrees. Citations were tracked from one study to another. Unpublished papers were secured from scholars working in the same research areas. Known completed studies that were not included in the retrieval system were secured. Additionally, ideas formulated by nurse scholars were included as sensitizing concepts to enrich the conceptual composition of the research topic. In short, every attempt was made to review as many referenced sources as possible, including books, journal articles, monographs, and published and unpublished manuscripts.

HISTORICAL DEVELOPMENT STUDIES

The first doctoral program for nurses was established in 1924 at Teachers College, Columbia University. The Ed.D. degree was awarded to nurses preparing to teach at the college level. According to the American Nurses' Foundation (1969) *Directory of Nurses with Earned Doctoral Degrees,* Edith S. Bryan was the first American nurse to earn a doctoral degree. She graduated in 1927 from Johns Hopkins University with a Ph.D. in psychology and counseling. The first Ph.D. program in nursing was established in 1934 at New York University in the School of Education.

Foundation of Doctoral Education

Matarazzo and Abdellah (1971) traced this country's founding of higher education at Harvard College in 1636 to the establishment of the first American study program for an earned Doctor of Philosophy degree at Yale University in 1861. From their analysis of a variety of historical documents, they determined that the changing status and the dramatic upgrading of educational preparation for nurses began almost a century later in the early 1950s. Drawing from the *Directory of Nurses with Earned Doctoral Degrees* (American Nurses' Foundation [ANF], 1969), Matarazzo and Abdellah (1971) described a pattern of nurses with earned doctorates between 1956 and 1970 by type of degree (Ed.D., Ph.D., and other) and by institution from which the degrees were granted. They documented the assistance of the United States Public Health Service (USPHS) regarding financial support of nursing research conferences, research training grants, nurse scientist graduate training programs, nurse research predoctoral fellowships, and faculty research development grants. A major contribution of their research on the early development of doctoral preparation in nursing was the tabular presentation of USPHS support of research training in nursing from 1956 to 1970. Matarazzo and Abdellah (1971) concluded that nursing had an adequately developed impetus and sufficient resources to offer a substantive Ph.D. in nursing. This study was important and timely in that established nursing doctoral education programs were expanding rapidly; new nursing doctoral education programs were being developed; and the nurse scientist programs were being phased out. The inclusion of data in relation to the support of USPHS gave an additional perspective for interpreting the past development of nursing doctoral education and for strategic planning for the future.

Historiographic methodology, generally, has two primary weaknesses: (a) the authenticity of documents used as the data base are questionable, and (b) the interpretation of data or information from documents tends to be subjective. At the time of the above report, both Matarazzo and Abdellah were in positions in which USPHS documents were readily available to them and to the general public. Availability of original public documents minimizes the question of authenticity for the Matarazzo and Abdellah (1971) report. Data from the documents were presented with meager interpretation other than the conclusion that there were sufficient momentum and resources to offer a substantive Ph.D. in nursing (Matarazzo & Abdellah, 1971). The researchers' conception and execution of the study were imaginative in that both primary and secondary sources of data were woven selectively into a conclusive interpretation of data. Although the methods for secondary data selection and for data analysis were not included in the report, the competency with which the study was conducted and reported repudiates the potential internal and external criticism of the meaning and value of the data and the interpretation given the data.

Links Between the Past and the Future

In an analysis of nursing doctoral education of the past, present, and future, Grace (1978) proposed three stages of development that nursing had experienced. Spanning the years 1926 to 1959, the first stage was the era of functional specialists during which nurses received doctoral degrees primarily in the field of education. Grace described the second developmental stage from 1960 to 1969 as the nurse scientist era. During this decade a large number of nurses obtained doctoral education in scientific disciplines related to nursing. Options for nurses to obtain doctoral education expanded tremendously when 10 universities were awarded funds from the Division of Nursing, USPHS, to establish Nurse Scientist Training Programs. Financial assistance was available also through the Division of Nursing's Special Predoctoral Research Fellowship Program.

Grace (1978) proposed that the third stage of development was best denoted as doctorates in and of nursing. The 16 nursing doctoral programs established during the 1970s resulted from the diverse doctoral preparation of nurses who developed these programs. This diversity also resulted in varying degrees of integration and synthesis of related scientific fields into what is now a substantive field of nursing. Grace did not clarify the concepts of diversity or of varying degrees of integration and synthesis.

This analysis and interpretation of the past, present, and future of nursing doctoral education (Grace, 1978) was another example of the use of primary and secondary sources of historical documents as the data base for the study. Grace did not identify the data source, method for selecting relevant documents as data, or means of data analysis. She assumed that there was evidence that the described events had occurred. Her most important scientific contribution was the conceptualization of three stages of development of nursing doctoral education. She identified factors and events that seemed to be associated with the conceptualizations and presented her analysis and results in a readable and understandable manner. She accomplished the relevant objective of extending knowledge of past events. Additionally, she provided a perspective for contemporary and future analysis of trends in nursing doctoral education.

On the basis of a survey conducted between 1972 and 1974, Leininger (1976) concluded that there would be 35 doctoral programs in nursing by the end of the decade. The data were collected from most nursing programs that either had or were planning a nursing doctoral program. An advantage of Leininger's survey was the obtaining of a great deal of information from the sample; a disadvantage of the survey was the lack of depth in the information gathered. The lack of depth in the data and the analysis of the data led Leininger to the erroneous conclusion that there would be 35 doctoral programs in nursing by 1980. In this study Leininger did not give sufficient detail regarding design, methodology, or data analysis and interpretation. However, the reported findings formed the basis for faculty to project and establish future nurse doctoral programs and question the substantive content of existing and projected programs.

The Emerging Nature of Nursing Doctoral Education

Matarazzo and Abdellah (1971) concluded that there were adequately developed nurse educators and nurse researchers to offer a reputable Ph.D. in nursing. Grace (1978) identified the relevant areas for concern as (a) the nature of research and theory development, (b) the distinctions between professional and academic doctorates in nursing, and (c) the definition of clinical and research components. Leininger (1976) expressed concern regarding (a) the future financial uncertainty in nursing education, (b) the need to prepare nurses at the doctoral level for leadership positions in nursing service and education, and (c) the need to examine and to clarify the need for both practice-oriented and research-oriented doctoral programs.

These issues and concerns prompted Murphy (1981) to explore the substantive nature of doctoral programs in nursing. She analyzed the philosophical perspectives, the objectives and conceptual frameworks, the criteria for admission of students, and the course descriptions of the 22 doctoral programs that admitted students during the 1981 to 1982 academic year. Murphy (1983) found that the designated degree of the various programs did not differentiate between professional and research degrees. Instead, Murphy reported that the philosophical stance of the graduate program of a university was the prime determinant of the conceptual nature of the nurse doctoral program within the university. There was little agreement among the materials received from the 22 respondents as to the nature of the scientific base of nursing. Research conducted by faculty tended to focus on the particular faculty member's area of interest rather than reflecting a central guiding theme, conceptual framework, or paradigm.

The problem under study was stated clearly in the research reports by Murphy (1981, 1983). Most course descriptions secured for this study were general and there was a high degree of variability among courses. A lack of rigor in the study design led to the collection of qualitative data that could be analyzed only at a nominal level. Reconceptualization of the course content into relevant categories was not accomplished. Murphy (1983) concluded that (a) the substantive content of nurse doctoral programs was pluralistic in nature, and (b) inductive generalizations were not derived appropriately from the use of course descriptions as the data base.

Beare, Gray, and Ptak (1981) developed a more quantitatively rigorous approach to examine the content being taught in nursing programs at the doctoral level. Subjects were asked to ascertain whether individual items on a list of subject content actually were required versus ideally required. Among the respondents, there was agreement that nursing theory, theory development, concept formulation, and quantitative analysis were required both actually and ideally. Beare et al. (1981) concluded that doctoral programs in nursing were set up for the preparation of scholars and researchers rather than for leaders in education and administration, as was called for by Leininger (1976).

Three major concerns were derived from an analysis of the Beare et al. report (1981): (a) There was a lack of clarity in operationalizing the concept of essential content, (b) the use of unvalidated techniques in data collection resulted in a compromise of the rigor of proof, and (c) the limited response rate of 12 out of 20 doctoral program respondents decreased confidence in the findings and results. The collection of quantifiable data permitted statistical analysis of the data, but the conclusions were questionable due to the lack of rigor in instrument development.

An ad hoc advisory group, selected by the National Research Committee on a Study of National Needs for Biomedical and Behavioral Research Personnel, was directed to describe developments in graduate education for nurses. The ad hoc advisory group conducted two surveys of a selected number of schools of nursing which either had or were developing doctoral programs for nurses (National Academy of Science, 1978). Site visits were conducted at 10 of the 16 established programs and at five institutions where preparations to initiate doctoral programs were under way during 1976 and 1977. The questionnaire for these surveys was designed to procure (a) graduate program enrollments, criteria for admission, and number of degrees awarded; (b) sources of doctoral and postdoctoral support for training; (c) faculty characteristics; and (d) amount and types of research activities by the faculty.

One of the findings of the study was the high degree of variability for research impetus among the institutions. The advisory group was of the opinion that research involvement by faculty was critical for the existing and proposed doctoral programs in schools of nursing. The group urged the professional community of nursing to consider a voluntary and sizable reduction in the projection of new programs for doctoral training in nursing until existing programs acquired additional strength in those aspects which contribute to the quality of doctoral education (National Academy of Science, 1978).

Site visits to 15 institutions included in the study sample added to the depth of data procured. The study was conducted to provide an improved data base for future planning of graduate education for nurses. A formulation of recommendations followed the evaluation of findings. An evaluation of follow-up action stemming from the recommendations would be an important next step. The research report (National Academy of Science, 1978) contained meager information about the development of the instruments, the design of the study, and the techniques used in data analysis. The findings were formulated well and have been used to develop public policy positions.

In summary, doctoral education for nurses was slow in developing. During the 1960s there were several routes available to nurses for earning a doctoral degree. Not until the middle 1970s did the Ph.D. in nursing emerge as the most desired degree.

In both historiographic and survey research reports investigators described the beginning endeavors, the various alternatives, and the assistance of the USPHS in the development of nursing doctoral education. The findings of the survey research reports provided a broad perspective for describing the early and recent program developments and for the planning and implementation of new doctoral programs. Findings from the reports, however, provided little guidance for the qualitative aspects of program development and monitoring. The next section contains a review and analysis of studies focused primarily on the quality of doctoral programs in nursing.

PROGRAM AND OUTCOME STUDIES

By the middle 1970s the discussion of doctoral programs had shifted from types of degrees offered and the mechanisms, strategies, and problems of program planning and implementation to concerns for substantive issues of quality. Several scholars developed sensitizing concepts that provided the conceptual base for the examination and evaluation of nursing doctoral programs from the perspective of quality.

Sensitizing Concepts

Armiger (1974) maintained that university nursing faculty should assume responsibilities as scholars and as mentors of student scholars. She distinguished between faculty with a scholarly commitment and those who are not so committed. Cleland (1976) pointed out that it is not enough to have a critical mass of doctorally prepared faculty to develop a doctoral program. There must also be a sufficient number of doctorally prepared faculty with recognized postdoctoral research experience to guide and direct students' research toward a dissertation.

Benoliel (1977) maintained that nurse scholars and researchers need to be able to move back and forth between the empirical world of nursing practice and the abstract world of theory development. Donaldson and

Crowley (1978) called for multiple methodological approaches for expanding further the scientific knowledge of nursing. Downs (1978) pleaded for a focus on the practical application of scholarship and research.

Meleis, Wilson, and Chater (1980) developed an analytic model that explicated the essential ingredients of scholarliness in relation to the dissertation. In another exposition, Meleis and May (1981) emphasized the prerequisite need for a scholarly milieu for the development and teaching of theory in doctoral programs. Curran, Habeeb, and Sobol (1981) suggested that for those nurses seeking a doctoral degree the overall quality of the school and faculty and the nature of the research programs were prime factors to be considered in selecting the appropriate program.

These scholars assisted in developing the conceptual base for clarifying the focus of doctoral education of nurses. If doctoral education programs were to produce nurse scholars and nurse researchers, faculty teaching in those programs must have been involved actively in scholarly research activities. The need for research to evaluate the scholarly milieu of nursing doctoral education programs was emerging.

Building the Research Base

Program analysis approaches developed by Clark, Hartnett, and Baird (1976) assisted Barhyte and Holzemer (1981) in developing the methodological design for the Cooperative Program Evaluation of Doctoral Education in Nursing Project. The cooperative project was established by support of 18 of the 22 doctoral programs that were in existence in 1978. The purpose of the project was to provide an evaluation of the quality of doctoral education in nursing. The unit of analysis was the program.

To assess and analyze the 18 participating programs, Barhyte and Holzemer sent three questionnaires to students, faculty, and alumni. The first questionnaire consisted of 16 dimensions of quality of doctoral education developed by Clark et al. (1976). Items pertaining to program characteristics were the content of the second questionnaire, and items dealing specifically and uniquely with nursing comprised the third instrument. The issue of instrument validity and reliability was not addressed in the report (Barhyte & Holzemer, 1981). The response rate was reported to range between 57% and 64% and no significant differences were found among the response rates by programs. Due to the small sample size of alumni, data from this group were not presented in the report. Barhyte and Holzemer used two different approaches for reporting findings from the data. The first approach included confidential data regarding individual programs. Responses of respective program's faculty, students, and alumni were compiled, analyzed, and submitted to the individual program's administrator. Each program administrator could compare the composite findings of his or her program with composite findings from other anonymous participating programs. A program administrator could use the findings from the report as a basis for management and modification of the program.

The second approach for reporting data was to compare data from Barhyte and Holzemer's (1981) study with data collected by Clark et al. (1976) in their analysis of doctoral programs in chemistry, history, and psychology. Barhyte and Holzemer (1981) reported that (a) nursing faculties' perceptions of their programs tended to be more positive than nonnursing faculties' perceptions of their programs, (b) nursing students' perceptions of their programs tended to be slightly higher than comparative students' perceptions of their respective nonnursing programs, (c) nursing faculty tended to perceive their respective programs more positively than did the nursing students, and (d) nursing students' mean for quality of faculty teaching was lower than the comparative students' mean for the same measure.

Among the limitations of this study, the question of validity was foremost. Holzemer (1982) proposed a multidimensional analytical model that included additional conceptional approaches that were focused on measures of program quality that had been validated.

Development of Analytical Models

Holzemer (1982) proposed a model by operationally dividing standards, criteria, and indicators into more discrete variables. He proposed standards for the areas of (a) domain of nursing, (b) scholarship, (c) professionalism, (d) collegiality, (e) productivity, and (f) propriety. He included the variables of faculty, students, academic program, and resources as criteria in the analytical model, and developed indicators for measuring each criteria. Holzemer posited the model within a systems framework consisting of context, environment, and the product of education. It was Holzemer's contention that the concept of quality must be extended to include a range of indicators of program processes and program outcomes for a more comprehensive description and analysis of the phenomenon.

The Holzemer (1982) model, though not tested at this time, may be useful in (a) a comprehensive description of nursing doctoral education programs and their products, (b) the examination and specification of relationships among the various concepts included in the model, (c) the prediction of different outcomes associated with various programs, and (d) program management and decision making based on data. The focus of the

Cooperative Program Evaluation of Doctoral Education in Nursing Project is now that of description and explanation rather than evaluation.

It is premature to delineate the weaknesses of the Holzemer model since there has been no research based on the conceptual model. Caution should be exercised by researchers who use this model regarding tendencies to (a) attempt to fit all data into a preestablished set of categories, (b) make the data fit the model, (c) develop measurement tools that lack validity and reliability, and (d) overgeneralize the findings beyond the scope of the model. As with all conceptual models, this model will have limited research potential until the underlying phenomena are identified, explicated, measured, and empirically tested.

In summary, there have been many persons concerned about the process and outcomes of nursing doctoral education. Relevant publications of scholars assisted in delineating the parameters of this concern, and their delineations were included as sensitizing concepts in this section. Few researchers have studied the process and outcomes of nursing doctoral education, particularly from the perspective of quality. An analytical model was developed by Holzemer (1982) that has potential for describing and explaining some of the relationships between process and outcomes. This model was derived from the research findings of scholars who examined similar phenomena in other disciplines. Research based on the Holzemer model has not been reported at this time.

In studies included in the next section, investigators described the characteristics and activities of nurses who have completed doctoral education programs. An essential focus of these studies was to provide a general description of doctorally educated nurses as one of this country's salient health care resources.

PRODUCT STUDIES

Boyle (1954) conducted a descriptive study of the similarities and differences in graduate education programs designed to prepare nursing instructors. Included in her sample were faculty members who had earned doctoral degrees. As part of this comprehensive study, Boyle made site visits to 19 nursing schools that offered educational programs for nursing instructors and were located in university settings. Two aspects of the final report are noteworthy. First, Boyle provided a detailed analysis of characteristics of teachers of nursing and the teaching programs in which they were involved. Second, she recommended that future research should include descriptions and evaluations of problems that graduates encountered in the employment arena. Boyle's work was used as a foundation by later investigators.

Developing the Design

Almost a decade later Cleino (1965) developed and used a questionnaire to survey 94 nurses holding doctoral degrees and teaching in baccalaureate or higher degree programs regarding their educational background and their teaching role. The educational backgrounds of the 94 nurses who held doctorates were so varied that few commonalities could be ascertained. Of the 94 nurses, 81 majored in professional education or in nursing education. Twenty-seven different institutions granted the degrees. Of the 94 nurses, 63 held the Ed.D. degree, 30 held the Ph.D. degree, and 1 held the D.S. degree.

Most of the respondents had previous teaching experience, but few had taught in a university setting prior to receiving their doctorates. Of the 94 respondents, 60 indicated that they had published. More than half of the group guided students in the preparation of master's theses, and 32 served as the head of at least one research project. On the basis of the findings, Cleino noted that nurse faculty members with an earned doctorate comprised 4.6% of the total nursing faculty in baccalaureate and higher degree programs compared to 40.5% nonnursing faculty with doctoral degrees in the colleges and universities.

Cleino (1965) presented a straightforward description of 94 nurse faculty members with doctoral degrees. She selected nurses who were holding faculty positions in baccalaureate and higher degree programs from the total universe of nurses with doctoral degrees. Of the 115 who were listed as holding such positions, 94 responded to the mailed questionnaire. Cleino did not generalize the findings of the study beyond the set of respondents. The study lacked the depth of the Boyle (1954) study since Cleino did not interview study subjects but relied solely on data from a mailed questionnaire.

ANF conducted a survey to assess the extent of research talent available for research and to monitor trends in the production and employment of doctorally prepared nurses. A questionnaire was mailed to all nurses who were known to have an earned doctoral degree. Data collected from the survey were compiled as a *Directory of Nurses with Earned Doctoral Degrees* (ANF, 1969).

Taylor, Gifford, and Vian (1971) analyzed selected information from the survey. In their report of findings, they described the methods employed by ANF in identifying nurses with earned doctoral degrees and concluded that (a) every effort was made to find and list all eligible subjects and (b) there was no way to ascertain those that were missed. In their analysis of the 676 subjects, Taylor et al. (1971) found that (a) most were female, (b) a high percentage was employed full time in some nursing activity, (c) most had earned their doctoral degree sometime during the past 10 years, (d) the

Western and Southern regions educated and employed fewer nurses with doctoral degrees than the Middle Atlantic and Midwestern regions, (e) most had earned a Ph.D. degree in an area of the behavioral sciences, and (f) most had received support from either the Nurse Research Fellowship Program or the Nurse Scientist Program of the U.S. Department of Health, Education and Welfare.

Expanding the Design

Data gathered by ANF was expanded to include 165 variables in the 1973 study. Nurses who had earned their doctoral degrees in foreign countries were included in the 1973 survey. Responses were obtained from 1,020 subjects. Pitel and Vian (1975) analyzed selected data from the 1973 survey and reported a continuing trend of nurses to earn the Ph.D. degree. Unexpected findings were that (a) only 3.5% classified their primary position as researchers, (b) less than half were engaged in research, (c) only 31.5% perceived research as a major responsibility in their present position, and (d) 20.8% had not engaged in any type of research for the previous five years. Finally, there was a major shift in dissertation topics toward research that could be classified as nursing. Most of the nurses with earned doctoral degrees were in academic settings with heavy teaching and administrative responsibilities. Most were promoted to the rank of professor or associate professor (Pitel & Vian, 1975).

Nurses earned doctoral degrees in 115 universities in the United States, 6 in Canada, and 11 in foreign countries. The highest number of nurses earned their doctoral degree in the Middle Atlantic region of the United States, but the highest number were employed in the Midwestern region. Only 9% of the subjects engaged in any form of postdoctoral training. A large number (43%) received predoctoral training support from the Division of Nursing, USPHS. Pitel and Vian (1975) indicated that, as a group, nurses with doctoral degrees exemplified occupational stability and minimal geographic mobility.

Both the Taylor et al. report (1971) and the Pitel and Vian report (1975) were based on the analysis of selected data that were available from surveys conducted by the ANF (1969, 1973). The primary purpose of the 1969 and 1973 ANF surveys was the compilation of a directory of nurses with earned doctoral degrees. Taylor et al. (1971) and Pitel and Vian (1975) used data that were placed in the directory along with available sociodemographic data for their reports.

The universe surveyed was well-defined, and the scope of both surveys (ANF, 1969, 1973) was extensive. Taylor et al. (1971) reported sample bias considering that there was a greater probability to include in the survey nurses who maintained visibility in nursing-related activities or who were employed. Information was not available regarding the evaluation of returned questionnaires for spurious answering and reporting. The ANF surveys (1969, 1973) relied heavily on self-reporting of personal items and information. The reliability of reporting personal information is high according to Kerlinger (1964).

There was no indication that the validity of the survey data was checked. Although it was quite simple to ascertain whether an individual respondent received a doctoral degree from a specific university in a designated field of study during a particular year, it was more difficult to ascertain the validity of self-reporting of research activities. Ordinarily, individual behavior is not checked for validity, but group behavior is available for external validating sources. For example, the group report of receipt of support for doctoral study could be validated by securing information from the Division of Nursing, USPHS, for specific years. This information could be used to check corresponding responses from subjects.

As in most surveys, the ANF surveys (1969, 1973) provided extensive data, but the cursory depth of the data did not allow for intensive analysis. For example, the relevance of the research reported by respondents to the profession was not addressed. In short, the scope of the data secured from the surveys and the analysis of the data provided descriptive trends of the characteristics and employment activities of doctorally prepared nurses. The relationship between some of the variables included in the study was explored. Findings were not generalized beyond the limitations of the surveys.

An Update

The American Nurses' Association's (ANA) Commission on Nursing Research developed a study to (a) update the directory of nurses with earned doctorates in the United States, (b) analyze the educational and professional work climate of doctorally prepared nurses, and (c) develop a national informational system that will serve as a model for the provision of periodically current data about nurses with earned doctoral degrees (ANA, 1981). A questionnaire was developed to elicit data regarding the three dimensions of the project, and the questionnaire was mailed to 2,596 nurses during Autumn of 1979 and Spring of 1980. A response rate of over 80% was obtained, and the data were analyzed and reported in two major sections. One section dealt with a comprehensive description of the study subjects and the other dealt with a description and an analysis of their professional productivity.

The background for the study was well-developed, and pertinent findings from other studies of doctoral education in nursing and nonnursing areas were summarized. Conceptualization and measurement of professional productivity were based on a review of the literature related to scholarly productivity of other disciplines. Factors that affected or were associated with productivity in other fields were examined from the perspective of changes occurring in nursing that relate to the development of a scientific base for nursing practice. The findings of the study were limited because the dimensions of administrative and teaching productivity were not included (ANA, 1981). There was a logical continuity between the work completed earlier in relation to subjects' sociodemographic characteristics, particularly the work completed by ANF (1969). The report (ANA, 1981) contained a detailed description of how the study was conducted. The design of the self-reporting survey was appropriate for the study questions, but less so for the productivity section of the study. Methods for selecting the subjects were described sufficiently. Adequate information was included in the discussion of the instruments and the methodology for comprehension and replication of the study.

Due to the intent and magnitude of the study (ANA, 1981), a large portion of the report dealt with summaries of the data collected, the statistical treatment of the data, and presentation of the results of the study. Eighteen figures and 148 tables were included in the report for detailed clarity in the summary of the data analysis and results. Directions were provided for reading the detailed summaries of data in the tables. Missing data were acknowledged, and the statistical methods selected for data analysis were incorporated into the text or table, as appropriate. Appropriate methods were employed for statistical analysis of the data.

The conclusion section was presented in three pages which do not describe, evaluate, or interpret the implications of the study sufficiently. Significant associations between variables were addressed generally in this section and included an association between professional productivity and several socialization experiences. In the report, readers are cautioned to interpret these associations with discretion because the data analysis was rudimentary.

Two models for describing the doctoral career among nurses were proposed as the *career-directing doctorate* and the *career-accommodating doctorate*. The utility of the conceptual model merits future examination and analysis. Several questions for further investigation were included in the last page of the report. The questions pertaining to the relationship between types of programs and adequacy of graduates to do research and publish findings are akin to questions that were posed by Holzemer (1982).

Overall strengths of the ANA study (1981) were that (a) the study was comprehensive in scope, (b) the study can be replicated, and (c) provision for periodical updates of the sociodemographic data have been incorporated in future planning. Overall weaknesses were that (a) the study was expensive, (b) the study was limited in scope in that it did not include in-depth questions related to administrative and teaching activities, (c) the reliability and validity of the data were not ascertained, and (d) the data base of the study was so mammoth that thorough data analysis will not be completed before new data are elicited. Furthermore, the questionnaire was lengthy. Response rates are likely to decrease due to the time required to complete the lengthy, 13-page questionnaire, and missing data are likely to increase for the same reason.

Micro Studies

In an attempt to ascertain the impact of doctoral education on graduates, Crowley (1976) informally interviewed nurse colleagues having doctoral degrees. This sample of convenience indicated that as a result of completing a doctoral program they all experienced material, professional, and personal gains. Contributions to the profession and to society were made through their leadership roles in nursing education and research.

The study was lacking in methodological sophistication, but it had two aspects that were not addressed by other macro-survey researchers. First, the subjects were interviewed, which enhanced the depth of responses. Second, the subjects reported personal gains as a result of earning a doctoral degree. Perceived personal gains was a concept that had not been included previously in research endeavors regarding nurses with doctoral degrees.

Downs (1976) assessed the impact of the educational program in a follow-up study of all graduates of the doctoral program in the Division of Nursing at New York University from 1964 through 1974. Of the 81 graduates, 68 (81%) returned a completed questionnaire that elicited their opinions about student life, faculty competency, course content, and dissertations. In general, the dissertation was deemed an essential part of doctoral education even though, for many, the process of preparing it was painful and frustrating. The respondents reported a high level of involvement in numerous professional activities including publication of books and articles, as well as completed research. On the basis of these findings, Downs questioned the inferences drawn that nurses with doctorates were not prepared for, committed to, and involved in research and scholarship.

Downs' report (1976) of her research contained insufficient information about the study design, methodology, data collection, and data analysis. Even though the respondents reported high involvement in research and scholarly activities, the actual level of involvement was not addressed. In short, the findings did not support sufficiently the generalization that all doctorally prepared nurses are prepared for, committed to, and involved in research and scholarship.

In general, for studies included in this section investigators documented with a high degree of accuracy the number of doctorally prepared nurses, the types of degrees they earned, the fields of study in which they earned their respective degrees, and their current employment patterns and activities. Weaknesses of the studies were that (a) the data from the respondents were self-reported and were treated at face value, (b) the macro surveys (ANA, 1981; ANF, 1969, 1973) were expensive and lacking in depth, and (c) the analysis of secondary data (Pitel & Vian, 1975; Taylor et al., 1971) was beset with methodological difficulties. Strengths of the studies were that (a) survey methods allowed the collection of a wide scope of data, (b) survey methods were less expensive than interviewing the entire population or a random sample of the population, (c) baseline data on nurses with doctoral degrees have been established, and (d) the data base could be updated periodically.

CONCLUSIONS AND FUTURE RESEARCH RECOMMENDATIONS

Doctorally educated nurses are one of the profession's most valuable resources. Because of this importance, research in the domains of programs that prepare nurses at the doctoral level and of nurses who have earned a doctoral degree is essential.

The development of the doctoral education of nurses, spanning the period from the 1950s to the 1980s, was described in some of the research presented in this review. Sociodemographic descriptions of nurses with earned doctoral degrees and the educational work climates in which they were employed were the target of other relevant research. Generalizations were that (a) over 2,500 nurses earned doctoral degrees from a variety of universities and in a variety of fields during the past three decades, (b) nurses with doctoral degrees were firmly entrenched in university settings and spent most of their time in teaching and administration but proportionately less time conducting research, and (c) the degree designation did not reflect accurately the type of program in which the nurse was involved.

Relevant trends identified during the past three decades were (a) an increase in the number of nurses who completed a doctoral degree, (b) an increase in the number of nursing education programs that offer a doctoral degree, (c) a preference for the Ph.D. over the Ed.D., (d) an increase in the number of nurses who completed a doctoral degree before the age of 40, (e) an increased concern for research involvement and scholarliness among both doctoral faculty and students, and (f) a relatively low level of active involvement in research by nurses with earned doctoral degrees. Events and situations, such as the Division of Nursing's USPHS support, that appeared to be related to or to influence these trends were identified and examined for associations.

Recommendations for future research include the development and initiation of a comprehensive study of a randomly selected sample of nurses enrolled in a variety of doctoral programs. Antecedent conditions such as previous degrees attained and work experience could be used for the identification of subsets in the sample. The variables included in the Holzemer (1982) model and the ANA (1981) study could be examined during the socialization process in doctoral study. After completion of the doctoral program, subjects could be followed to examine professional productivity and other relevant variables. Hypotheses could be generated from this comprehensive approach regarding the relation of programs to products.

The data on nurses with doctoral degrees that were obtained by the ANA (1981) survey should be expanded periodically. Access to these data should be expanded to include regional centers. The data should be circulated widely for future policy formulation at the state, regional, and national levels.

Programs within regional centers could be established to begin strategic planning for the future of nursing doctoral education for the remainder of this century. From the strategic planning that is developed from each of the regions, the number and types of programs needed and the number and differentiated competencies of graduates needed could be projected nationally. These projections could be analyzed in relation to the nursepower needs–analysis studies that deal with need for doctorally prepared nurses. National policy regarding need for and support of doctorally prepared nurses would be influenced by these systematically derived projections.

For the future, attention must be given to the validity of data for studies regarding nurse doctoral education. The use of interviewing techniques and authentic public documents are helpful in the exploration of the nature of data and for suggesting and testing hypotheses. Building a research foundation will require the tenacity and creativity found in many of the doctorally prepared scholars and researchers in nursing.

REFERENCES

American Nurses' Association. (1981). *Nurses with doctorates*. Final report on Grant No. (5R01-NU00661-02), Division of Nursing, U.S. Department of Health and Human Services. Kansas City, MO: Author.

American Nurses' Foundation. (1969). Directory of nurses with earned doctoral degrees. *Nursing Research, 18,* 465–480.

American Nurses' Foundation. (1973). *International Directory of Nurses with Doctoral Degrees*. New York: Author.

Armiger, B. (1974). Scholarship in nursing. *Nursing Outlook, 22,* 160–164.

Barhyte, D. Y., & Holzemer, W. L. (1981, June). *Cooperative program evaluation of doctoral education in nursing*. Paper presented at the Forum on Doctoral Education in Nursing, Seattle, WA.

Beare, P. G., Gray, C. J., & Ptak, H. F. (1981). Doctoral curricula in nursing. *Nursing Outlook, 29,* 311–316.

Benoliel, J. Q. (1977). The interaction between theory and research. *Nursing Outlook, 25,* 108–113.

Boyle, R. (1954). A study of programs of professional education for teachers of nursing in nineteen selected universities. *Nursing Research, 2,* 100–125.

Clark, M. J., Hartnett, R. T., & Baird, L. L. (1976). *Assessing dimensions of quality in doctoral education: A technical report of a national study in three fields*. Princeton, NJ: Educational Testing Service.

Cleino, E. (1965). Profile of 94 nurse faculty members with doctoral degrees. *Nursing Outlook, 13*(10), 37–39.

Cleland, V. (1976). Developing a doctoral program. *Nursing Outlook, 24,* 631–635.

Crowley, D. (1976). *Why doctoral education for nurses?* (NLN Publication No. 15-1639). New York: National League for Nursing.

Curran, C. L., Habeeb, M. C., & Sobol, E. G. (1981). Selecting a doctoral program for a career in nursing. *Journal of Nursing Administration, 11,* 35–40.

Donaldson, S., & Crowley, D. (1978). The discipline of nursing. *Nursing Outlook, 26,* 113–120.

Downs, F. S. (1976). Doctoral preparation in nursing: Is it worth it? *Nursing Outlook, 24,* 375–377.

Downs, F. S. (1978). Doctoral education in nursing: Future directions. *Nursing Outlook, 26,* 56–61.

Grace, H. D. (1978). The development of doctoral education in nursing: In historical prospective. *Journal of Nursing Education, 17,* 17–29.

Holzemer, W. L. (1982). Quality in graduate nursing education. *Nursing and Health Care, 3,* 536–542.

Kerlinger, F. N. (1964). *Foundations of behavioral research*. New York: Holt, Rinehart & Winston.

Leininger, M. (1976). Doctoral programs for nurses: Trends, questions, and projected plans. *Nursing Research, 25,* 201–210.

Matarazzo, J. D., & Abdellah, F. G. (1971). Doctoral education for nurses in the United States. *Nursing Research, 20,* 404–414.

Meleis, A. I., & May, K. (1981). Nursing theory and scholarliness in the doctoral program. *Advances in Nursing Science, 4*(1), 31–41.

Meleis, A. I., Wilson, H. S., & Chater, S. (1980). Toward scholarliness in doctoral dissertations: An analytical model. *Research in Nursing and Health, 3,* 115–124.

Murphy, J. F. (1981). Doctoral education in, of, and for nursing: An historical analysis. *Nursing Outlook, 29,* 645–649.

Murphy, J. F. (1983). *Doctoral education for nurses: Some substantive issues.* Unpublished manuscript.

National Academy of Sciences. (1978). *Personnel needs and training for biomedical and behavioral research.* Washington, DC: Commission on Human Resources, National Research Council.

Pitel, M., & Vian, J. (1975). Analysis of nurse-doctorates. *Nursing Research, 24,* 340–351.

Taylor, D. D., Gifford, A. J., & Vian, J. (1971). Nurses with earned doctoral degrees. *Nursing Research, 20,* 415–417.

PART IV

Research on the Profession of Nursing

CHAPTER 9

Ethical Inquiry

Susan R. Gortner
School of Nursing
University of California, San Francisco

CONTENTS

Appreciation is expressed to several individuals who made substantial contributions to the preparation of this chapter. Ida Marie Moore, research assistant for the chapter, reviewed and abstracted the articles. Christine Solis, National Institutes of Health Minority High School Student Research Apprentice (2 S03 RR03278-01), carried out the library searches and abstracted articles. Mary Kawahira, secretary for the Nursing Research Emphasis Grant (5 R21 NU00828-03), funded by the Division of Nursing, typed and helped revise the final manuscript. Susan Karpuk was most helpful in the task of editing the final version.

Most ethical inquiry in nursing remains philosophical in nature rather than empirical. This observation does not negate the importance of philosophical analysis, but rather underscores the recency of ethics as an object of research and the difficulty investigators have had with the measurement of ethical principles and concepts. For example, White (1983) noted insufficient appreciation in nursing of the continuing debate in philosophy over the nature and meaning of "ought" language, of value-laden words such as "good," and of the difference between surveys of moral development and philosophical analysis. Further, a potpourri of situations involving legal, social, and personal belief issues in nursing has led to an overexpansion of ethical dilemmas and application of formula ethics. White (1983) suggested "the construction of ethical positions supported by coherent and detailed philosophical reasoning" (p. 43), using ethical judgments, rules, and principles rather than whole theories; such positions should be combined with clinical nursing research to ask what moral matters actually mean to individuals. Thus, one might expect in future reviews an increased reporting of investigations of the patient and family as the unit of analysis and of the clinical and research environment, rather than conceptualizations of ethical dilemmas by nurses or studies of moral reasoning. It can be expected that future reviewers may identify key issues other than those chosen for this first chapter on ethics in this *Annual Review* series.

Because of the paucity of research on the topic of ethical inquiry in nursing, this chapter is intended to serve both as a stimulus to future research through identification of selected issues and as a review of nursing research on ethics published through 1982 on the nurse, the patient, and the clinical environment. Specifically, three issues confronting clinical investigators in nursing were identified for introductory comments in order to cast the framework for the critical review of the limited research that follows. The first issue deals with the combined roles of healer or nurturer and scientist, the second with the protection of human subjects, and the third with peer and institutional review.

THE NURSE AS PRACTITIONER AND AS SCIENTIST

Beecher's (1970) classic work on the investigator generally is considered to be the most authoritative reference on the clinician turned investigator. Among the topics raised were the difference between practice, therapy, and research; the extent of informed consent on the part of research subjects; the nature and conduct of clinical trials; the values of the investigator; and the conduct of unethical research. In a presentation before the New York Academy of Sciences, Ellis (1970) addressed the role of the nurse in medical research involving patients under her or his care, as well as areas of research interest to the nurse clinician-investigator. The Kantian imperative that human beings be treated as ends and not as means to ends is in keeping with nursing's intrinsic humanitarianism; research objectivity does not require that the subject be seen as object or means to a scientific or utilitarian end (Aroskar, 1980b; Ellis, 1970; Gortner, 1974; Lumpp, 1979; May, 1979).

The ethical value system of the investigator is seen by authorities as an essential ingredient in the conduct of clinically relevant research. So pervasive is this point that it is acknowledged to guide the design of research as well as the choice of research topic.

Increasing professional concern about flagrant abuses of human rights and the potential for severe conflict of interest have led to increased documentation of ethical topics in the nursing literature since the late 1960s. In the first major review of nursing ethics research, Armiger (1977) revealed only three citations dealing with ethics during the first 25 years of *Nursing Research,* 1952 to 1977. The establishment of the clinician as an investigator in his or her own right has been acknowledged for the field of medicine for some time but was first acknowledged formally in nursing's *Guidelines on Ethical Values: The Nurse and Research* (American Nurses' Association [ANA], 1968). Two roles for nurses in the research setting were noted: practitioner and investigator. In the *Human Rights Guidelines for Nurses in Clinical and Other Research* (ANA, 1975), again one saw the changing responsibility of nurses in relation to the conduct of research and participation in medical and other health-related research. For the first time, the importance of ethics in the conduct of socially and clinically important research to the profession and to the public was addressed. While the relationship of trust between patient and nurse always has been an essential element of professional ethics, a particular point was made that the relationship of trust between subject and investigator must be assured in research. This safeguarding of rights, together with the guarantee that no risk, discomfort, or threat would evolve from participation in the research, was emphasized. The nature of the healing relationship between clinician and client also was discussed by Pellegrino (1980). The patient sees the nurse more than the physician as an advocate, surrogate, and interpreter of the system. The nurse as clinical scientist is obliged to make the dual role clear to patients and to be aware of distinctions between science and practice. The former demands objectivity and delay of intervention or therapy until evidence is accumulated, as well as protection of the research and the integrity of the research design. The latter demands empathetic identification with the person under care, prompt intervention in order to prevent further harm, and protection of the integrity of the person who is at risk.

The potential for conflict of interest in the clinical investigator role is considerable. The position was held by some, in particular by Beecher (1970), that the clinician should not be allowed to conduct other than therapeutic research on his or her patients, while Levine (1981) no longer made the distinction between therapeutic and nontherapeutic research. Engelhart (1978) reemphasized the deontological ethic, that is, respect for persons as free agents regardless of societal benefits. Thus, the obligation of the clinician-investigator is to foster the best interests of individual human subjects in research that may have societal benefits and to avoid experimentation upon unwilling subjects. Protection of the patient or subject is necessary at all times.

The boundaries between practice and research are not well defined. The National Commission for the Protection of Human Subjects of Biomedical and Behavioral Research (1978a) in its *Belmont Report* characterized research as an activity undertaken to test an hypothesis, permit conclusions to be drawn, and develop generalized knowledge. Practice refers to those interventions or activities that are designed solely to enhance the well-being of an individual patient or client. Research and practice may be carried on together when research is designed to evaluate the safety and efficacy of therapy. Recent categorizations of nursing science and research are consistent in describing an area of activity known as clinical therapeutics or clinical interventions. For research to be conducted within a healing relationship, the National Commission (1978a) enumerated three principles: (a) respect for persons as autonomous agents, including the protection of those with diminished autonomy; (b) beneficence—the obligation to do no harm, to maximize possible benefits, and to minimize harm; and (c) justice—an adequate assessment of burdens and benefits.

Peculiar to the problems of establishing boundaries between therapy and research are what Levine (1978) called boundary problems, or those problems associated with determining who is client and who is subject, and clarifying the intent of both the client and the professional. The intent of the professional must be made explicit in order to determine whether the proposed activity falls within the category of therapy or research. Here again the conscience or moral perspective of the clinician is a major factor in the conduct of research (ANA, 1975; Armiger, 1977; Ellis, 1970). The intent of the client, whether to remain patient or become subject, also needs to be addressed in establishing boundaries between practice and research. The direct and derivative benefits to the client-patient must be assessed according to the best tenets of informed consent. Thus, the importance of the research plan, its timing, the efficacy of the care system, and the skill of the clinician-investigator all must be considered in the assessment process.

Given the ethic of harm avoidance as well as the protection of rights and welfare of those entrusted to care, the clinician is committed to follow a course of action that will result in positive well-being for others. This commitment may suggest that when there is a conflict between the research protocol and treatment plans, research ought to be put aside and treatment plans carried out (Gortner, 1982).

PROTECTION OF HUMAN RESEARCH SUBJECTS

Protection of human research subjects represents a considerable body of information over the past 15 years that is beyond the scope of this chapter, but as a special issue provides part of the framework for research on ethics in nursing. Human experimentation is age-old, having been carried out on those who were considered to be of no human value, such as prisoners or slaves, or by investigators on themselves in an effort to understand better certain basic phenomena. Not until the Nuremberg trials of military war criminals after World War II was public attention focused on the abuses of human beings in the name of research and science. Those trials resulted in what has become a major code of ethics, the Nuremberg Code, for the conduct of research (Nuremberg Military Tribunals, 1949). In 1964, the World Medical Assembly ratified these ethical guidelines for research involving human subjects as the Declaration of Helsinki (World Medical Association, 1966).

During the next decade, guidelines were developed at the National Institutes of Health Clinical Center for the participation of human subjects in research. They were enlarged and formalized to extend to all research supported by the then United States Department of Health, Education, and Welfare (1971). Technical amendments to the guidelines were announced in 1974 and commented on by Bloch, Phillips, and Gortner (1977), followed by the publication of new rules for the protection of human subjects (Basic HHS policy, 1981).

Certain classes of research were seen to involve less potential risk to human subjects, and these have received special consideration for expedited or exempted review in the regulations. Continued interest in the topic of protection of human subjects centers around the promotion of informed consent and subject autonomy, as well as the protection of subjects at risk, particularly those vulnerable groups or populations in which the capacity to give consent may be compromised.

Informed consent is given knowingly and voluntarily by a research subject who has been informed of risks, benefits, and purposes of the research. The right to withdraw from the research at any time without prejudice to treatment is also implicit (ANA, 1975; Armiger, 1977; Basic HHS policy, 1981; Davis, 1979; Hayter, 1979; Notter, 1969). The explanation of a proposed study and its attendant risks and benefits must be in language understandable to the lay person; otherwise the subject will give uninformed and uneducated consent (Ingelfinger, 1972). The requirement of signed consent may be inappropriate to the elderly with impaired memory or other functional disability. Yet institutional review boards require written consent. What alternatives may be appropriate in lieu of a signature to represent understanding and voluntary consent in an elder needs "immediate and careful study" in order not to exclude elders as potential subjects in nursing research (Robb, 1983), while assuring them protection.

Informed consent as a major dimension of patient rights and medical practice was reviewed by Rosoff (1981). A state-by-state review of case law emphasized the responsibilities of the provider, as well as the institution, in assuring informed consent in the conduct of patient care. Rosoff (1981) surveyed over 3,000 practicing physicians to learn what steps physicians took in obtaining informed consent, to learn what they knew and thought about the subject, and to raise the level of awareness indirectly as a result of the survey. The low response rate (24%) of the survey made it difficult to generalize the findings. However, the survey results suggested that the topic itself could become a fruitful area for investigation, particularly with regard to state law and interpretation. For example, what is the standard of disclosure and what are the conditions under which withholding of information is justified?

Promoting subject autonomy and the protection of subjects at risk were addressed repeatedly by the National Commission (1978a, 1978b). Other documents from this National Commission (1976, 1977, 1978c) pertained to the participation of prisoners, children, and the mentally infirm in behavioral and biomedical research. Recently Watson (1982) reviewed the literature of the historical development of informed consent as an issue in research with special subjects. Watson took the position that persons in whom voluntary consent was compromised were the least preferred research subjects and need special protection by nurse investigators.

PEER AND INSTITUTIONAL REVIEW

The requirement of peer review, that is, the scrutiny by others of a proposed research plan that will involve human subjects, is relatively recent in nursing research. It is one of the major accomplishments in the ethics of research of the past decade (Bloch et al., 1977; Fletcher, 1980; Hayter, 1979; National Commission, 1978b). Until 1971, when such peer review was required for health-related research supported by the United States government (U.S. Department of Health, Education, and Welfare, 1971), the standard had been only the conscience of the investigator as sole determiner of the ethics of the proposed study (Levine, 1981). As a result of the large federal subsidization of basic and applied biomedical and health-related research in this country, and as a result of certain studies that were publicized for their abuses of human subjects, particularly with regard to informed consent and protection of autonomy and privacy, most research, whether governmentally supported or not, now is subjected to scrutiny by a group of institutional peers. The conscience of the individual investigator no longer suffices as the sole determinant of what constitutes moral protection of human subjects in the conduct of scientific inquiry. Rather, the judgment of "reasonable persons" is used as a standard in determining how much and what sort of information should be provided to patients, so they may make a decision about participating in research (Rosoff, 1981). The National Commission (1978a) suggested that a standard of the "reasonable volunteer" might be proposed to characterize what information prospective volunteers should have in order to make a decision about participating in research (Levine, 1981).

While the major purpose of peer or institutional review is to assure adequate protection of human subjects, the importance of the research question, adequacy of the design, and the societal benefits of research generally also are reviewed in the process (McNemar & Simmons, 1980; Northrop, 1980; Pellegrino, 1980). To ignore the canons of science is to start out immorally (Levine, 1981; Pellegrino, 1980), to violate the ethical principle of beneficence (Beauchamp & Childress, 1979), and to defy both the Nuremburg Code (Nuremburg Military Tribunals, 1949) and Declaration of Helsinki (World Medical Association, 1966). These codes state that research on human subjects should be preceded by animal studies and that there should be adequate justification for the need to involve human subjects. Northrop (1980) addressed the need for self-regulation of research by the nursing profession and urged as measures toward that end participation in the federal regulatory process (e.g., public comment), membership on institutional review boards, and promulgation of institution-wide practices regarding ethics in nursing research.

With this brief overview of major accomplishments in the history of research with human subjects, one cannot hope to provide a definitive treatment of the subject. Those interested in historical accounts have access to excellent works by Armiger (1977), Beecher (1970), Bloch et al. (1977), Hayter (1979), and Levine (1981). The past 15 years of experience with clinical research involving human subjects has resulted in the following accomplishments: (a) increased public awareness of the welfare and protection of human beings as research subjects; (b) the establishment of peer review and institutional boards as a mechanism to allow public scrutiny of research in advance of its initiation; (c) the development of the concepts of risk and benefit in research, with the former seen as probability ratios, and the latter seen, not as measures of probability, but rather as the good accruing to society, the individual, or both; and (d) a clear definition of the principles of informed consent and protection from harm (Gortner, 1982).

THE NURSE AS THE UNIT OF ANALYSIS IN ETHICAL INQUIRY

Conceptualization of Ethical Dilemmas

The nursing perspective in ethical inquiry has been addressed by a number of writers, among them Davis and Aroskar (1978), Benoliel (1983), Curtin and Flaherty (1982), Gadow (1982), and Mahon and Fowler (1979). If there is such an entity or disciplinary field as nursing ethics, it is the result of the distinctiveness of nursing as a clinical and moral art practiced in bureaucratic settings, and, as such, constrained in its effectiveness by institutional policies. Benoliel (1983) referred to hypothetical models of practice in medicine, that is, the engineering, priestly, and contractual models, which may or may not have relevance in nursing and still await research. Gadow's (1982) proposed use of existential advocacy as a basic philosophy of nursing has not been tested empirically but is in keeping with the contractual model of Benoliel. Curtin and Flaherty (1982) used a detailed case analysis approach to ethical problems in nursing practice. It is possible that investigators seeking systematic data on such topics as cardiopulmonary resuscitation, abortion, refusal of treatment for minors, and interpersonal conflicts of providers might find these analyses useful.

The conceptualization of the ethical dilemma in nursing has been the subject of the Davis and Aroskar text (1978), as well as writings by Smith and Davis (1980), Aroskar (1980a), and survey research by Davis (1981). The conceptualization of an ethical dilemma as conflict between two ethical principles (Smith & Davis, 1980) is a definition that White (1983) supported as well. An example of such a dilemma would be between principles of patient autonomy and provider beneficence. Other Smith and Davis conceptualizations were: (a) a conflict between two possible actions in which there were some persuasive but inconclusive arguments favoring a particular course of action, and equally persuasive but inconclusive arguments against the same course of action; (b) a conflict between the necessity for action and the need for reflection in a situation for which ethical training gave insufficient precedent or preparation; (c) a conflict between two equally unsatisfactory alternatives; and (d) a conflict between one's ethical principles and one's role obligations.

Relationship Between Moral Reasoning and Decision Making in Ethical Dilemmas

Aroskar (1980a) defined a dilemma as a choice between equally unsatisfactory alternatives or a difficult problem that seemed to have no satisfactory solution. Ethical dilemmas are those situations in which moral principles and ethical theories such as utilitarianism are involved. She suggested an analytic process not unlike that of Curtin and Flaherty (1982): (a) determine the situational facts or data base for moral inquiry; (b) consider the questions that come from decision theories; and (c) articulate the moral approaches, positions, or theories to be used in considering alternative action.

While these conceptualizations of what constitutes an ethical dilemma on the part of nurse ethicists are of interest, actual definitions proposed by or solicited from nurses may be of greater interest. Two such investigations were noteworthy. The first was a survey of subscribers conducted through

Nursing '74, in which 11,000 nurses responded to a standard set of 55 questions dealing with physician–nurse conflict, petty theft, difficult patients, heroic treatment, patient confidentiality, and so forth (What are your ethical standards, 1974). As an attempt to define personal ethical standards, the survey was conceptually inadequate, since no theoretical guidelines were provided respondents. Many survey questions did not fall within the domain of formal ethics; those that did used situational ethics (i.e., "What would you do if . . .") and posed some traditional ethical dilemmas regarding abortion, letting die, telling on other professionals, and tattling (whistle blowing). The reported findings based on cross tabulations and cluster analyses did not provide other than descriptive information on the opinions of the survey respondents, of whom 50% were diploma prepared, 22% baccalaureate prepared, and almost two thirds under the age of 35 (Nursing ethics, 1974a; Nursing ethics, Part 2, 1974b).

Criticizing the use of predetermined categories of response that limit the nature of the question as well as the type of response, Davis (1981) reported a survey of 205 registered nurses from the San Francisco Bay Area in California. The respondents represented 50% of a random sample of nurses who were members of a local nursing organization. The investigator deliberately excluded any definition of ethical dilemma in the survey tool, since the intent of the study was to determine the understanding that staff nurses had of this concept and how they defined ethical dilemma from their own experience. The definition of an ethical dilemma by the respondents was primarily in general terms and in terms of a situation in which the respondent was forced to act against principles. When asked to describe incidents in which ethical dilemmas were faced, the most frequently described categories were (a) prolongation of life with heroic measures, (b) unethical or incompetent activity of colleagues, (c) confidentiality, (d) violation of patient autonomy, and (e) withholding treatment. Ethnicity and religion showed no association with any of the empirical variables. Education was a significant factor in that diploma nurses gave fewer general definitions of ethical dilemmas than did baccalaureate nurses and more often cited disagreement with physicians than did the baccalaureate graduates. Future investigators might examine the underlying ethical principles, theories, and rules for action that practicing nurses articulate, since the conceptualization of the ethical dilemma in relation to staff nursing appears adequate.

Schroeck (1980) solicited identification of moral issues of importance to nursing from 83 undergraduate nursing students and 48 postbasic students who were participating in nursing course work in Scotland. These included abortion, resuscitation, organ transplantation, euthanasia, and psychosurgery. It was not possible to determine whether moral or sociocultural issues predominated in unspecified areas. In an attempt to deal with a moral issue in depth, the author provided a close examination of truth-telling, using selected literature in the health professions and in ethics. The analysis was conceptual rather than empirical and provided a thoughtful review of this one topic.

Role of Educational Preparation in the Development of Moral Judgment and Critical Thinking

All nursing authors writing on this topic agreed on the need for formal education in ethics for nurses yet recognized that moral learning is a personal experience. Implicit in this consensus was the assumption of relationships between educational preparation, critical thinking, and levels of moral reasoning. Cognitive developmental psychological theory as cited by Ketefian (1981a, 1981b) formed the rationale for an empirical test of that assumption with a volunteer sample of 79 practicing nurses from three major medical centers. The Watson-Glaser (1964) Critical Appraisal Test and the Defining Issues Test (Rest, 1974) were used. A positive relationship was found between critical thinking and moral reasoning ($r = .5326$; $p < .001$) and between level of formal education and moral reasoning ($F = 9.644$; $p < .01$). Multiple correlation supported the relation of the predictor variables of level of formal education and critical thinking on the dependent variable of moral reasoning. According to Ketefian, findings were consistent with existing theory and empirical data on moral development, but not consistent with unpublished dissertation research in nursing. To account for these differences Ketefian suggested that nursing's rapid professionalization may account for the differences found in critical thinking and levels of moral reasoning among diploma and baccalaureate nurses. No critique was made by the author of the Kohlberg (1976) levels or stages of moral development, which provided the basis for the judgments on ethical behavior. The stage assessment procedures have been criticized (Clay, Povey, & Clift, 1983) for reliability and validity, with questions raised as to whether a person can be described as being in a given stage.

With the same 79 practicing nurses, Ketefian demonstrated weak relationships among moral reasoning, knowledge and valuation of ideal moral behavior, and perception of realistic moral behavior. Ideal and realistic moral behavior was appraised through an author-designed instrument; for details on the instrument see Ketefian (1981b). Unlike Davis' (1981) findings, ethnic differences were found, with higher idealized behavior exhibited by nonminority nurses, while younger nurses exhibited more idealized moral behavior. There were no differences in realistic moral behavior among groups. Since the respondents were the same in both Ketefian studies (1981a, 1981b), these data should be cross-validated.

The relationship between cognitive theory, moral development, and level of education also was demonstrated by Crisham (1981) in a sample of 225 staff nurses with associate degrees ($n = 57$) and baccalaureate degrees ($n = 85$), nurses with master's degrees ($n = 10$), college junior prenursing students ($n = 36$), and graduate level nonnurses ($n = 37$). A low positive correlation was found between moral judgment regarding hypothetical and real-life nursing dilemmas. Because of the inclusion of nonprofessionals in this study, comparative displays of moral judgment and principled thinking were possible. Further examination is needed of idealized versus realistic moral reasoning and action on the part of professionals.

THE PATIENT AND FAMILY AS THE UNIT OF ANALYSIS IN ETHICAL INQUIRY

Values Associated with Decision Making Regarding Treatment

Illustration of patient and family situational crises during life-sustaining therapy are common in the nursing literature, yet surprisingly little research has been done on the motives and beliefs of persons seeking or refusing treatment, and on family advocacy on behalf of patients. Gortner, Shortridge, Baldwin, and Sparacino (1980) and Gortner, Hudes, and Zyzanski (1984) examined ethical influences on family decision making regarding medical and surgical treatment for coronary artery disease, and they demonstrated the feasibility of such an approach in the elective treatment situation. Values examined for 100 patients and 100 family members were those of autonomy, beneficence, nonmaleficence, and justice. Findings supported the hypothesis of shared values among family members and provided support for the ethical constructs of autonomy and beneficence or nonmaleficence, but not for justice. Patient autonomy in the decision-making process was a shared family value on the part of patients and spouses. The decision for surgery, once made, could be supported by family members; but before the decision was made, families tended to respect the patient's right to autonomy within the context of the family (Gortner et al., 1984).

How have patient and family decision making varied within a treatment situation and between treatment situations, and to what extent could case experience with refusal of treatment be generalized? Paradigm cases have been useful devices in surveying clinician attitudes toward continuation of therapy. Cogliano (1980) reported the use of six hypothetical situations in a survey of 134 elderly senior center members and nursing home residents to determine which of a number of medical procedures were seen as acceptable and ordinary and which were seen as extraordinary measures. The agreement among respondents in classifying all procedures as ordinary and preferred, except when death was imminent, suggested that there may be treatment preferences within age-groups and that some issues may be more important than others, for example, control of pain and patient rights.

Patient Advocacy Within the Context of the Family

The autonomy principle was explicated by Gadow (1982) as a key philosophical position in nursing practice, if not in research generally. Patient self-interest was defined as the *best interest* for that person; that is, only the patient could determine what constituted his good health. The advocacy model proposed by Gadow (1982) had an existential as well as a right-to-self-determination basis. Existential advocacy in contrast to paternalism or laissez-faire assists patients in determining how much information they want about treatment. This remains to be examined empirically in both the patient–nurse interaction and the patient–family interaction. These questions will intrigue investigators in the future in their efforts to further understand both patient autonomy and treatment decisions.

THE CLINICAL AND RESEARCH ENVIRONMENT AS THE UNIT OF ANALYSIS IN ETHICAL INQUIRY

The Research Environment

Research is extremely limited at present on both the clinical and research environments and on the social, cultural, and technological factors affecting nursing care. In a unique study, Gunter and Loehning (1971) documented the milieu of the nursing care unit in order to gain insight into the occurrence of therapeutic and nontherapeutic effects. The object of analysis was a research unit which was among the first of its kind to be developed with support from federal funds and in which patients and volunteers were exempted from regular hospital charges. Findings revealed the ambivalent feelings of nurses toward the motives of medical personnel in the conduct of research, as well as toward their own legal and moral obligations to patients, especially those children and adults whose competency to make informed decisions was in doubt. Because of the descriptive and exploratory design as well as the small number of respondents—15 full-time and 4 part-time registered nurses—the findings must be considered suggestive of further research. The investigators posed as a future hypothesis that there is a relationship between satisfaction of the nurse and the ability to state values and to translate values into practices. Philosophically, a close correlation of stated values and actual practices might clarify the essence of nursing.

The hypothesis generated for further study should be viewed within the context of this historic article reported in the first year of published federal guidelines for the protection of human subjects and during a period when the medical and nursing literature first began to show an increase in the number of articles on the issues of informed consent and research environments. However, 10 years later Crisham (1981) propounded the hypothesis of milieu effects, specifically those of the patient care unit, on the socialization of staff nurses and their value judgments and interpretation of ethical dilemmas in nursing.

The Clinical Environment

In a more recent study, Germain (1980) addressed the clinical rather than the research environment. The unit of analysis was a 23-bed adult oncology unit and related departments in a large accredited urban community hospital. The study sample included (a) hospital administrators; (b) members of various levels of the nursing administration; (c) three medical oncologists; (d) support staff such as social workers, chaplains, and various therapists; and (e) patients and their families. During a 12-month period of extensive field study and ethnography using participant observation methods, a number of ethical dilemmas arising in the subculture of the cancer unit and in the clinical investigator role were revealed. Among the subcultural or environmental ethical issues were (a) absence of a well-established evaluative program for management of a patient's pain; (b) absence of strict informed consent procedures and precise research designs; (c) philosophical differences between physicians in their approaches to the medical management of malignant disease; (d) consent to treatment predicated primarily on faith in the physician rather than informed knowledge of the treatment; and (e) need for greater regard for patients' rights to treatment and privacy. Suggested areas for further research included subject privacy and protection, the confidentiality of research reports versus the need for publication of such reports, objectivity versus subjectivity with regard to selection and reporting phenomena, and intervention versus nonintervention by the participant-observer investigator in the subculture of the unit. These last ethical issues were among those that confront the participant-observer as investigator, as well as the clinician turned investigator.

DESIGN OF RESEARCH

The influence of personal values in the selection of problems and in design and conduct of research has been acknowledged. Fry (1981) commented on the relation of scientific and moral values, noting that professional accountability (the response to scientific values of competence) was grounded in personal accountability (the response to humanistic values of moral concern). Whether research design and methods must be in complete accord with professional orientation, that is, whether the scientific method is compatible with a humanistic philosophy of practice, is a matter of some debate. These are philosophical issues and not ones that should be resolved empirically.

Protection of Vulnerable Subjects

Several topics are of interest in regard to research design and human subjects. The first is whether certain classes of persons are too vulnerable to be considered research subjects. While the National Commission (1976, 1977, 1978c) considered carefully the vulnerability of prisoners, children, and the mentally infirm and suggested special precautions for each to protect autonomy, it did not consider clinical populations separately. Are some patients too ill and at too great a risk because of treatment to be considered potential research subjects? Is research involving the questioning of motivation and decision making about treatment intrusive or therapeutic, in that it provides an opportunity for persons to ventilate feelings (Gortner, 1982)?

A second question is whether there is intended or unintended coercion, that is, infringement on self-determination and freedom to choose because of the nature of the clinical relationship of researcher with patients and clients? A related question deals with the nature of the investigator role in field research: To what extent does one present oneself as friend or one of the group to be studied (Davis, 1980)? Finally, to what extent are requirements of the research plan subjected to variations and limitations imposed by daily treatment plans and procedures? How is the validity of the plan affected, and when should research be stopped?

Determination of Risk

Research risks and benefits have been studied extensively by the National Commission for the Protection of Human Subjects of Biomedical and Behavioral Research (1976, 1978a), and by its successor, the President's Commission for the Study of Ethical Problems in Medicine and Biomedical and Behavioral Research (1981, 1982, 1983). Present federal regulations (Basic HHS policy, 1981) clearly were written with the concept of variable risk in mind. In an empirical study of no-risk research, Gortner, Heath, and Sanders (1981) used the case of the University of California, San Francisco Committee on Human Research, and its review actions that resulted in the decision "no subjects at risk" over two consecutive time points. The purpose of the investigation was to describe the nature of no- or low-risk research in one setting, and to determine whether certain fields of science and certain research techniques might be so characterized. This study yielded 562 cases for study, of which a small proportion resulted in the no-subjects-at-risk decision. These, then, were examined further, and it was found that for the majority, little or no direct subject involvement was required, subject anonymity was assured uniformly, and laboratory studies of tissue specimens or body fluids were involved. These kinds of studies at present undergo an exempt or expedited institutional review as a result of new federal regulations (Basic HHS, 1981) exempting from peer review certain classes of research because of low or minimal risk.

Can risk be determined other than through peer review, such as through institutional review boards (IRBs)? Through what rationale and criteria are investigators making risk or benefit estimates, and to what extent are these employed by their IRBs (Gortner et al., 1981)? There appears to be little merit in continuing the argument that certain fields of social science, such as sociology and anthropology, should not be subjected to the same reviews as biomedical research. Nursing as a health science field uses human subjects in research and, thus, must bear scrutiny on ethical issues similar to those of biomedicine. Similarly, nurse membership on IRBs is desirable if not essential from a number of perspectives (Robb, 1981).

MEASUREMENT OF ETHICAL CONSTRUCTS

Measurement of values employing ethical constructs such as autonomy, beneficence, nonmaleficence, and justice for patient populations and of nurses' moral judgment regarding actual clinical situations has been reported by several investigators. The work of Gortner et al. (1984) on the appraisal of patient and family values in the choice of treatment has been ongoing for four years and has produced a 15-item Inventory of Values in the Choice of Treatment that has validity and reliability for cardiac surgery populations. Crisham (1981) described the Nursing Dilemma Test with regard to psychometric development and properties and its relation to a more general appraisal of moral judgment (the Defining Issues Test). The decision-making process employed by volunteer staff nurses to resolve six recurring nursing dilemmas was explored through interviews with the nurses in a series of pilot studies. Content validity was determined through expert opinion and the Defining Issues Test. It was then administered by mail to a convenience sample of 225 staff, faculty, and students. The sequence of psychometric development employed by Crisham was impressive. The tool has promise as a measure of moral judgment in nursing in that it uses real-life nursing dilemmas and confirms the relation between moral reasoning and level of education.

The Beauchamp and Childress (1979) bioethical framework provided the theoretical basis for the work of Gortner et al. (1984), while cognitive-developmental theories and situationally determined ethical issues provided the base for Crisham's (1981) tool. Ketefian (1981b) developed a tool, Judgments about Nursing Decisions, containing seven stories depicting nurses in ethical dilemmas and requiring respondents to indicate whether the nurse in the story should or should not engage in a specified action (ideal moral behavior) and whether she or he was likely to engage in the nursing action. In the pilot testing, Ketefian found that the instrument had content validity and reasonable consistency ($\alpha = .70$). Construct validity should be determined. These instruments are illustrative of the promising opportunities ethical theory and reasoning offer to investigators interested in instrument development. As reviewed here, much of the instrumentation in nursing research was reported within the past five years, and it can be expected that activity will increase in the measurement field pertinent to ethics.

CONCLUSIONS AND RESEARCH DIRECTIONS

Ethical inquiry, as opposed to ethical reasoning and debate, is relatively new in the field of nursing research, as well as in other health fields, as revealed in this review covering the period 1968 through early 1983. Characteristically, the conduct of studies dealing with ethical issues and questions in nursing has been centered on the documentation of dilemmas in nursing practice. Most investigators used case description through presentation of the nursing perspective on such issues as abortion, care of the defective newborn, or prolongation of life. They solicited the opinions of clinicians with regard to many of these issues primarily through interview or survey research techniques. Studies in which concerns or opinions of clients are solicited, those under treatment, or those considering treatment or who have withdrawn from it, have been underrepresented. Those questions raised in the studies reviewed suggested (a) the importance of determining standards of disclosure and conditions for withholding information, (b) alternatives to the signed consent for elderly persons, (c) what constitutes a reasonable volunteer for research, (d) further study of patient and family values and decision making in treatment situations, and (e) preference for paternalistic versus existential advocacy models of care by patients and families.

Another area for research is the clinical environment and, in particular, the conduct of research during the course of therapy. A number of investigators have pointed out the need to examine milieu effects on both clients and clinicians in order to determine the patient care unit variables that may affect moral judgment and decisions.

Finally, though the topic of ethics has become well recognized in the past decade, the appraisal of the moral judgment of clinicians and clients has just been started. Several instruments appear to have promise, and nurses can look forward to reports by investigators in nursing in this important area.

REFERENCES

American Nurses' Association. (1968). *Guidelines on ethical values: The nurse and research*. Kansas City, MO: Author.

American Nurses' Association. (1975). *Human rights guidelines for nurses in clinical and other research*. Kansas City, MO: Author.

Armiger, B. (1977). Ethics of nursing research: Profile, principle, perspective. *Nursing Research, 26*, 330–336.

Aroskar, M. A. (1980a). Anatomy of ethical dilemmas: The theory. *American Journal of Nursing, 80*, 658–663.

Aroskar, M. A. (1980b). Four imperatives for ethical consideration in nursing research. *Proceedings of the First Annual Scholarly Nursing Leadership Conference: Ethical Dimensions of Nursing Research* (pp. 1–11). Baltimore: University of Maryland School of Nursing.

Basic HHS policy for protection of human research subjects. (1981, January 26). *Federal Register, 46*, 8366–8392.

Beauchamp, T. L., & Childress, J. F. (1979). *Principles of biomedical ethics*. New York: Oxford University Press.

Beecher, H. K. (1970). *Research and the individual: Human studies*. Boston: Little, Brown.

Benoliel, J. Q. (1983). Ethics in nursing practice and education. *Nursing Outlook, 31*, 210–215.

Bloch, D., Phillips, T. P., & Gortner, S. R. (1977). Protection of human research subjects. In M. H. Miller & B. C. Flynn (Eds.), *Current perspectives in nursing: Social issues and trends* (pp. 14–31). St. Louis: Mosby.

Clay, M., Povey, R., & Clift, S. (1983). Moral reasoning and the student nurse. *Journal of Advanced Nursing, 8*, 297–302.

Cogliano, J. F. (1980). Extraordinary measures in terminal illness: Issues in nursing ethics, research and practice. *Proceedings of the First Annual Scholarly Nursing Leadership Conference: Ethical Dimensions of Nursing Research* (pp. 134–148). Baltimore: University of Maryland School of Nursing.

Crisham, P. (1981). Measuring moral judgement in nursing dilemmas. *Nursing Research, 30*, 104–110.

Curtin, L., & Flaherty, M. J. (1982). *Nursing ethics, theories and pragmatics*. Bowie, MD: Robert J. Brady.

Davis, A. J. (1979). Ethical issues in nursing research: Informed consent. *Western Journal of Nursing Research, 1*, 145–147.

Davis, A. J. (1980). Ethical issues in nursing research. *Western Journal of Nursing Research, 2*, 760–762.

Davis, A. J. (1981). Ethical dilemmas in nursing: A survey. *Western Journal of Nursing Research, 3*, 397–407.

Davis, A. J., & Aroskar, M. (1978). *Ethical dilemmas and nursing practice*. New York: Appleton-Century-Crofts.

Ellis, R. (1970). The nurse as investigator and member of the research team. *Annals of the New York Academy of Sciences, 169*, 435–441.

Engelhart, H. T. (1978). Basic ethical principles in the conduct of biomedical and behavioral research involving human subjects. In National Commission for the Protection of Human Subjects of Biomedical and Behavioral Research, *The Belmont report: Ethical principles and guidelines for the protection of human subjects of research* (Appendix, Vol. I, pp. 8–1 to 8–45) (DHEW Publication No. OS 78-0013). Washington, DC: U.S. Government Printing Office.

Fletcher, J. C. (1980). History of the development of policy to protect human subjects in research. *Proceedings of the First Annual Scholarly Nursing Leadership Conference: Ethical Dimensions of Nursing Research* (pp. 49–58). Baltimore: University of Maryland School of Nursing.

Fry, S. T. (1981). Accountability in research: The relationship of scientific and humanistic values. *Advances in Nursing Science, 4,* 1–13.

Gadow, S. (1982). Philosophical foundations of nursing ethics. *Proceedings of Encounter with Ethics: Dilemmas and Directions in Nursing* (pp. 20–41). Chicago: Rush-Presbyterian-St. Luke's Medical Center.

Germain, C. P. (1980). Anthropologic research in health care facilities: Ethical dilemmas of the nurse-ethnographer. *Proceedings of the First Annual Scholarly Nursing Leadership Conference: Ethical Dimensions of Nursing Research* (pp. 82–93). Baltimore: University of Maryland School of Nursing.

Gortner, S. R. (1974). Scientific accountability in nursing. *Nursing Outlook, 22,* 764–768.

Gortner, S. R. (1982). The role of research in ethical inquiry. *Proceedings of Encounter with Ethics: Dilemmas and Directions in Nursing* (pp. 146–161). Chicago: Rush-Presbyterian-St. Luke's Medical Center.

Gortner, S. R., Heath, E., & Sanders, P. (1981). The institutional review board: A case study of no risk decisions in health-related research. *Nursing Research, 30,* 21–24.

Gortner, S. R., Hudes, M., & Zyzanski, S. (1984). Appraisal of values in the choice of treatment. *Nursing Research, 33,* 319–324.

Gortner, S. R., Shortridge, L., Baldwin, A., & Sparacino, P. (1980). Ethical influences on family decisions regarding election of treatment. *Proceedings of the First Annual Scholarly Nursing Leadership Conference: Ethical Dimensions of Nursing Research* (pp. 114–133). Baltimore: University of Maryland School of Nursing.

Gunter, L. M., & Loehning, E. L. (1971). Medical research and nursing unit milieus: Values related to protection and emotional support. In M. Batey (Ed.), *Communicating nursing research (Vol. 4): Is the gap being bridged?* (pp. 31–50). Boulder, CO: Western Interstate Commission for Higher Education.

Hayter, J. (1979). Issues related to human subjects. In F. S. Downs, & J. W. Flemming (Eds.), *Issues in nursing research.* New York: Appleton-Century-Crofts.

Ingelfinger, F. J. (1972). Informed (but uneducated) consent. *New England Journal of Medicine, 287,* 465–466.

Ketefian, S. (1981a). Critical thinking, educational preparation, and development of moral judgment among selected groups of practicing nurses. *Nursing Research, 30,* 98–103.

Ketefian, S. (1981b). Moral reasoning and moral behavior among selected groups of practicing nurses. *Nursing Research, 30,* 171–176.

Kohlberg, L. (1976). Moral stages and moralization. In T. Likona (Ed.), *Moral development and behavior*. New York: Holt, Rinehart & Winston.

Levine, R. J. (1978). The boundaries between biomedical and behavioral research and the accepted and routine practice of medicine. In National Commission for the Protection of Human Subjects of Biomedical and Behavioral Research, *The Belmont report: Ethical principles and guidelines for the protection of human subjects and research* (Appendix, Vol. I, pp. 1–4 to 1–44) (DHEW Publication No. OS 78-0013). Washington, DC: U.S. Government Printing Office.

Levine, R. J. (1981). *Ethics and regulation of clinical research*. Baltimore: Urban Press.

Lumpp, S. F. (1979). The role of the nurse in the bioethical decision-making process. *Nursing Clinics of North America, 14,* 13–21.

Mahon, K. A., & Fowler, M. P. (1979). Moral development and clinical decision-making. *Nursing Clinics of North America, 14,* 3–12.

May, K. A. (1979). The nurse researcher: Impediment to informed consent. *Nursing Outlook, 27,* 36–39.

McNemar, A., & Simmons, S. (1980). Ethical concerns in the research review process. *Proceedings of the First Annual Scholarly Nursing Leadership Conference: Ethical Dimensions of Nursing Research* (pp. 66–72). Baltimore: University of Maryland School of Nursing.

National Commission for the Protection of Human Subjects of Biomedical and Behavioral Research. (1976). *Report and recommendations: Research involving prisoners* (DHEW Publication No. OS 76-131). Washington, DC: U.S. Government Printing Office.

National Commission for the Protection of Human Subjects of Biomedical and Behavioral Research. (1977). *Report and recommendations: Research involving children* (DHEW Publication No. OS 77-0004). Washington, DC: U.S. Government Printing Office.

National Commission for the Protection of Human Subjects of Biomedical and Behavioral Research. (1978a). *The Belmont report: Ethical principles and guidelines for the protection of human subjects of research* (DHEW Publication No. OS 78-0012). Washington, DC: U.S. Government Printing Office.

National Commission for the Protection of Human Subjects of Biomedical and Behavioral Research. (1978b). *Report and recommendations: Institutional review boards* (DHEW Publication No. OS 78-0008). Washington, DC: U.S. Government Printing Office.

National Commission for the Protection of Human Subjects of Biomedical and Behavioral Research. (1978c). *Report and recommendations: Research involving those institutionalized as mentally infirm* (DHEW Publication No. OS 78-0006). Washington, DC: U.S. Government Printing Office.

Northrop, C. (1980). Promotion of ethical conduct in nursing research through legislation and self-regulation. *Proceedings of the First Annual Scholarly Nursing Leadership Conference: Ethical Dimensions of Nursing Research* (pp. 59–65). Baltimore: University of Maryland School of Nursing.

Notter, L. E. (1969). Protecting the rights of research subjects. (Editorial). *Nursing Research, 18,* 483.

Nuremberg Military Trials: U.S. v. Karl Brandt. (1949). *Trials of War Criminals before the Nuremberg Military Tribunals* (Vol. 2, pp. 181–182). Washington, DC: U.S. Government Printing Office.

Nursing ethics. (1974a). *Nursing '74, 4*(9), 34 – 48.

Nursing ethics, Part 2. (1974b). *Nursing '74, 4*(10), 56–66.

Pellegrino, E. D. (1980). The ethics of nursing research: Some special aspects. *Proceedings of the First Annual Scholarly Nursing Leadership Conference: Ethical Dimensions of Nursing Research* (pp. 20–32). Baltimore: University of Maryland School of Nursing.

President's Commission for the Study of Ethical Problems in Medicine and Biomedical and Behavioral Research. (1981). *Protecting human subjects: The adequacy and uniformity of federal rules and their implementation.* Washington, DC: U.S. Government Printing Office.

President's Commission for the Study of Ethical Problems in Medicine and Biomedical and Behavioral Research. (1982). *Implementing human research regulations: The adequacy and uniformity of federal rules and their implementation.* Washington, DC: U.S. Government Printing Office.

President's Commission for the Study of Ethical Problems in Medicine and Biomedical and Behavioral Research. (1983). *Summing up: Studies of the ethical and legal problems in medicine and biomedical and behavioral research.* Washington, DC: U.S. Government Printing Office.

Rest, J. (1974). *Manual for the Defining Issues Test.* (Mineographed). Minneapolis: University of Minnesota.

Robb, S. S. (1981). Nurse involvement in institutional review boards: The service setting perspective. *Nursing Research, 30,* 27–29.

Robb, S. S. (1983). Beware the "informed" consent. (Editorial). *Nursing Research, 32,* 132.

Rosoff, A. (1981). *Informed consent: A guide for health care providers.* Rockville, MD: Aspen Systems.

Schroeck, R. A. (1980). A question of honesty in nursing practice. *Journal of Advanced Nursing, 5,* 135–148.

Smith, S. J., & Davis, A. J. (1980). Ethical dilemmas: Conflicts among rights, duties, and obligations. *American Journal of Nursing, 80,* 1463–1466.

U.S. Department of Health, Education, and Welfare. (1971). *The institutional guide to DHEW policy on protection of human subjects* (DHEW Publication No. NIH 72-102). Washington, DC: U.S. Government Printing Office.

Watson, A. (1982). Informed consent of special subjects. *Nursing Research, 31,* 43–47.

Watson, G., & Glaser, E. M. (1964). *Critical thinking appraisal manual.* New York: Harcourt, Brace, and World.

What are your ethical standards? (1974). *Nursing '74, 4*(3), 29–34.

White, G. (1983). Philosophical ethics and nursing: A word of caution. In P. L. Chinn (Ed.), *Advances in nursing theory development* (pp. 35–46). Rockville, MD: Aspen Systems.

World Medical Association. (1966). Declaration of Helsinki: Recommendations guiding doctors in clinical research. *Journal of the American Medical Association, 197*(11), 32.

CHAPTER 10

Cost-Effectiveness Analysis in Nursing Research

CLAIRE M. FAGIN
AND
BARBARA S. JACOBSEN
SCHOOL OF NURSING
UNIVERSITY OF PENNSYLVANIA

CONTENTS

This chapter includes a review of nursing research dealing with the cost effectiveness of a wide variety of nursing practices. In a previous article Fagin (1982) summarized unpublished as well as published nursing research that implied, as well as explicitly provided, evidence of cost savings. No attempt was made in that summary to examine the methods used to arrive at conclusions nor to determine whether cost-effectiveness or cost–benefit analyses (CEA or CBA) had been documented. In order to judge future research needs in this important area, the authors of this chapter examined critically the methods and use of CEA or CBA in recently published research. Following the model used in the earlier publication, studies again were grouped into four areas:

1. Organization of nursing services—studies in which investigators examined cost when changes were made in the ratio of registered nurses to other nursing personnel, the weekly or daily working schedules of nurses, and the style or pattern of nursing care used.
2. Testing specific nursing interventions—studies in which investigators examined the cost of new nursing interventions in direct patient care, patient education, and innovative uses of nurse practitioners.
3. Substitution of nurses for other providers—studies in which investigators examined cost when nurses were used in areas more customarily employing medical providers.
4. Testing alternative models of practice—studies in which investigators examined cost when changes were introduced in customary modalities of health and illness care or in the system of delivering such care.

DESIGN ISSUES FOR COST-EFFECTIVENESS AND COST–BENEFIT ANALYSIS

Formal economic analyses of cost benefits or effectiveness in the health field were not common until this generation. During the past few years there has been heightened interest in these techniques. Cost-effectiveness analysis and cost–benefit analysis both require economic and efficacy evaluation. For *cost-effectiveness* analysis (CEA), the effectiveness of a particular intervention is assessed using explicit, quantitative methods to measure its net cost. For *cost–benefit* analysis (CBA), costs and benefits must be valued in monetary terms. Therefore, CBA usually requires placing a monetary value on all the consequences—tangible and intangible, direct and indirect—of a possible course of action (Klarman, 1974). Life expectancy, potential employment, secondary diseases, pain, grief, and the value of life are areas that were debated in attempting to solve methodological problems of CBA in health care (Hodgson & Meiners, 1982). Thus, CEA is likely to be more common, since specific dollar costs of alternative programs could be compared with specific measures of outcome without assigning a dollar value to the latter.

Since CEA appears more easily understood, there has been heavy reliance on this technique. As its popularity has increased, however, inadequate methodology and technically low-quality analyses have been noted in some of the current literature (Warner & Hutton, 1980). Prescott and Sorenson (1978) pointed out that an analysis of costs *assumes* that the changes in clients between pre- and posttreatment can be attributed to the effect of the treatment program. Thus, an elegant cost analysis of an innovation evaluated by a poor design may be meaningless.

An experimental design generally is agreed to be the desired model for evaluating the impact of new services or techniques (Kerlinger, 1973). Such designs are prospective, implying pretreatment planning and deliberate control over the protocol for intervention. The particular experimental design considered to offer the best possibility of support for the assumption of causality is the randomized, controlled trial (RCT) (Fisher, 1966). Simply because investigators describe their study as an RCT is, however, an insufficient basis for evaluating the design. The quality of each RCT must be assessed because these trials can vary from very imperfect to almost perfect in their implementation (Chalmers et al., 1981).

Certain other experimental designs represent compromises with the ideal of the RCT. The most common compromise is the nonrandomized trial (NRT) in which pretreatment equivalence of the groups may be at risk. If the groups are also nonconcurrent, then comparisons across groups are even more difficult because of the potentially different historical events that might have affected each group. Noncontrolled trials (NCT), that is, experiments without a control group, are labeled "inadequate" for drawing causal inferences by Kerlinger (1973); however, investigators can suggest causal relationships by comparing baseline measures to outcome measures or by comparing outcome measures with available norms. If no deliberate controlled intervention occurs, the study is nonexperimental. Causal attributions can be problematic for such designs.

Some reviewers have implied that concerns about design quality might be irrelevant when combining results (Devine & Cook, 1983); others have noted that findings varied according to design quality (Chalmers, Celano, Sacks, & Smith, 1983). Since the issue of whether results of various studies may be combined regardless of design quality has not been settled, we have chosen not to aggregate all of the data, but to consider design quality in our review. Of course, this issue might have been decided by reviewing only

RCTs and NRTs with careful matching, as in the review by Mumford, Schlesinger, and Glass (1982), but prior acquaintance with studies of cost effectiveness led us to believe this review would have been very brief!

METHOD OF LITERATURE SEARCH, SCREENING, AND CLASSIFICATION

A search for recent nursing publications relevant to CEA or CBA was conducted in four ways. First, a MEDLARS search was carried out for articles published since 1975. Second, the references of reviewed publications were examined. Third, authors of unpublished manuscripts listed by Fagin (1982) were contacted to determine publication status. Fourth, a call for notification about publications was placed in the American Nurses' Association *Council of Nurse Researchers' Newsletter*. The search yielded 213 publications, which then were screened for inclusion in the final sample.

On initial review, a decision was made about whether the article included the analysis of a set of data to answer a research question. If a reasonable doubt existed as to whether the report was research, it was not included in the final sample. A decision was also made as to whether the study was about nursing, that is, whether nurses were involved in the substitutive or alternative care, the organization of nursing care, or the design and delivery of an intervention. Third, the article was examined to see whether it contained a cost analysis that placed an actual monetary value on the innovation. Many studies simply implied cost savings and were not included in this review. The final sample consisted of 52 articles. Since one article (Spitzer, Roberts, & Delmore, 1976) contained reports on two projects, the total number of projects reviewed was 53.

The 53 projects then were classified according to the previously given taxonomy of principal designs. Of the 53 studies reviewed, 35 (66%) were classified as experimental. The remaining 18 studies were nonexperimental. One difficulty should be noted: Some reports classified as experimental actually may have been evaluation studies planned and conducted after the fact of the intervention. Occasionally, such studies have been written for journals as though they were prospective experiments. Fletcher and Fletcher (1979) also alluded to this particular problem in classifying research designs. Our estimate of the percentage of studies that were experimental was, therefore, probably an overestimate.

In addition to design, two other factors were considered as critical to the evaluation of research in the CEA or CBA area: (a) the set of alternatives to which the innovations were compared, and (b) the clarity and appropriateness of the variables contributing to the identification of costs.

REVIEW OF MAJOR AREAS

Organization

Eleven studies met the criteria for review in this category. They were focused on four different organizational systems for the delivery of nursing care: (a) primary nursing (Betz, 1981; Fairbanks, 1981; Felton, 1975; Giovannetti, 1980; Jones, 1975; Marram, Flynn, Abaravich, & Carey, 1976); (b) all RN primary nursing (Osinski & Powals, 1980; Shukla, 1983); (c) all RN nursing (Forster, 1978; Hinshaw, Scofield, & Atwood, 1981); and (d) the 12-hour shift (Ganong, Ganong, & Harrison, 1976).

The phrase "all RN" actually meant *almost all*. Hinshaw et al. (1981) and Shukla (1983) appeared to come closest to "all RN." All definitions of primary nursing included the essential idea that patients were assigned a primary nurse on admission to the hospital, and that nurse continued to be accountable for that patient on a 24-hour basis until discharge.

Ten of the 11 studies reviewed here included measures that related to quality of care. Osinski and Powals (1980) did not provide data on quality of care. Seven investigators examined attitudes of either nurses, patients, or physicians relative to satisfaction with care, perception of quality of care, or variables such as group cohesion. Five studies included global or specific measures of the quality of nursing care. Four investigators examined behavioral measures such as direct patient care hours, turnover, infection rate, length of stay, and complications.

None of the 11 studies was an RCT. Of the six studies of primary nursing, two were NRTs, one was an NCT, and three were not experiments. The two NRTs are examined first. Jones (1975) studied the effect of primary nursing on renal transplant patients by following patients admitted to either a primary nursing unit or a team nursing unit. Nineteen patients were admitted to the units according to "randomized, alternating assignment," with no further details given about the assignment method. Since alternation is not a method used in randomized trials, this study was classified as an NRT. No mention was made of how nurses were assigned to units. Jones provided strong evidence that the two groups of patients were similar initially. Patients on the primary nursing unit were discharged, on the average, 21 days earlier, probably because they had fewer complications after surgery. Jones then calculated the cost savings of primary nursing by multiplying the average cost per day at that hospital for renal transplant patients by the number of patient days "saved" in the experimental group.

A second NRT comparing primary and team nursing was conducted by Felton (1975). This investigator found quality higher and costs lower on the primary unit. Unfortunately, the evidence provided for the initial similarity of the two units was weak. Further, in a replication of the Felton study, but without a cost analysis, Shukla (1981) found no significant differences in quality of care.

Fairbanks (1981) reported the only other experimental (NCT) study of primary nursing included here. The cost analysis was focused entirely on the variable of turnover. Comparisons were made between the primary nursing unit and the entire hospital. Since turnover was much lower on the experimental unit, Fairbanks implied savings by pointing to the estimated costs of hiring new graduates.

None of the other three studies of primary nursing can be considered experimental (Betz, 1981; Giovannetti, 1980; Marram et al., 1976). All three of these studies were comparative surveys of primary versus team nursing. In each study, evidence for equivalence of the units to assure a valid comparison was either flawed or missing. It is not surprising, then, that the results were inconsistent. Marram et al. claimed that quality of care was higher and costs were lower on the primary nursing unit. In contrast, Giovannetti claimed that primary nursing was not cost effective because quality of care was the same but costs were higher. Betz, on the other hand, claimed that both quality of care and costs were lower on the primary unit; these results do not satisfy our definition of cost effectiveness.

A variation of primary nursing, all RN primary nursing, was examined in two nonexperimental studies (Osinski & Powals, 1980; Shukla, 1983). Shukla studied a primary nursing unit that was operating before the research was started. This investigator compared three units: all-RN staffing for primary nursing, team nursing, and modular (subunit) nursing. A strong effort was made to offer evidence of similarity across the units in numerous key variables. Shukla judged the cost of care per patient day to be highest for the primary unit (about $2 per day more than team nursing).

The design of the second study of all RN primary nursing was much weaker. Osinski and Powals (1980) mailed a questionnaire to 110 hospitals asking about their mode of nursing. After a rate of return of only 32%, they compared costs per day for each mode to one surgical unit with all RN staffed primary nursing in a hospital where costs were known but which did not participate in the mailed questionnaire survey. Costs were reported to be lower for this one all RN primary nursing unit.

Several investigators studied all RN staffing without combining such a staffing pattern with primary nursing. The two studies included in this review were nonexperimental. Hinshaw et al. (1981) conducted a longitudinal evaluation of an administrative change to all RN staffing on one medical unit where patient care requirements were consistently high. In this study, changing to all RNs also meant having fewer staff. Hinshaw et al. stated that quality of care was maintained, while costs were contained and even seemed to drop slightly. In another survey of the same type, Forster (1978) reported cost savings for an all RN unit.

In the final study to be considered in this section, the 12-hour shift was evaluated in a survey (Ganong et al., 1976). Administrators of one hospital instituted a two-shift daily schedule—seven days on and seven days off. The investigators claimed that the change resulted in patient care of comparable quality, fewer staff, and reduced costs.

The variables most commonly used in the cost analyses in this section by their frequency of use were: salaries—7; total number of patient days—4; beds—3; extra hours (e.g., overtime, absenteeism)—3; nursing care hours—3; and turnover—3. The type of measurement was invariably the cost of care for the innovation (usually the cost per patient day or cost per bed), which then was compared to the costs for different units in the same hospital, units in different hospitals, or the cost of care before the innovation was implemented. Two investigators collected data on only one variable for the cost analysis, turnover, which was then compared to orientation costs. In the typical study four variables were considered for analysis of costs. Only Jones (1975) examined length of stay and related it to costs.

Interventions

Ten studies on interventions met the criteria for review. Six of these reports involved nurses as members of a team for an innovative method of patient care (Cintron, Bigas, Linares, Aranda, & Hernandez, 1983; Giordano et al., 1977; Kane, Jorgensen, Teteberg, & Kuwahara, 1976; Komrower, Sardharwalla, Fowler, & Bridge, 1979; Linn & Taylor, 1979; Zwaag, Mason, Joyner, & Runyan, 1980). In four studies, the investigators tested equipment or methods used by nurses in direct patient care (Chavigny & Nunnally, 1975; Field et al., 1982; Steffel, Schenk, & Walker, 1980; Stronge & Newton, 1980).

The six studies of nurses functioning on a team of providers are examined first. Linn and Taylor (1979), in an RCT conducted in Australia, assigned 150 patients randomly to one of two groups: regular home care or regular home care plus a monthly visit by a nurse who focused on the topic of medications and communicated with a physician about medication problems. Linn and Taylor provided no information on the preintervention similarity of the groups. After 12 months, they found more correctly labeled medicine containers and 12% lower costs for medicines in the experimental group than in the control group. Linn and Taylor did not report the cost of nurse visits, but claimed that the reduction in the cost of medication offset that expense to some extent.

Kane et al. (1976) assigned 13 nursing homes at random to receive primary care from one of three teams: (a) nurse practitioner, supported by physician and pharmacist; (b) nurse practitioner and social worker, supported by physician and pharmacist; and (c) whatever form of care existed previously plus a social worker. Since the unit of analysis in this study was the patient, not the nursing home, the design of this project was judged to be an NRT. The investigators provided no evidence of the initial similarity of the groups, nor did they adjust for possible pretreatment differences. In view of their weak design, Kane et al. were wise simply to suggest the cost effectiveness of the nurse practitioner–social worker team.

Three of the studies of nurses as members of a team for an innovative method of patient care were classified as NCTs: nurses giving continuing care to chronic disease patients in decentralized clinics (Zwaag et al., 1980), nurse practitioners providing care in a clinic for heart disease patients in Puerto Rico (Cintron et al., 1983), and pediatric nurse practitioners functioning as pivotal professionals in an outreach program for juvenile diabetics (Giordano et al., 1977). In each of these studies, nurses were judged to deliver care that was cost effective.

The sixth study in this group was a nonexperimental evaluation of a regional screening program in England to detect phenylketonuria (PKU) (Komrower et al., 1979). A liaison nurse, working with a pediatrician and a dietician, conducted the screening, communicated the results, and instructed families about treatment. Over a 10-year period, more than 500,000 persons were screened, and 69 cases of PKU were found. The general health of the 69 patients (emotional, physical, and intellectual) was described as good. Costs of detecting and treating these cases included salaries, equipment, indirect costs, hospital stay, lab tests, diet, and the costs of education at a regular school. For comparison, the investigators surveyed long-term mental hospitals and located 54 untreated PKU patients, whose average length of stay was 22 years. The cost of looking after patients with untreated PKU proved to be far greater than the cost of the regional screening and treatment program.

In the last four reports, investigators studied specific methods or equipment used by nurses in direct patient care. In the only RCT, Field et al. (1982) examined the effects of nonnutritive sucking on preterm neonates in an intensive care unit. They randomly assigned 57 infants to receive or not to receive pacifiers during all tube feedings. These investigators stratified their assignments on gestational age and birth weight, and, in addition, provided evidence of the similarity of the groups on other key variables. After blind evaluation, the clinical findings replicated those of Measel and Anderson (1979) in that the infants were ready for bottle feeding earlier, gained more weight, and were discharged earlier. Field et al. provided the additional information that the average hospital costs of the experimental group were approximately $3,500 less, strongly suggesting the cost effectiveness of this intervention.

Chavigny and Nunnally (1975) compared methods for collecting clean-catch urine specimens in a clinic population of 1,350 obstetric patients. These investigators, in an NRT with nonconcurrent groups, studied three cleansers, patient self-care versus nurse care, and group versus individual teaching. The groups were similar in age and percentage of symptomatic patients at the diagnostic level. There were no differences between levels of bacteriuria in specimens collected by patients and those collected by nurses, nor were there differences in specimens between patients taught in groups and patients taught individually. Since a nurse-collected specimen was four times as expensive as one collected by a patient, and a specimen from a patient taught individually was 10 times more expensive than a specimen from a patient taught in a group, Chavigny and Nunnally concluded that group teaching and patient-collected specimens were cost effective. They decided that the cleansers required further study.

In another NRT with nonconcurrent groups, Stronge and Newton (1980) compared glass thermometers to electronic thermometers in hygiene, operational errors, and costs. Observation on a surgical ward indicated that the electronic thermometers were more hygienic, led to fewer operational errors, and took less nursing time. Electronic thermometers were more expensive, but were cost effective in that the time saved on the unit equaled one extra nurse per week.

The last study (Steffel et al., 1980) also was considered an NRT with nonconcurrent groups in which 13 patients and three nurses each rated 5 of 10 pressure-reducing devices. Each device was tested at least four times. No evidence was given of randomization or counterbalancing. The investigators presented the ratings and the costs of the 10 devices without commenting on cost effectiveness. Of the four top-rated devices, two were the cheapest, and two were the most expensive.

Substitution

Eighteen studies met the criteria for review in this category; two of the studies were reported in one article (Spitzer et al., 1976). Record, McCally, Schweitzer, Blomquist, and Berger (1980) noted that the term "substitutability" implies that quality of care is not threatened. Eleven of the 18 studies reviewed here included an examination of quality of care prior to the presentation of cost analysis data (Brodie, Bancroft, Rowell, & Wolf, 1982; Burnip, Erickson, Barr, Shinefield, & Schoen, 1976; Chambers, Bruce-Lockhart, Black, Sampson, & Burke, 1977; Komaroff, Sawayer, Flatley, & Browne, 1976; Salkever, Skinner, Steinwachs, & Katz, 1982; Schultz et al., 1977; Soghikian, 1978; Spector, McGrath, Alpert, Cohen, & Aikins, 1975; Spitzer et al., 1976; Thompson, Basden, & Howell, 1982). In each case, the investigators concluded that the quality of care given by nurse practitioners was at least comparable to the care provided by physicians. The investigators of the other seven studies assumed comparable quality of care, either commenting that they made this assumption from their literature review or implying that the physicians involved already were convinced of the comparability of care (Briggs, Hickok, Rassier, Brickell, & Kakar, 1980; Draye & Stetson, 1975; Greenfield, Komaroff, Pass, Anderson, & Nessim, 1978; Heagarty, Grossi, & O'Brien, 1977; Muller et al., 1977; Reid, Eberle, Gonzales, Quenk, & Oseasohn, 1975; Tennant, Sorenson, Simmons, & Day, 1980).

Only two of the studies of substitution were RCTs. The first one to be considered, often referred to as the "Burlington trial" (Spitzer et al., 1974), is included in this review because the cost analysis was not published until after 1975 (Spitzer et al., 1976). Within the suburban group practice of two physicians in Canada, families were assigned randomly to receive primary care conventionally (physician only) or from a nurse practitioner, with physician consultation available. All families were given the opportunity to refuse their assignment and thus opt out of the trial; only 7 of 1,598 families did so. Spitzer et al. (1974) provided evidence that randomization worked by pointing out that the groups did not differ in blind evaluation of baseline health status.

A random sample of 817 patients was interviewed before and after the trial about their use of health services to provide estimates of the annual units of use of each of 12 types of services. Each estimate was then multiplied by the average cost per unit for each service for the entire province of Ontario. These costs were then combined in a weighted sum (Utilization and Financial Index, Spitzer et al., 1976), indicating the cost of health care per patient per year. This comprehensive composite index showed an 11% decrease in one year. The main sources of the reduction were costs for physician services and changes in hospital utilization (i.e., fewer admissions and decreased length of stay).

In the second RCT, Schultz et al. (1977) used a 2 × 3 factorial design and randomly assigned ambulatory, homebound, and nursing home patients to receive health care from a physician only or from an adult health nurse practitioner–physician team. These investigators provided strong evidence for pretreatment equivalence of the patient groups, and evaluators were blind to group assignment. Each of the nurse practitioner–physician teams, however, decided for themselves how to share the responsibilities for initiating, coordinating, supervising, treating, and evaluating care. After a comprehensive cost analysis, the authors concluded that the physician-only pattern was cost effective for ambulatory elderly patients, but for homebound and nursing home patients, the nurse practitioner–physician team was more cost effective. Thus, through two well-designed RCTs convincing demonstrations of the economic value of nurse practitioners were provided. The question of the generalizability of the results remains.

Spitzer et al. (1976) evaluated two nurse practitioners and two physicians in one suburban group practice in Canada where only .4% of the patients refused their random assignments to provider. Schultz et al. (1977) studied 167 elderly patients, but they were classified into small subgroups for analysis. In addition, process data on how the team functioned were lacking.

It might be argued that since both Spitzer et al. (1976) and Schultz et al. (1977) demonstrated the economic value of nurse practitioners, the fact that the bulk of the other investigators also indicated the positive economic value of nurse practitioners serves to extend the external validity of those two RCTs. The diverse circumstances of the other 16 studies certainly lend credence to this argument. The samples consisted of people of all ages, representing both the healthy and the sick. Some of the studies were focused on specific illnesses, such as otitis media, while others admitted anyone who called for an appointment. Most of the studies took place in urban areas, but suburban and rural areas were represented too. The typical study involved two nurse practitioners (range: 1 to 44). The estimated total number of nurse practitioners involved in the studies reviewed here was more than 80. They tended to work in health maintenance organizations or community clinics, but a few worked in hospital clinics or private practices.

For the most part, the samples of patients were large. The median sample size was approximately 1,000, so lack of statistical power was generally not a problem. Few samples were chosen randomly, but the investigators usually included all available patients over, on the average, a period of six months. The quality of the designs of the 16 remaining studies, however, varied greatly.

Six studies were NRTs involving concurrent groups. Although the quality of the investigators' attention to pretreatment equivalence varied, the cost of care was judged to be less with a nurse practitioner in five of the six studies. The strongest evidence for initial similarity of groups was given by Salkever et al. (1982) and Batchelor, Spitzer, Comley, and Anderson (1975); in the second study, Spitzer et al. (1976) analyzed for costs. Thompson et al. (1982) noted differences between groups in age and sex, but adjusted the data statistically before making cost comparisons. In two other NRTs, part of the sample was assigned randomly to provider and part of the sample was not. Greenfield et al. (1978) provided evidence of similarity between randomly and nonrandomly allocated patients for each provider, except for sex. Burnip et al. (1976) assigned to provider at random, but allowed patients to change their assignment. Burnip et al. provided no evidence of the prior similarity of groups. Since both Greenfield et al. and Burnip et al. studied large samples, it would have been worthwhile in each study to analyze separately those who were assigned randomly.

Soghikian (1978) described his design as an RCT and stated that 225 hypertensive patients were assigned randomly to either a physician or a nurse practitioner. These reviewers, however, classified the design as an NRT. For the cost analysis part of the study Soghikian removed patients who had diseases besides hypertension so that patient use of service could be compared. The physician group then consisted of 45 patients and the nurse practitioner group had 94 patients left. Soghikian offered no comment about the significant difference between groups in the percentage of patients with other diseases, 56% in the physician group versus 24% in the nurse practitioner group ($p < .001$, chi square analysis calculated by these reviewers). Soghikian was the only investigator using an NRT with concurrent groups who reported that costs were higher for nurse practitioners.

In the remaining three NRTs, the investigators used nonconcurrent groups. In one study the investigators reported a decrease in costs (Komaroff et al., 1976), in a second a slight increase in costs was reported (Chambers et al., 1977), and in the third results were indeterminate (Muller et al., 1977). The seven other studies were NCTs or were nonexperimental and will not be discussed here, except to note that five of them indicated the positive economic value of the nurse practitioner (Briggs et al., 1980; Brodie et al., 1982; Draye & Stetson, 1975; Heagarty et al., 1977; Tennant et al., 1980). In contrast, Reid et al. (1975) found that costs were competitive, while Spector et al. (1975) found that costs were higher.

In 15 of the 18 studies, costs were examined as costs for the patient over a specific time interval or as costs per visit. In two studies, however, the investigators used unit costs per service (Spitzer et al., 1976), and in one study the investigators used costs per episode (Salkever et al., 1982). Costs in studies without a comparison group or a baseline measure tended to be analyzed in terms of profitability (income minus expenses).

On the average, investigators used six variables in their cost analyses. The most frequently used ones were: salaries—15; laboratory tests—10; return visits—9; consultation time—9; indirect costs—8; time with patient—7; equipment—6; and medication charges—6.

Alternatives

Fourteen studies met the criteria for review in this category. Nine of the studies were focused on the alternative of home care (Amado, Cronk, & Mileo, 1979; Colt, Anderson, Scott, & Zimmerman, 1977; Creek, 1982; Gerson & Hughes, 1976; Gibbins et al., 1982; Kassakian, Bailey, Rinker, Stewart, & Yates, 1979; Martin & Ishino, 1981; Martinson et al., 1978; Widmer, Brill, & Schlosser, 1978). Two studies were focused on an alternative entry system for health care (Garfield et al., 1976; Hodgson & Quinn, 1980). The remaining three studies were focused on adult day care (Weissert, 1978), midwifery (Reid & Morris, 1979), and the alternative nursing care offered in a rehabilitation center (Alfano, 1982).

The alternative of home care is examined first. Hammond (1979) noted that in most studies of the cost effectiveness of home health care, the health outcomes of patients were assumed to be the same as for other treatment modes. Five of the nine studies of home care reviewed here contained measures that related to quality of care (Creek, 1982; Gibbins et al., 1982; Kassakian et al., 1979; Martin & Ishino, 1981; Martinson et al., 1978). In general, these measures involved self-reports by patients (or their care givers) of satisfaction with home care. In each study subjects were well satisfied. A few investigators supplied behavioral information, such as number of bedsores, return to work, and continuation of hobbies. In only one instance was the quality of home care less than for institutional care.

While Kassakian et al. (1979) reported that quality for home care patients was higher in general, they found that home care patients reported more pain; however, more than half of the sample did not answer this question. In contrast, Creek (1982) found that home care patients were well satisfied with pain control.

None of the studies of home care was an RCT, and only one was an NRT (Gerson & Hughes, 1976). These investigators described their study as an RCT to evaluate a home care nursing program for patients in Newfoundland who normally would have had a short hospital stay; however, physicians did not cooperate with the experiment. More than half of the patients randomly assigned to home care never received that care, but instead stayed in the hospital as long as the control group. Gerson and Hughes tried to overcome this flaw by providing evidence that the groups were similar, but sizable amounts of data were missing. Gerson and Hughes concluded that costs for total episodes were roughly equivalent for each group.

Of the eight remaining studies of home care, five might be considered NCTs. A study of home care for 32 dying children will serve as an example here (Martinson et al., 1978). The families were assigned a primary nurse who gave both technical and emotional support by means of home visits, phone visits, and being on call at all times. The investigators then compared the estimated average cost of home care per day to the average cost per day for local hospitals. They also compared the average cost per episode for the 32 families with the average cost per episode for 22 "similar" children not part of the project who died of cancer in a hospital. No details were provided about the 22 children used for comparison. By their judgment, home care resulted in reduced costs.

Investigators of three other NCTs of home care also claimed reduced costs (Amado et al., 1979; Gibbins et al., 1982; Widmer et al., 1978). In addition, one investigator (Creek, 1982) stated that the economic value of a home care hospice varied according to the comparison made. His evaluation indicated that home care was less expensive than local hospitals, but more expensive than skilled care at a nursing home in a private room. In the three nonexperimental studies of home care, investigators agreed concerning its positive economic value (Colt et al., 1977; Kassakian et al., 1979; Martin & Ishino, 1981).

In seven of the studies of home care, investigators compared the average costs per unit of time for a group receiving home care with the average costs in local institutions for the same unit of time. In three investigations, costs for a group of home care patients were compared to costs for similar groups of patients not receiving home care. Three cost analyses were focused on the cost savings from institutional days prevented. Several investigators offered more than one type of cost analysis. The variables most commonly used for cost analyses of home care by their frequency of use were: salaries (or fees)—nine; transportation and communication—five; and equipment—three. It was frequently very difficult to tell just what variables were being used. Some investigators referred to total program costs or visit costs without giving any further details.

In two studies, the investigators examined alternative entry systems for the delivery of health care. Garfield et al. (1976) described their study as an RCT of a new entry system at a health maintenance organization versus their traditional system. The new system involved an assessment on entry to one of several health status groups, and then a matching of the needs of each group with appropriate services and providers (nurse practitioners or physicians). The investigators did not defend the similarity of the two groups, nor did they mention whether clients were permitted to change their assignment. They claimed the cost of care was less for the new system, regardless of initial health status.

Another alternative entry system (Hodgson & Quinn, 1980) was evaluated in a nonexperimental study. This system, called Triage, involved a single entry model combining assessment, coordination and monitoring of appropriate care, reassessment, and claims or reimbursement. The professional team included nurse clinicians. After following 2,128 patients for three years, Hodgson and Quinn inferred improved quality of care from the increased percentage of those placed in nursing homes who returned home as compared to the national rate. A detailed cost analysis provided evidence that total costs were comparable to the cost of services under Medicare.

Alfano (1982) compared the alternative nursing care given at a rehabilitation center to that offered in a general hospital environment with an RCT design. Patients were assigned at random to agencies, but no evidence was given for the initial similarity of groups. Nurses (all RNs using the case method) provided patients with interim care during the postcritical phase of their illness and prepared them for discharge into the home, with physician consultation available. Measures relating to quality of care indicated comparable or better quality of care at the rehabilitation center. Length of stay was longer for those assigned to the rehabilitation center, but the cost per day was half that of the cost per day at a hospital; therefore, the average costs for the control group exceeded those of the experimental group. No data were given in the article on the variables used in the cost analysis, and apparently these details also were lacking in the final unpublished report examined by Prescott and Sorenson (1978).

The alternative of adult day care was examined by Weissert (1978) in a nonexperimental study. Ten of a population of 18 adult day-care centers were chosen deliberately for the sample to represent a broad mix. This investigator conducted a comprehensive cost analysis, but did not examine quality of care. The cost of two types of adult day-care programs, day hospitals and multipurpose centers, were compared to nursing homes. Weissert admitted that the chief problem with his design was the comparability of the day-care and nursing home populations, and was appropriately cautious in his conclusions. Since the costs for adult day care were less than the costs of nursing home care, even when out-of-pocket costs for living at home were considered, Weissert simply suggested that adult day care was a promising candidate for further investigation.

Finally, alternative perinatal care offered by nurse-midwives in four counties in Georgia was analyzed for cost effectiveness by Reid and Morris (1979) in a retrospective survey. Two comparisons were made: (a) a before-and-after comparison of the four counties, and (b) comparison with seven adjacent counties not participating in the program. Both of these comparisons were marred by dissimilarities between the groups. Reid and Morris made no statistical adjustment prior to analysis. They claimed that quality of care was better after the introduction of nurse-midwives and that expenditures decreased.

DISCUSSION

All of the researchers used the approach of cost-effectiveness analysis. In each study some change in practice was compared with another form of practice from the standpoint of costs; most investigators also measured quality of care. Evidence for cost effectiveness was claimed in 41 of 53 studies. Thus, conclusions about the cost effectiveness of nursing practices tended to be positive, regardless of design quality.

None of the investigators used cost–benefit analysis. It is conceivable that such a technique might have been useful in several categories. Such dimensions as nurse satisfaction, turnover, and quality of clients' lives in home versus hospital would have had to be valued in monetary terms to make comparisons between one form of care and another.

We have noted the relative absence of RCTs. This finding was not surprising. First, the use of such a design in health care research is relatively recent (approximately 30 years old according to Gehlbach, 1982), and RCTs still make up only a small percentage of published research (Wortman, 1981). Second, RCTs may be ethically impossible in a free society, especially for the study of alternative methods of health care. Patients prefer to choose their alternative rather than to be assigned randomly. Also, randomized trials may be impractical for the study of different ways of organizing nursing care. Nurses may not appreciate being assigned at random to units, nor may nurse researchers have the power to assign patients at random to units. Third, occasionally, researchers did assign at random, but a comparison of the groups revealed that the procedure went awry. Perhaps some researchers lack knowledge of accepted methods of random assignment or lack knowledge of the fundamental importance of randomization in controlling variables.

We do not wish to imply that RCTs are the only route to truth; many major advances in health care have arisen from NRTs. If, however, a RCT is judged to be an impossible method for a particular research question or situation, than researchers should be willing to use those statistical and design techniques which at least can begin to compensate for potential pretreatment differences. Many of the experiments and the surveys reviewed here would have benefited from techniques such as analysis of covariance, stratification, matching, partial correlation, and control by sample criteria.

These questions about appropriate designs are of more concern in some of the four groups of studies reviewed than others. Further, as we indicated earlier, it is also important to note the clarity and appropriateness of the variables contributing to the identification of costs and the set of alternatives to which the innovations were compared.

The weakest group of studies from the standpoint of design and completeness of information on these two factors was in the area of *organization of nursing services*. None of the 11 studies reviewed was a RCT and few of them provided sufficient information on which to make the judgments stated, positive or negative. We concluded, therefore, that definitive judgments about cost effectiveness of innovations in organization of nursing services, a critical area for nursing practice, could not be made on the basis of the research so far.

The second group of projects dealing with *specific nursing interventions* was extremely diverse. The procedures in each of the 10 studies were quite specific and there was a clear description of outcomes. In 9 of the 10 studies the authors concluded that the innovations introduced were cost effective. Special attention must be given to the outcomes of the study done by Field et al. (1982), which replicated those of Measel and Anderson

(1979). This RCT showed lower costs in the experimental group and, because of the quality of the design and the replication of previous results, provided strong evidence of the cost effectiveness of the innovation studied. Overall, this group of articles provided impressive evidence of nursing's professional development in studying new nursing interventions and suggested the importance of continuing the study of the costs of numerous and varied techniques and processes of nursing practice.

Nineteen studies were reviewed in the category of *substitution*. We have already mentioned some methodological problems in these studies; however, overall the designs and cost analyses were the strongest of the four areas. Most of the investigators judged their results as providing evidence of the positive economic value of the nurse practitioner.

Nine of the 14 studies reviewed in the category of *alternatives* focused on home care. While most investigators reported reduced costs, some methodological weaknesses in these studies were noted. It was also in the home care alternative that qualitative variables appeared extremely important but were not measured in terms of cost. Thus, positive results may have been underestimated in the home care alternative by the CEA technique. There was lack of clarity in the cost-effectiveness analyses, leaving us with questions about procedures, alternatives studied, and comparability of groups.

Researchers studying alternatives other than home care concluded that the alternative model was cost effective. The quality of the designs, the specificity with which variables were described and controlled for, the comparability of groups, and the criteria used in cost analysis varied in this diverse group of articles. Here, too, many authors claimed improved quality of care but did not assign a monetary value to this outcome. Thus, the general findings of cost effectiveness, despite methodological problems in some studies, might be seen as possible underestimations of positive potential outcomes.

In sum, while we are pleased to report positive results for cost effectiveness in 77% of studies reviewed, we must remind the reader that there was a variety of possible explanations for this unity. On the negative side, in addition to the methodological problems discussed earlier, three other possibilities should be mentioned. First, publishing bias may have been operating and authors were unwilling to share negative findings that conflicted with cherished beliefs. Or, journal editors were not interested in articles describing negative results that went against prevailing trends. Second, experimenter bias may have existed. In examining why so many hypotheses in educational research were supported, Cohen and Hyman (1979) pointed out that some studies served only to illustrate experimenter bias by offering results that were foreordained. We urge that high standards for research designs not be abandoned in the search for a quick answer. This pressure may result in studies that are political rather than scientific in approach. Third, an interpretative bias may have been present. "If the design of an experiment is faulty, any method of interpretation which makes it out to be decisive must be faulty too" (Fisher, 1966, p. 3). Fourth, no bias may have existed and the positive result indeed may have been entirely correct. Even in this event, which we hope is the case in the majority of studies, caution should be exercised in considering the innovations described as prescriptive for the future. Downs (1979) pointed out that applied research has a shorter life span than basic research; therefore, these studies may serve only to suggest interim actions.

RECOMMENDATIONS FOR RESEARCH DIRECTIONS

Many of the studies reviewed here would have profited from improved designs. Greater control of pertinent variables is needed so that meaningful cost comparisons can be made. In before-and-after studies, multiple measures of costs before the innovation begins as well as afterwards would be helpful in establishing better baselines. Improved reporting of research designs and methods, so that readers could tell more clearly just what procedures were followed, might have been all that was necessary in some of the reviewed articles.

It is possible that studies with negative results (or with results favoring the control group) may never have been submitted or accepted for publication. This possibility has been noted by others (Chalmers, Matta, Smith, & Kunzler, 1977). In this regard, we urge researchers with such results to submit them for publication or for presentation at research conferences which may result in published proceedings. If the study is well designed, we urge editors of research journals to publish such articles even though they present results against the mainstream.

All future studies that have implications for cost effectiveness must have the most sophisticated designs for analyzing cost benefit or cost effectiveness. Authors must define and state clearly the dollars and cents effects, so that any reader may obtain the full and correct impact of the work.

When applying for funding, nurse researchers should include monies for design, statistical, measurement, and cost-analysis collaborators (as opposed to consultants). Collaborators are accountable participants in planning and implementation of the study, not merely advisers at the start or critics after the data have been collected. Finally, we would like to remind nurses of the value of qualitative research in studying the effectiveness of various innovations. In the love affair with quantitative results, which has led to almost total reliance on statistical studies, nurses have downplayed qualitative research. The reporting of case studies and the use of an ethnographic approach, for example, would increase the body of knowledge and provide substantive questions for further investigation. Cost effectiveness analysis would benefit from both quantitative and qualitative research.

REFERENCES

Alfano, G. J. (1982). Hospital-based extended care nursing: A case study of the Loeb Center. In L. H. Aiken (Ed.), *Nursing in the 1980s: Crises, opportunities, challenges* (pp. 211–228). Philadelphia, PA: Lippincott.

Amado, A., Cronk, B. A., & Mileo, R. (1979). Cost of terminal care: Home hospice vs. hospital. *Nursing Outlook, 7,* 522–526.

Batchelor, G. M., Spitzer, W. O., Comley, A. E., & Anderson, G. D. (1975). Nurse practitioners in primary care. IV. Impact of an interdisciplinary team on attitudes of a rural population. *Canadian Medical Association Journal, 112,* 1415–1420.

Betz, M. (1981). Some hidden costs of primary nursing. *Nursing and Health Care, 2,* 150–154.

Briggs, R. M., Hickok, D. E., Rassier, D. S., Brickell, N. J., & Kakar, S. R. (1980). Midlevel personnel in obstetrics and gynecology practices: Cost-effectiveness and consumer benefits. *The Western Journal of Medicine, 132,* 466–470.

Brodie, B., Bancroft, B., Rowell, P., & Wolf, W. (1982). A comparison of nurse practitioner and physician costs in a military out-patient facility. *Military Medicine, 147,* 1051–1053.

Burnip, R., Erickson, R., Barr, G. D., Shinefield, H., & Schoen, E. J. (1976). Well-child care by pediatric nurse practitioners in a large group practice. *American Journal of Diseases of Children, 130,* 51–55.

Chalmers, T. C., Celano, P., Sacks, H. S., & Smith, H. (1983). Bias in treatment assignment in controlled clinical trials. *The New England Journal of Medicine, 309,* 1358–1361.

Chalmers, T. C., Matta, R. J., Smith, H., & Kunzler, A. (1977). Evidence favoring the use of anticoagulants in the hospital phase of acute myocardial infarction. *New England Journal of Medicine, 297,* 1091–1096.

Chalmers, T. C., Smith, H., Blackburn, B., Silverman, B., Schroeder, B., Reitman, D., & Ambroz, A. (1981). A method for assessing the quality of a randomized control trial. *Controlled Clinical Trials, 2,* 31–49.

Chambers, L. W., Bruce-Lockhart, P., Black, D. P., Sampson, E., & Burke, M. (1977). A controlled trial of the impact of the family practice nurse on volume, quality, and cost of rural health services. *Medical Care, 15,* 971–981.

Chavigny, K. H., & Nunnally, D. S. M. (1975). A comparison of methods for collecting clean-catch urine specimens in a clinic population of obstetric patients. *American Journal of Obstetrics and Gynecology, 122,* 34–42.

Cintron, G., Bigas, C., Linares, E., Aranda, J. M., & Hernandez, E. (1983). Nurse practitioner role in a chronic congestive heart failure clinic: In-hospital time, costs, and patient satisfaction. *Heart and Lung, 12,* 237–240.

Cohen, S. A., & Hyman, J. S. (1979). How come so many hypotheses in educational research are supported? *Educational Researcher, 8,* 12–16.

Colt, A. M., Anderson, N., Scott, H. D., & Zimmerman, H. (1977). Home health care is good economics. *Nursing Outlook, 25,* 632–636.

Creek, L. V. (1982). A homecare hospice profile: Description, evaluation and cost analysis. *Journal of Family Practice, 14,* 53–58.

Devine, E. C., & Cook, T. D. (1983). A meta-analytic analysis of effects of psychoeducational interventions on length of postsurgical hospital stay. *Nursing Research, 32,* 267–274.

Downs, F. S. (1979). Clinical and theoretical research. In F. S. Downs & J. W. Fleming (Eds.), *Issues in nursing research.* New York: Appleton-Century-Crofts.

Draye, M. A., & Stetson, L. A. (1975). The nurse practitioner as an economic reality. *Nurse Practitioner, 1,* 60–63.

Fagin, C. M. (1982). The economic value of nursing research. *American Journal of Nursing, 82,* 1844–1849.

Fairbanks, J. E. (1981). Primary nursing: More data. *Nursing Administration Quarterly, 5,* 51–62.

Felton, G. (1975). Increasing the quality of nursing care by introducing the concept of primary nursing: A model project. *Nursing Research, 24,* 27–32.

Field, T., Ignatoff, E., Stringer, S., Brennan, J., Greenberg, R., Widmayer, S., & Anderson, G. C. (1982). Nonnutritive sucking during tube feedings: Effects on preterm neonates in an intensive care unit. *Pediatrics, 70,* 381–384.

Fisher, R. A. (1966). *The design of experiments* (8th ed.). New York: Hafner.

Fletcher, R. H., & Fletcher, S. W. (1979). Clinical research in general medical journals. *The New England Journal of Medicine, 301,* 180–183.

Forster, J. F. (1978). The dollars and sense of an all-RN staff. *Nursing Administration Quarterly, 3,* 41–47.

Ganong, W. L., Ganong, J. M., & Harrison, E. T. (1976). The 12-hour shift: Better quality, lower cost. *Journal of Nursing Administration, 6,* 17–29.

Garfield, S. R., Collen, M. F., Feldman, R., Soghikian, K., Richart, R. H., & Duncan, J. H. (1976). Evaluation of an ambulatory medical-care delivery system. *The New England Journal of Medicine, 294,* 426–431.

Gehlbach, S. H. (1982). *Interpreting the medical literature.* Lexington, MA: D. C. Heath.

Gerson, L. W., & Hughes, O. P. (1976). A comparative study of the economics of home care. *International Journal of Health Services, 6,* 543–555.

Gibbins, F. J., Lee, M., Davison, P. R., O'Sullivan, P., Hutchinson, M., &

Murphy, D. R. (1982). Augmented home nursing as an alternative to hospital care for chronic elderly invalids. *British Medical Journal, 284,* 330–333.

Giordano, B., Rosenbloom, A. L., Heller, D., Weber, F. T., Gonzalez, R., & Grgic, A. (1977). Regional services for children and youth with diabetes. *Pediatrics, 60,* 492–498.

Giovannetti, P. (1980). A comparison of team and primary nursing care systems. *Nursing Dimensions, 7,* 96–100.

Greenfield, S., Komaroff, A. L., Pass, T. M., Anderson, H., & Nessim, S. (1978). Efficiency and cost of primary care by nurses and physician assistants. *The New England Journal of Medicine, 298,* 305–309.

Hammond, J. (1979). Home health care cost effectiveness: An overview of the literature. *Public Health Reports, 94,* 305–311.

Heagarty, M. C., Grossi, M. T., & O'Brien, M. (1977). Pediatric nurse associates in a large official health agency: Their education, training, productivity, and cost. *American Journal of Public Health, 67,* 855–858.

Hinshaw, A. S., Scofield, R., & Atwood, J. R. (1981). Staff, patient, and cost outcomes of all-registered nurse staffing. *Journal of Nursing Administration, 11*(11 & 12), 30–36.

Hodgson, J. H., & Quinn, J. L. (1980). The impact of the triage health care delivery system upon client morale, independent living, and the cost of care. *The Gerontologist, 20,* 364–371.

Hodgson, T. A., & Meiners, M. R. (1982). Cost-of-illness methodology: A guide to current practices and procedures. *Milbank Memorial Fund Quarterly, 60,* 429–462.

Jones, K. (1975). Study documents effect of primary nursing on renal transplant patients. *Hospitals, 49,* 85–89.

Kane, R. L., Jorgensen, L. A., Teteberg, B., & Kuwahara, J. (1976). Is nursing-home care feasible? *Journal of the American Medical Association, 235,* 516–519.

Kassakian, M. G., Bailey, L., Rinker, M., Stewart, C. A., & Yates, J. W. (1979). The cost and quality of dying: A comparison of home and hospital. *Nurse Practitioner, 4,* 18–19, 22–23.

Kerlinger, F. N. (1973). *Foundations of behavioral research* (2nd ed.). New York: Holt, Rinehart & Winston.

Klarman, H. E. (1974). Application of cost-benefit analysis to the health services and the special case of technologic innovation. *International Journal of Health Services, 4,* 325–352.

Komaroff, A. L., Sawayer, K., Flatley, M., & Browne, C. (1976). Nurse practitioner management of common respiratory and genitourinary infections, using protocols. *Nursing Research, 25,* 84–89.

Komrower, G. M., Sardharwalla, I. B., Fowler, B., & Bridge, C. (1979). The Manchester regional screening programme: A 10-year exercise in patient and family care. *British Medical Journal, 2,* 635–638.

Linn, J. T. B., & Taylor, W. B. (1979). Medications for the elderly. *Medical Journal of Australia, 1,* 315–316.

Marram, G., Flynn, K., Abaravich, W., & Carey, S. (1976). *Cost effectiveness of primary and team nursing.* Wakefield, MA: Contemporary.

Martin, M. H., & Ishino, M. (1981). Domiciliary night nursing service: Luxury or necessity? *British Medical Journal, 282,* 883–885.

Martinson, I. M., Armstrong, G. D., Geis, D. P., Anglim, M. A., Gronseth, E. C., MacInnis, H., Kersey, J. H., & Nesbit, M. E. (1978). Home care for children dying of cancer. *Pediatrics, 62,* 106–113.

Measel, C. P., & Anderson, G. C. (1979). Nonnutritive sucking during tube feedings: Effects upon clinical course in premature infants. *Journal of Obstetric, Gynecologic, and Neonatal (JOGN) Nursing, 8,* 265–272.

Muller, C., Marshall, C. L., Krasner, M., Cunningham, N., Wallerstein, E., & Thomstad, B. (1977). Cost factors in urban telemedicine. *Medical Care, 15,* 251–259.

Mumford, E., Schlesinger, H. J., & Glass, G. V. (1982). The effects of psychological intervention on recovery from surgery and heart attacks: An analysis of the literature. *American Journal of Public Health, 72,* 141–151.

Osinski, E. G., & Powals, J. G. (1980). The cost of all R.N. staffed primary nursing. *Supervisor Nurse, 11,* 16–21.

Prescott, P. A., & Sorenson, J. E. (1978). Cost-effectiveness analysis: An approach to evaluating nursing programs. *Nursing Administration Quarterly, 3,* 17–40.

Record, J. C., McCally, M., Schweitzer, S. O., Blomquist, R. M., & Berger, B. D. (1980). New health professions after a decade and a half: Delegation, productivity, and costs in primary care. *Journal of Health Politics, Policy and Law, 5,* 470–497.

Reid, M. L., & Morris, J. B. (1979). Perinatal care and cost effectiveness: Changes in health expenditures and birth outcome following the establishment of a nurse-midwife program. *Medical Care, 17,* 491–500.

Reid, R. A., Eberle, B. J., Gonzales, L., Quenk, N. L., & Oseasohn, R. (1975). Rural medical care: An experimental delivery system. *American Journal of Public Health, 65,* 266–271.

Salkever, D. S., Skinner, E. A., Steinwachs, D. M., & Katz, H. (1982). Episode-based efficiency comparisons for physicians and nurse practitioners. *Medical Care, 20,* 143–153.

Schultz, P. R., McGlone, F. B., Kinderknecht, E., Morton, L. L., Eylar, S. A., & Monley, S. M. (1977). *Primary health care to the elderly: An evaluation of two health manpower patterns.* Denver, CO: Medical Care and Research Foundation.

Shukla, R. K. (1981). Structure vs. people in primary nursing: An inquiry. *Nursing Research, 30,* 236–241.

Shukla, R. K. (1983). All-R.N. model nursing care delivery: A cost-benefit evaluation. *Inquiry, 20,* 173–184.

Soghikian, K. (1978). The role of nurse practitioners in hypertension care. *Clinical Science and Molecular Medicine, 55*(4), 345–348.

Spector, R., McGrath, P., Alpert, J., Cohen, P., & Aikins, H. (1975). Medical care by nurses in an internal medicine clinic: Analysis of quality and its cost. *Journal of the American Medical Association, 232,* 1234–1237.

Spitzer, W. O., Roberts, R. S., & Delmore, T. (1976). Nurse practitioners in primary care. VI. Assessment of their deployment with the Utilization and Financial Index. *Canadian Medical Association Journal, 114,* 1103–1108.

Spitzer, W. O., Sackett, D. L., Sibley, J. C., Roberts, R. S., Gent, M., Kergin, D. J., Hackett, B. C., & Olynich, A. (1974). The Burlington randomized trial of the nurse practitioner. *The New England Journal of Medicine, 290,* 251–256.

Steffel, P. E., Schenk, E. A. P., & Walker, S. L. (1980). Reducing devices for pressure sores with respect to nursing care procedures. *Nursing Research, 29,* 228–230.

Stronge, J. L., & Newton, G. (1980). Electronic thermometers: A costly rise in efficiency? Research reports. *Nursing Mirror, 151*(8), 29.

Tennant, F. S., Sorenson, K., Simmons, C., & Day, C. M. (1980). A study of the economic viability of low-cost, fee-for-service clinics staffed by nurse practitioners. *Public Health Reports, 95,* 321–323.

Thompson, R. S., Basden, P., & Howell, L. J. (1982). Evaluation of initial implementation of an organized adult health program employing family nurse practitioners. *Medical Care, 20,* 1109–1127.

Warner, K. E., & Hutton, R. C. (1980). Cost-benefit and cost-effectiveness analysis in health care. *Medical Care, 18,* 1069–1084.

Weissert, W. G. (1978). Costs of adult day care: A comparison to nursing homes. *Inquiry, 15,* 10–19.

Widmer, G., Brill, R., & Schlosser, A. (1978). Home health care: Services and cost. *Nursing Outlook, 26,* 488–493.

Wortman, P. M. (1981). Randomized clinical trials. In P. M. Wortman (Ed.), *Methods for evaluating health services: Vol. 8. Sage Research Progress Series in Evaluation*. Beverly Hills, CA: Sage.

Zwaag, R. V., Mason, W. B., Joyner, M. B., & Runyan, J. W. (1980). Cost of chronic disease care. *Journal of Chronic Diseases, 33,* 713–720.

PART V

Other Research

CHAPTER 11

Philosophy of Science and the Development of Nursing Theory

FREDERICK SUPPE
PROGRAM IN HISTORY
AND PHILOSOPHY OF SCIENCE
AND SCHOOL OF NURSING
UNIVERSITY OF MARYLAND
AND
ADA K. JACOX
SCHOOL OF NURSING
UNIVERSITY OF MARYLAND

CONTENTS

This chapter incorporates portions of Suppe (1982). Some of the material here was developed in courses the authors have co-taught with Beverly Baldwin and Glenn Webster. We wish to thank them for their influence on our work.

During the past 30 years nurses have devoted considerable attention to defining nursing and developing its scientific knowledge base to reflect the distinctness of nursing as a profession. The work in the 1950s and the early 1960s was largely on concept identification and formation, and nurses generally did not characterize their efforts as theory development. In the later 1960s and 1970s nurses began to propose theories and to focus specifically on theory construction. Philosophy of science sometimes was consulted, though as Silva and Rothbart (1984) noted, those developing nursing theories and those writing on metatheoretical issues in nursing were essentially two different groups. Thus, some nursing theories have not been based on concepts from philosophy of science. Additionally, there has been delay in the dissemination of recent changes in philosophy of science to those writing about theory development in nursing and to those developing nursing theory.

The central problem of philosophy of science is understanding the nature of scientific knowledge. Subproblems include analyzing the following scientific products and their contributions to knowledge: theory, law, explanation, concept, induction and confirmation, testing, intertheoretic reduction, measurement, discovery, experiment, and observation. The term *theory* in science is multivocal, encompassing both specific theories such as the theory of natural selection and broader entities that we will call conceptual models.

For this chapter, we reviewed the literature in philosophy of science and in the development of nursing theory for the past 30 years. When relevant, we have drawn on and given brief explanation of earlier works in philosophy to illustrate their influence on nursing theory development, as well as to indicate when the nursing literature has been inconsistent with ideas from philosophy of science. It was not our intent to review all aspects of nursing theory or all applications of philosophy in nursing. Rather we examine specifically the relationship between philosophy of science and nursing theory, citing nurse theorists to exemplify points in our analyses. After discussing the nature of concepts, theories, and conceptual frameworks and their use in nursing, specific approaches to the development of nursing theory are examined. Criteria for the evaluation of theory are considered and recommendations are made for the future development of nursing theory. Discussion of methodological issues relevant to various aspects of theory development is integrated throughout the chapter.

OVERVIEW OF PHILOSOPHY OF SCIENCE AND NURSING THEORY DEVELOPMENT

From the 1920s until the mid 1960s philosophy of science was dominated by logical positivism, which sharply distinguished the context of justification from the context of discovery in science. Dismissing the latter as psychology, not philosophy, positivists focused on the logical analysis of completed end-products of science. Thus those embracing the *Received View of Theories* (RV) analyzed the structure of logically ideal theories and paid no attention to the working versions of theories employed in the process of scientific discovery. The covering law model of explanation was used to analyze logically ideal causal and statistical explanations, and the ordinary sorts of informal explanations that frequently satisfy in science were ignored. The positivists' approach to testing, confirmation, and verification was to develop probabilistic-based inductive logics.

Beginning in the 1960s positivism came under increasing attack. Arguments were mounted that positivistic analyses of theories, explanation, and confirmation were fundamentally defective, and that insistence on analyzing the logically ideal resulted in accounts that had little to do with actual science, its theories, explanation, and confirmatory procedures. Specifically it was maintained that the contexts of discovery versus justification distinction was artificial and that theories and explanations could be understood only within their discovery contexts. Positivism succumbed to these attacks, and in the 1970s and 1980s many new treatments were witnessed which attempted fidelity to actual practice and placed a high premium on understanding the role of theories, explanation, and rationality in the growth of scientific knowledge.

In nurses' attempts to establish a science base, the 1950s and 1960s were characterized by a search for relevant concepts from the basic sciences, especially the behavioral sciences (e.g., National League for Nursing, 1958). Little explicit focus on the use of knowledge from the philosophy of science helped guide this work. Rather, nurses working alone or with biological or behavioral scientists identified concepts and principles from the basic sciences that could be used in nursing practice.

The early work by nurses in defining nursing, articulating nursing's philosophical base, and identifying the knowledge necessary for nursing practice was not viewed by them as nursing theory development. As Peplau (1983) noted recently in a discussion of her work, "It's a set of concepts, a framework that you can apply to various kinds of nursing situations, but to call it a nursing theory, I wouldn't." Nurses' efforts represented a wide variety of philosophical beliefs, and they drew from multiple sources in identifying relevant knowledge. Much of the work done in the 1950s and early 1960s formed the basis for later attempts to develop nursing theories.

Starting in the mid 1960s, conferences were held to discuss the nature of theories needed in nursing, and nurses began to publish accounts of their own attempts to develop theories. Much of the nursing theory literature has focused on how theories are constructed. The extent to which philosophy of science has been relied upon in the discussion of nursing theory construction and the development of specific nursing theories has varied widely.

Courses in philosophy of science seldom have been part of nursing curricula. In the last two decades, nurses interested in theory studied independently, enrolled in philosophy courses, or, more commonly, learned about theory development in sociology, psychology, or education courses and through the literature of those disciplines. Some philosophers have contributed in important ways to the nursing literature (e.g., Dickoff & James, 1968; Griffin, 1980; Suppe, 1982; Webster, Jacox & Baldwin, 1981), but, in general, nurses' direct exposure to philosophy of science ideas has not been common. No doubt this contributed to much of the discussion of nursing theory development not reflecting recent changes in philosophy of science. This changed gradually as more nurses studied philosophy of science and worked with philosophers in developing their ideas, as the literature of the 1980s (Jacox, 1984; Silva & Rothbart, 1984; Webster, et al., 1981) has begun to reflect.

CONCEPTS

Nursing theory is concerned, among other things, with concepts and their development. The most common nursing characterization of concepts is expressed by the Nursing Theories Conference Group (1980):

> Concepts are basically vehicles of thought that involve images. They are abstract notions and are similar in definition to ideas. Impressions received by sensing our environment evolve into concepts. (p. 2)

This view of concepts was first articulated by Arnauld (1662/1964) in *The Port Royal Logic;* it received its most extensive development by Locke in 1690 in his *Essay Concerning Human Understanding*. Locke's efforts were subjected to extensive criticism by his contemporaries, especially Berkeley

(1734/1901), whose main criticism was that if concepts were images or sense impressions, then there could be no abstract concepts. For instance, it would be impossible to have an image or an impression of the abstract concept of a triangle without visualizing a particular triangle. Thus, the notion of abstract concepts and the requirement that concepts be visualizable images were incompatible.

The definition of concepts as evolving from sensory impressions leads to concern for how they are operationalized. Strict operational definition is based upon positivism's RV. With the RV the vocabulary of a scientific language is divided into *logical terms* (including the terms of mathematics), *observational terms* (describing directly observable phenomena), and *theoretical terms* (descriptive of nonobservable phenomena). Validation of statements using only logical and observational terms is nonproblematic; reason suffices for the former and observation for the latter. Verification of theoretical term assertions, however, is problematic, so the RV restricts theoretical terms to those that have been defined operationally in terms of the observation vocabulary.

It was found later that legitimate physical science theories employed theoretical concepts that could not be defined operationally in terms of the observation vocabulary, but that added to the testable observable content of the theory. Interpretive systems were introduced to allow a much broader range of definitional forms for theoretical terms. Additionally, key terms in physics, for example, almost never were defined operationally.

While nurses writing about concept development often embraced a version of Locke's imagistic view of concepts and insisted on precise operational definitions of all concepts, the actual development of concepts in nursing has not been strictly the imagistic characterization. What nurses commonly did in the development of concepts was attempt to specify the meanings of terms via operational definitions and literature summaries. Peplau's (1957) early work on concept development, for example, was not restricted to the narrow RV interpretation of operational definition, but reflected a much broader range of definitional forms for theoretical terms. Peplau's work (1957, 1968) has had a dominant influence on the development of concepts in nursing, especially psychiatric nursing. Norris (1982) provided rich examples of a broader approach to concept development in the general field of nursing. Forsyth (1980) discussed development of the concept of empathy using description and analysis of model cases, illustrating empathy as well as alternative cases that represent contrary concepts, extraction of meanings from the literature, and application of the concept in different social situations. Zderad and Belcher (1968) sensitively discussed the strengths and weaknesses of operational definitions in nursing practice.

Use of strict RV operational definition would restrict unnecessarily nurse theorists to using only a subset of the legitimate definitional forms encountered in science. Fortunately, many nurses have not accepted such restriction.

THEORIES

Received View and Semantic Conception of Theories

RV and positivistic notions of science have had a strong influence on those writing about metatheoretical issues in nursing, especially from the mid 1960s to the late 1970s. As noted above, the RV distinction between mutually exclusive observation and theoretical vocabularies was attacked in the 1960s as fundamentally inadequate. There is no natural rationale for dividing descriptive vocabulary into the observational and theoretical that coheres with our intuitions as to which terms are paradigmatically observational or theoretical. Terms which in one context are observable are theoretical in other contexts and vice versa. The observational/theoretical distinction was closely allied with the analytic/synthetic distinction. A sentence is analytic if it is true or false in virtue of the meanings of its terms and its grammatical structure. A sentence is synthetic if empirical evidence is necessary to determine its truth or falsity. Every sentence is analytic or synthetic. The latter distinction was rejected because many sentences were found to be neither analytic nor synthetic, and confidence in the observational/theoretical distinction waned.

Further, based on the RV, theories and hypotheses containing theoretical terms had to be confirmed or refuted solely on the basis of directly observable evidence. This precluded empirically evaluating the truth of interpretive systems, even though such evaluation was crucial to their assessment. Finally, it was shown that the definitional forms allowed to mediate observational and theoretical concepts or terms failed to capture or do justice to the complexity of empirical relationships characteristic of the most impressive theories of, say, physics. The RV did not illuminate what was epistemologically most distinctive of scientific theories. Thus, philosophers of science rejected the RV as fundamentally inadequate. More recently, virtually no leading philosopher of science has subscribed to the RV.

After the RV rejection, philosophers explored alternative analyses. Hempel (1970) proposed a variation on the RV in which the observational/

theoretical distinction was replaced by an "antecedently available" and "theoretical" vocabulary distinction, whereby the former vocabulary could grow as science advanced. Operational definitions and interpretative systems were replaced by "bridge principles." This view provided for operational definitions divorced from the discredited observational/theoretical distinction. Gortner (1984) espoused use of Hempel's analysis in developing nursing theories.

The most widely used analyses of theories today are versions of the *Semantic Conception of Theories* (SC). On the SC, phenomena of kind K are viewed as state-transition systems. Parameters or variables characteristic of the type of phenomena are selected and the simultaneous values of these parameters for a phenomenon constitute the *state* of the system. No observational/theoretical distinction is employed to classify parameters. The behavior of the system constitutes its changes in state over time. Thus a phenomenon can be viewed abstractly as a system possessing a mechanism which produces state-transition behavior. The job of a theory is to characterize all and only those state-transition behaviors characteristic of the entire class of systems of kind K. A theory does so by specifying an abstract structure which specifies via its laws a class of allowable behaviors, that is, changes in state of phenomena for systems of kind K. In asserting a theory one claims that this abstract structure stands in some representing relationship with the behaviors of all physically possible phenomena of kind K. The SC provided an account of theories that was quite faithful to actual theories in much of science and provided philosophical illumination about theories and their epistemological roles (Suppe, 1972, 1974b, 1977).

Conceptions of Theory in Nursing

The influence of the RV on nursing theory was pervasive, yet influence did not always constitute slavish adherence. Thus, Hardy (1974) presented an RV treatment that adhered to the observational/theoretical distinction, required operational definitions, and so forth. Jacox (1974) presented and applied to nursing a version of the RV and associated positivistic doctrines. On the other hand, Bohny (1980) presented a hypothetical-deductive view of theory which, while strongly influenced by the RV and positivism, did not subscribe explicitly to many details of the RV in that it seemed equally compatible with the RV's observational/theoretical distinction and Hempel's (1970) alternative antecedent/theoretical distinction.

Many writers, such as Diers (1979), Donaldson and Crowley (1978), Wald and Leonard (1964), and Wooldridge, Schmitt, Skipper, and Leonard

(1983) stressed that nursing theories should be practice oriented. Dickoff and James (1968) are philosophers who have contributed substantially to the nursing literature and have had a major influence on many nurses, including those writing on metatheory and those conducting research on nursing practice. They identified four levels of theory: factor-isolating, factor-relating, situation-relating, and situation-producing theories. The second and third correspond to theories as analyzed by the RV and SC. Dickoff and James maintained that nursing practice theories are situation-producing and are a distinct kind of theory, although based on lower level theories. Key to a situation-producing theory is the imposition of goal states that one desires to achieve and the possibility of manipulating input variables so as to affect whether or not goal states are achieved. In nursing contexts the selected goal states are normative; their selection or justification cannot be accomplished by purely scientific procedures. Nonscientific normative or ethical assumptions play an essential role in selecting or justifying goal states, and considerations of moral and political philosophy are crucial for evaluation of such assumptions. Situation-producing theories are a species of teleological theory. Work on the SC has shown that teleological theories are regular theories with laws of quasi-succession on which goal states have been imposed (Suppe, 1976).

Not all nursing authors characterize theories in accordance with the RV. As noted earlier, this is in part because the term theory in science is multivocal. The term encompasses both specific theories, such as the theory of natural selection and quantum theory, which may be analyzed as related to the RV and SC, and also broader entities called conceptual frameworks or conceptual models. A conceptual framework is based on certain assumptions about the phenomena with which it is concerned and provides a broad perspective or world view of those phenomena. Attempting to characterize theory to encompass conceptual models, some nurse theorists provided broad descriptions. Stevens (1979) for example, included as nursing theories all theses on the nature of nursing and noted that theory development extends from the most primitive to the most sophisticated formulations. Other nurse theorists made the same distinction between theories and conceptual frameworks that we make here (Fawcett, 1980; Rogers, 1982). Rogers, for example, noted that "A science will have many theories, but the theories don't come out of the blue. They derive from an organized conceptual system" (1982, p. 248).

It is not only nurses, of course, who have used the term theory to analyze conceptual frameworks or models and simple propositions asserting relationships between concepts. Debates in sociology, for example, over the nature of sociological theory reflected similar practices. Merton's (1968) work was a classic attempt to sort out the confusion by distinguishing between simple propositions, middle range theories, and grand theories. When nurses call for theories *for* nursing they frequently refer to practice-oriented middle range theories. When speaking of theories *of* nursing, they commonly refer to grand theories, which we call conceptual frameworks.

CONCEPTUAL FRAMEWORKS

Philosophers of science increasingly are concerned with the dynamics of theorizing and rationality in the growth of scientific knowledge. They recognize that development of theory (in the RV, SC senses) does not proceed in a vacuum, but rather is guided by some extratheoretical entities. The work of Kuhn (1970), Hanson (1958), and Feyerabend (1970) can be construed as conceptual frameworks or grand theories. As with Merton's grand theories, these conceptual frameworks characteristically are not empirically testable directly; rather, they provide a perspective from which specific theories or hypotheses are developed and evaluated.

Much of nursing theory has been focused on the development of conceptual frameworks for nursing. The National League for Nursing framework (1978) as well as the theories of Johnson (1974), King (1981), Orem (1980), Rogers (1970), and Roy (1976) are paradigmatic conceptual frameworks that by themselves do not allow direct empirical testing. Rogers (1970) claimed the principles of her theory were verifiable and surveyed various studies she said tested her theory. Such "tests" only test the theory if augmented by auxiliary claims that provide most of the testable content. This is precisely how Merton understood grand theories as not testable. The value of Rogers' and others' conceptual frameworks is to provide a broad perspective within which specific theories can be developed and tested. As discussed below, one aspect of evaluation of conceptual frameworks is the adequacy of the specific theories they spawn.

The analyses of Toulmin (1972), Laudan (1978), Lakatos (1970), and Shapere (1983, in press) introduced such extratheoretical entities as research programs, research traditions, explanatory ideals, and domains; these investigators attempted to show how theories could be evaluated rationally as to their adequacy. Only some of these entities plausibly are construed as conceptual frameworks, and such rational evaluation generally does not constitute testing in the positivistic sense but does involve using empirical evidence. While such work has not produced a definitive account of conceptual frameworks or their evaluation, it did provide valuable insights for assessing and rethinking current nursing discussions of conceptual frameworks and their evaluation.

Taxonomies: A Type of Conceptual Framework

Taxonomies and classification schemes are a type of conceptual framework that function to organize phenomena systematically. In science, taxonomies usually contain hierarchically organized concepts (such as species, genus, family, phylum, kingdom), and there is some underlying theory, collection of theories, or empirically established propositions that provide the basis for so organizing the taxa and for explaining and predicting relationships between entities or organisms in different taxa. In medical nosology, for example, various disease entities are classified into diseases (e.g., serum hepatitis), disease types (hepatitis), and more general classifications (diseases of the liver) organized hierarchically. At the disease level at least, entities ideally are lumped together on the basis of theories or confirmed propositions that establish a common etiology. Scientific classification is not arbitrary but is based on known connections between the properties of entities being classified and characteristic features of the various level taxa (Suppe, 1974a).

Nurses recently have devoted considerable effort to developing conceptual frameworks or taxonomies for nursing diagnosis. Gordon and Sweeney (1979) summarized the variety of approaches taken in developing taxonomies for nursing diagnosis, and Kritek (1982) observed that the classification of nursing diagnoses represents a form of theory development. Kritek, influenced by RV accounts of theory (Dickoff, James, & Wiedenbach, 1968; Jacox, 1974), unfortunately argued that a classification of nursing diagnoses represents theory at the factor-isolating level and should be completed before higher level theories are developed. This argument ignored the intertwining of concept and theory development that actually occurs as theories are developed and also reflected the continuing influence of RV conceptions of theory on nurses.

Bircher (1975) argued for the need of a taxonomy for nursing diagnoses, noting that it facilitates communication, articulates and focuses attention on essential nursing concerns, and provides a view of the world specific to nursing. She clearly saw a taxonomy for nursing as a conceptual framework. For development of a nursing taxonomy she proposed a 10-step inductive procedure reminiscent of Bacon's (1620) inductive and Glaser and Strauss' (1967) grounded theory approaches to concept and theory development.

One of the most sophisticated discussions of the connections between nursing diagnosis and taxonomies was by Douglas and Murphy (1981). Following the third Nursing Theories Conference Group's definition that "nursing diagnosis is a concise phrase or term summarizing a cluster of empirical indicators representing patterns of unitary man" (1980, p. 54), they developed a view of the development of taxonomies along the lines of Sokal's (1974) numerical taxonomy approach. Their approach was similar to Bircher's recommendations and posed the same problems as Sokal's. Sokal argued for an atheoretical approach to taxonomy which was based on cluster analysis (Sokal & Sheath, 1963). Promising as early attempts were, the cluster generated taxonomies they produced proved to be nonreplicable and idiosyncratic. Further, cluster analysis produced many candidate taxonomies and one had to resort to precisely the sorts of antecedent theory they eschewed in construct validation procedures used to evaluate the candidate taxonomies, and select which of them to adopt (Suppe, 1981).

These difficulties, together with problems we will discuss later with inductive and grounded theory approaches, strongly suggest that the atheoretical inductive approaches proposed in developing taxonomies for nursing diagnosis are not promising. It is preferable to approach taxonomies as conceptual frameworks which are to be evaluated much the same as other conceptual frameworks.

In taxonomy development, as in other theory development, the development of concepts (diagnoses in this case) is intertwined with the development of the conceptual framework, using both inductive and deductive processes. In giving the historical account of the work of the national conference for development of nursing diagnoses, Gordon (1982) reported an atheoretical beginning in the development of nursing diagnoses. A modification of Rogers' (1970) conceptual framework was then introduced and conference participants subsequently tried to reconcile their previously identified nursing diagnoses with a framework dealing with unitary man interacting with the environment. The question to be raised is whether or not there is sufficient consensus in nursing that Rogers' conceptual framework is the appropriate choice for organizing nursing diagnoses, or the problems with which nurses deal. We suggest that the choice was premature and that additional frameworks should be considered or developed.

APPROACHES TO NURSING THEORY DEVELOPMENT

Having discussed the main sorts of conceptual devices employed to formulate nursing knowledge—concepts, theories, and conceptual frameworks—we turn now to various overlapping approaches which maintain that nursing knowledge has special characteristics that affect how nurses should formulate theories and conceptual frameworks. The first of these is the systems approach, which represents primarily a deductive approach to theory in which a set of assumptions about how aspects of the world operate as applied to nursing.

Systems Approaches

Riehl and Roy (1980) construed Johnson (1974), Neuman (1982), Orem (1980), Rogers (1970), and Roy (1976) as taking systems approaches, as did the Chrisman and Riehl (1974) systems developmental stress model, and the holistic approaches of Brodt (1980), Levine (1971), Mathwig (1969), and Zbilut (1980). Yet there is disagreement among nurses as to what counts as a systems approach. For example, Stevens (1979, pp. 208–209) denied that Rogers, Chrisman and Riehl, or any holistic approaches wherein the whole is greater than the part, qualified as a systems approach under her own classification scheme for theories. Such use and disagreement reflects the fact that there are nearly as many meanings attached to "systems" as there are advocates of systems approaches (Suppe, 1978).

In nursing by far the most frequently cited systems theory sources are from General Systems Theory (GST). Putt's (1978) work was a particularly important example of GST applied to nursing. Beginning as a splinter movement within logical positivism, GST basically included acceptance of the RV. Unlike most positivists, who were persuaded that all of science ultimately could be reduced to physics and chemistry, developers of GST denied such reductionism. Rather, they claimed that there was a hierarchy of levels from the subatomic to the physical, biological, psychological, social, and suprasocial. Components at each level were systems, and the systematic organization of next-lower level constituents endowed the system with attributes that were emergent with respect to, rather than attributes reducible to, characteristics of lower level entities. Yet it was believed that radically different systems obeyed essentially the same laws. For example, locust migration behavior, epidemiology, and mob behavior were governed by laws expressible in the same formulae. GST's crucial reliance on the RV in arguing its holistic doctrines seriously undercuts many of its central claims, and the hierarchical structure underlying its emergentism doctrine is rather suspect (Suppe, in press). Donaldson and Crowley (1978) argued for the undesirability of nurses committing themselves to such hierarchies.

While the systems metaphor provided a useful way of looking at nursing phenomena, its utilization did not require buying into the metaphysical excesses and RV epistemological constrictions of GST. From an examination of the articles in Putt's (1978) collection, our impression is that GST approaches to nursing theory use the systems metaphor, espouse holism, and use some of the GST terminology without accepting the metaphysics or epistemology of GST. Questionable as this is, it is preferable to imposing GST's whole structure on nursing theory in an unduly constricting manner. At the same time, it is misleading since it claims allegiance to views it honors primarily by utilizing its terms and extensive flow charting.

A second systems approach was provided by the SC that views phenomena as systems and attempts to characterize classes of phenomenal behavior via state-transition laws. Unlike GST, the SC was not tied to the epistemology of the RV and was neutral with respect to the metaphysical controversies over emergentism versus reductionism and holism. Just because it was faithful to actual theories in the more developed sciences and did not represent a GST-like proposal for reforming science, the SC provided a better guide for approaching nursing theory from a systems perspective.

Holistic Approaches

Much of nursing theory is concerned with characterizing what is unique about nursing, and thus with showing how nursing is more than just attenuated medicine. A common approach is to construe medicine as concerned with the body and nursing as concerned with the integration of mind and body interacting and being interdependent with the environment (Levine, 1971). One can simply insist that nurses pay attention to and nurture the physical, mental, and environmental needs of the patient. Holistic approaches deny that this is enough, for they claim that the person is emergent with respect to physical, mental, and environmental constituents, being a synergistic entity, and that cooperation of discrete agencies or components is such that the total effect is greater than the sum of the constituent effects taken separately (Brodt, 1980). Thus, for nursing merely to concentrate separately on the physical, mental, and environmental needs of the patient ignores the needs of the emergent whole person.

The insistence in holistic nursing that the whole is greater than the sum of its parts is reminiscent of GST's emergentist doctrines. Yet holistic approaches are separable from GST. For example, Mathwig (1969) employed a systems holistic approach that did not commit itself to GST's metaphysics, and Levine (1971) similarly proposed an adaptational holistic perspective on nursing. Parse (1981) combined parts of Rogers' work with ideas from existentialism and phenomenology. Paterson and Zderad (1976) based their conception of holistic nursing on existential and phenomenological philosophy and emphasized the need to attend to reality as experienced by both patient and nurse. Rogers (1982), Chinn and Jacobs (1983), Fitzpatrick and Whall (1983), and Thibodeau (1983) all have noted that unitary man is distinct from the sum of the parts.

Beyond sensitizing us to aspects of nursing phenomena upon which to focus theoretical efforts, adopting a holistic approach has methodological implications. Historically, the problem of emergentism, of which holism is a contemporary version, has been intimately connected with the issue of whether the human sciences were methodologically distinct from the natural sciences. The controversy began in 1739–1740 when Hume published *A Treatise of Human Nature*. He argued that the moral sciences, concerned with human nature or activity, human conduct, social practices, and feelings, emotions, and thoughts could and should be investigated and understood via the same experimental methods employed in the physical sciences. In the 19th and early 20th centuries Durkheim (1895/1950) and Weber (1925/1947) took exception, arguing that if we are to understand people's behavior or social events, we must have access to their ideas. This would require the human sciences to be methodologically distinct from the natural sciences. That is, the human sciences required a different kind of *Verstehen* or understanding than has been provided by the natural science empirical methods (Levison, 1974). Emergentism frequently has been used as a basis for arguing that the human sciences require a distinct methodology.

The problem of *Verstehen* remains unresolved. Comptean positivism and early logical positivism were modern heirs to Hume's position, and various Wittgensteinian, phenomenological, ethnomethodological, and hermeneutical methodologies were current heirs to Weber's and Durkheim's positions (Dallmayr & McCarthy, 1977). Some, for example hermeneutics, maintain that the appropriate methods for the human sciences are more those of the humanities than those of the natural sciences.

Many nurses espousing or developing holistic theories have rejected positivistic and RV notions of science as adequate for the development and testing of theories. Munhall (1982), for example, proposed that qualitative research methods are more consistent with nursing's philosophical beliefs than is the scientific method, described by her in RV terms. Zbilut (1980) maintained that the philosophical-transcendental level of thought "confers a special meaning or significance . . . since it 'ties up' the holistic 'bundle' " (p. 177). Paterson (1971) and Paterson and Zderad (1976) advocated a humanistic approach to nursing which is methodologically distinct from the empirical sciences. Discussion and debates of the merits of quantitative and qualitative methods have increased in the nursing literature.

Inductive Approaches

Traditionally deductive and inductive approaches have been advocated for the development of scientific theory. In the 17th century, Descartes (1664) advocated the rationalistic approach wherein all of science would be obtained via deducing consequences of self-evident or indubitable truths. Such an approach proved incapable of providing any adequate role for observation and experimentation. While deductive reasoning plays a role in science, it alone is insufficient.

In 1620, Bacon proposed inductive empiricism as the scientific method. Through unbiased observation one would ascertain regularities among phenomena that inductively would yield lower level generalizations. Continuation of the inductive process would lead to higher level generalizations. Initially induction was presented as a method for scientific discovery which, if followed, would guarantee the truth of the resulting generalizations, laws, and theories. For Bacon this was only a theoretical ideal, since in practice one could not complete fully the inductive procedure and so the resulting inductions were fallible.

A serious blow to induction was struck by Hume (1739–1740), who argued as follows: All knowledge must be analytic or empirical. Induction reasons from particular observations (This swan is white) to empirical generalizations (All swans are white). The inference from observed instances to the generalization is invalid unless one adds the further assumption, called an induction hypothesis, that the observed instances are representative of the total population. Since this induction hypothesis is not logically true, it must be empirical. Since it is an empirical generalization, it must be established by induction. Repeating the argument applied to the induction hypothesis, we obtain the need for a new induction hypothesis that must be established by induction, and so on into an infinite regress. Thus there is no noncircular justification of induction.

One strongly inductivist view influencing nursing theory was grounded theory (Glaser & Strauss, 1967). The basic idea of grounded theory is that one approaches a body of phenomena without preconception to record observations, works out concepts and hypotheses, refines them in light of new observations, and continues the process until saturation occurs. Saturation is the point at which additional data no longer affect the theoretical outcome. The approach was anticipated by Bacon (1620) as his first method of induction. Bacon, however, was aware that the only guarantee that saturation would occur was that one had a complete catalog of unprejudiced data and such an exhaustive data base was impossible to obtain. More recent philosophy of science literature contained various attempts to develop epistemologies (e.g., Goodman, 1955; Peirce, 1931–1958) which presuppose that a saturation condition would obtain. Without exception such views failed because there was no guarantee that saturation would occur and there were no viable criteria for assessing when saturation did occur.

While there have been occasional examples of inductivist approaches (e.g., Atwood, 1977) and some involved in the development of taxonomies for nursing diagnoses advocated such an approach (Bircher, 1975; Douglas & Murphy, 1981), few nurses have taken a strict inductivist approach. Benoliel (1977), Norris (1982), and Wald and Leonard (1964) advocated inductive approaches to the development of nursing theory. None of these persons was committed to induction being sufficient for all general scientific knowledge, however. The thrust of their recommendations was that more relevant nursing theory would result from inductively studying nursing practice than would occur if nurses borrow theory from the biopsychosocial sciences and apply it to nursing contexts.

EVALUATION OF THEORIES AND CONCEPTUAL FRAMEWORKS

Rejecting on Humean grounds the possibility of inductively confirming theories, Popper (1959, 1965) argued that we can test theories by attempting to falsify them. Thus, empirically we can reject theories even though we cannot confirm them. Since failure to falsify does not imply the truth of a theory, we should not adhere dogmatically to a single theory. Rather we should proliferate boldly a plurality of theories and subject them to rigorous tests. However, Popper's view was unsatisfactory since falsification was as problematic as confirmation. For testing of theories inevitably required auxiliary hypotheses, and so the failure of a test did not show that the theory was false; rather it showed the theory *or* the auxiliary hypotheses were false.

The situation then is that we can test theories only relative to various presuppositions or assumptions that are not themselves subject to scientific tests at that time. According to many philosophers of science these assumptions are components of conceptual frameworks or other supratheoretical entities. Fawcett (1980) reflected this view in her claims that nursing conceptual frameworks/models/global theories cannot be compared externally:

> Evaluative questions allow one to draw judgmental conclusions by focusing on internal validity of a model, although not on external comparisons among various conceptualizations. . . . Since models explain the phenomena of district [*sic*] disciplines or schools of thought, we cannot make direct comparisons. Reese and Overton cautioned that "because of basic lack of communication, the partial overlap in subject matter, and the differences in truth criteria [each model] must be evaluated separately, and in obedience to its own ground rules. . . . Thus, judgments must be limited to the adequacy of each conceptual framework as it stands alone. (pp. 12–13)

Her basic view that conceptual models have their own presuppositions and internal evaluating criteria that preclude the objective and neutral external comparative evaluation of competing models is a specific instance of incommensurability claims, which the philosophers Kuhn (1970) and Feyerabend (1970) have made respectively for paradigms and global theories.

At the heart of Kuhn's and Feyerabend's defense of the incommensurability claim is a theory of meaning that says that a paradigm/grand theory/framework completely determines the meanings of all its constituent terms, and that any alteration in the theory changes the meanings of all its constitutent terms. The corollary is that no two distinct global theories can assign the same meanings to any terms they have in common, hence, that there can be no neutral data for testing competing paradigms or global theories. For data to be relevant to such a test, they must be expressed in the terms of the global theory. If expressed in the terms of one global theory, however, the meanings will be different from those of the competing global theory and hence not relevant to the latter. Critics have asserted that Kuhn's and Feyerabend's analysis of theoretical meanings is implausible and that the only arguments in its support presuppose their meaning analysis (see Suppe, 1977, pp. 135–151, 170–180, 199–208, 636–649). Stung by such criticisms, Kuhn, but not Feyerabend, retreated from both his incommensurability claims and the underlying meaning analysis to a translation thesis to allow some comparison between paradigms or global theories.

In Fawcett's (1984, pp. 47–48) discussion of analysis and evaluation of conceptual models of nursing, she noted that direct external comparisons cannot be made. She, however, referred to Jacobson's (1981) attempt to evaluate the impact of nursing conceptual models using parameters that apply to all models and stated that such work may increase understanding of the nature of comparison among models. Beyond this brief mention, Fawcett did not discuss explicitly the problem of incommensurability. In her scheme for evaluation of conceptual frameworks, Fawcett determined the extent to which several nursing frameworks met criteria related to making assumptions explicit—inclusion and linking of four concepts viewed by her as necessary for all nursing conceptual frameworks, logical congruence, social considerations, theory-generating capability, and contributions to nursing knowledge. In identifying these criteria for evaluating all conceptual frameworks, she seemed to have rejected the incommensurability thesis.

It appears that a primary benefit of conceptual models is to sensitize researchers to potentially important variables to include in local or middle-range testable theories. Thus, even though a conceptual model or framework is not adequately precise to afford direct test, it can be evaluated on the basis of the adequacy of the local theories it spawns. In this sense, Rogers (1970) was correct in claiming that the adequacy of testable research based upon her global theory constitutes a means for the latter's objective evaluation.

Not all supratheoretical entities that were introduced into philosophical analyses of the growth of scientific knowledge were tied to incommensurability views. Lakatos (1970) viewed theories as developed and evaluated within a research program that produced a sequence of theories, each a modification of prior ones consistent with the program's presuppositions. These theories are tested empirically and, depending on whether new theories in the sequence predict novel facts that are not refuted by testing, the research program could be judged as progressive or degenerating. According to Laudan (1978), science proceeds from within a research tradition, with both the tradition and the theories it produces evaluated on the basis of their problem-solving success. He developed a classification of scientific problems and a procedure for weighting these problems and evaluating overall problem-solving success. Shapere (1983, in press) emphasized that scientific research proceeds from a scientific domain of established theory and fact that generates problems to which theories are a type of answer.

Rather than there being a fixed set of methodological standards for evaluating theories, science evolves new methods and standards as it advances, and these standards are informed by what has been learned. There are emerging quite sophisticated and promising accounts of rationality in the growth of scientific knowledge, including the evaluation of nonabsolute presuppositions. Currently philosophers of science are concerned with detailing how the presuppositions necessary for evaluating theories are evaluated rationally. While none of the attempts is without its critics, they do provide considerable insight into the scientific evaluation of theories and supratheoretical entities. They also shed considerable illumination on such traditional standards for theory evaluation as Occam's razor. (All other things considered, the simpler of two theories is to be preferred.)

Nursing theory has a sizable literature devoted to the evaluation of theories and conceptual frameworks that reflects controversy over how these are evaluated most appropriately. We will confine our attention to nursing approaches not already discussed. Reflecting the fact that nursing practice theories are teleological and that evaluation of goal states in nursing theory must be done on the basis of normative, not scientific, considerations, Duffy and Muhlenkamp (1974), Ellis (1968), Fawcett (1980), and Stevens (1979) stressed that values should be made explicit. Fawcett (1980), Johnson (1974), and Stevens (1979) stressed that values (hence the goal states) in practice theory should be assessed on the basis of social congruence, social significance, and social utility. Such criteria, while clearly relevant to a caring discipline, also potentially are problematic. There is the possibility that such criteria can be interpreted so that nursing becomes an instrument for promoting social conformity in ways that jeopardize individual well-being. More sophisticated forms of normative evaluation, perhaps drawing from the resources of moral and social philosophy, are needed as Beckstrand (1980) and Donaldson and Crowley (1978) have noted.

Relative to a set of goals, theories may be more or less adequate in achieving those goals. Some writers (Dickoff et al., 1968; Ellis, 1968; Hardy, 1974; Stevens, 1979) imposed various criteria concerned with the pragmatic adequacy of theories in achieving those goals. Such criteria usually were presented as distinct from questions of the empirical truth or adequacy of theories. On the SC account of practice theories given above, in isolated circumstances the pragmatic adequacy of a theory in achieving its goals is nothing distinct from its empirical truth. Questions of pragmatic, as distinct from empirical, adequacy largely concern a theory's robustness or adaptability to nonisolated circumstances or its feasibility of implementation in realistic practice settings.

Many authors (e.g., Duffy & Muhlenkamp, 1974; Ellis, 1968; Fawcett, 1980; Fitzpatrick & Whall, 1983; Hardy, 1974; Stevens, 1979) imposed criteria such as internal consistency, conceptual adequacy, logical development, as well as considerations of simplicity (parsimony, fidelity to Occam's razor) and testability. While these may seem to be readily understood, absolute criteria shared by all of science, in fact all of these evaluative criteria have varied over the history of science and are not absolutes.

For example, the criteria of consistency in quantum theory are quite different from those of traditional deductive logic, and the notion of inductive consistency is controversial and problematic. We have encountered diverse views as to what constitutes testability and conceptual adequacy. The notions of simplicity used in theoretical physics have changed rather dramatically over the last few decades and have little to do with 19th century notions. Rather than being straightforward, absolute criteria for evaluation, these constitute rather specific presuppositions for doing science on a par with induction hypotheses. They are subject to rational evaluation as constituents of supratheoretical entities in ways philosophy of science is exploring today.

Other evaluative criteria stressed by Fawcett (1980), Stevens (1979), and others concern whether the theories or conceptual frameworks are appropriately nursing ones. For example, Fawcett (1980) was concerned that a conceptual framework contain the National League for Nursing's four essential concepts of nursing (Yura & Torres, 1975). Of course, other conceptions of nursing have their own different sets of concepts that define nursing (e.g., ANA, 1980; Donaldson & Crowley, 1978). If we broadly conceive a conceptual framework for nursing as including a conception of what nursing is, specification of values for nursing practice, methodological presuppositions for research and testing of theories, criteria for evaluating theories, a body of accepted background information or facts, and perhaps principles specifying broad constraints on the content of theories and procedures for generating problems, then there are and should be many different sets of criteria for evaluating nursing theory. Within such a framework, the criteria for evaluating theories may be fairly definite. The issue then becomes to evaluate the adequacy of competing frameworks. Any hope that there will be fixed criteria for evaluating the adequacy of frameworks is challenged seriously by Shapere's (1983, in press) work on rationality and the growth of scientific knowledge. Such evaluation is not arbitrary, however, and such frameworks are not incommensurable.

SUMMARY AND RESEARCH DIRECTIONS

Nurses' concern with theory development is very recent and occurred simultaneously with major changes in philosophy of science that are just beginning to be reflected in the nursing literature. In the past 30 years, nurses have made considerable progress in describing nursing's philosophical beliefs, identifying relevant concepts, becoming sensitive to the need to systematize knowledge by constructing and testing theories, and putting forward some preliminary conceptual frameworks and theories.

Though not the only one, the dominant view of theory development from philosophy of science to influence nurses has been the now largely discredited RV based in logical positivism. Refutation of the RV has been followed by new approaches to science and theory development. While no single approach has supplanted the RV and debate continues regarding how theories are evaluated, there is consensus that the conceptual framework within which specific theories are developed and tested must be taken into account and that positivistic research methods alone are inadequate.

The emerging views of science make clear that some of the issues debated in the development of nursing theory have been false and overly restrictive. Debate has focused on such issues as (a) Should there be one or many theories? (b) Should we have theories *of* or theories *for* nursing? (c) Do we use inductive or deductive methods? (d) Are quantitative or qualitative methods more appropriate for understanding human behavior? (e) How is the practice of nursing distinct from the science of nursing? (f) Can there be a science of nursing? Post-RV conceptions of science suggest different answers to these and related questions.

Considering the present stage of development of nursing theory and the recent changes in philosophy of science, we make the following suggestions.

1. Nurses seriously interested in theory development should seek direct exposure to the philosophy of science literature. Although gradually changing, the nursing literature continues to reflect ideas discredited by contemporary philosophers of science. With philosophy of science changing so rapidly, the timely transfer of its knowledge must be facilitated so that theory development in nursing is informed adequately. Doctoral students in nursing especially would benefit from taking courses in philosophy of science or nursing theory courses which integrate the philosophy of science, or otherwise having direct contact with ideas being developed and debates taking place within philosophy.
2. The formulation and comparison of several major conceptual frameworks (supratheoretical entities) should be encouraged. Further, within each framework, the development and evaluation of multiple specific theories should be promoted. There is need for creativity in the development and careful examination of the conceptual frameworks proposed for sensitizing nurses to phenomena of importance to consider in developing nursing knowledge. To a

large extent, what have been called theories of nursing are these conceptual frameworks (Johnson, 1974; King, 1981; Orem, 1980; Rogers, 1970). While not altogether absent, few specific theories have been derived from these conceptual frameworks and subjected to test. It may be that, as nurses define specialty areas more definitively, they will facilitate the development and testing of theories with a more limited focus and capability of being tested (e.g., Fawcett, 1975; Galligan, 1979; O'Toole, 1981; Riehl & Roy, 1980). At present, there is a gap between the loosely defined conceptual frameworks and the conduct of research.

3. Taxonomies of nursing diagnosis should be viewed as a form of conceptual framework. Some current attempts to develop nursing diagnoses advocate a strongly inductive and atheoretical approach shown to have many problems. Specification of a conceptual framework that would both guide the identification of nursing diagnoses (problems) and in turn be shaped by the developing diagnoses is needed.
4. Multiple approaches to theory development and testing should be encouraged. Debates about inductive versus deductive and qualitative versus quantitative approaches to theory development and testing are useful only insofar as they make clear that alternatives are available. All attempts to develop theory involve both deduction and induction as well as other modes of reasoning, though some may emphasize one approach more than the other. Different stages of theory development may require a greater emphasis on induction or deduction. Similarly, quantitative and qualitative methods of study are both appropriate, depending on the nature of the problem being addressed. Finally, use of strict RV operational definitions unnecessarily restricts theory development to a subset of legitimate definitional forms. There is need for greater tolerance of diversity in the development and testing of nursing theories. Additionally, more critical dialogue among groups concerned with theory development in nursing should be encouraged to promote cross-fertilization of ideas.
5. Discussions of theory development should include attention to methodological implications. There tends to be little overlap between those attracted to theory development and those attracted to the advanced study of research methods. Mechanisms to bridge this gap should be developed so that there is a closer match between the theories developed and the methods used to test them. Additionally, greater attention should be placed on methods for theory

development. While there has been work on concept formation (e.g., Norris, 1982; Peplau, 1957), Walker and Avant's (1983) suggested procedures for theory construction, including development of concepts, statements, and theories, represents one of the first comprehensive attempts in nursing to address primarily methodological rather than philosophical issues in theory development. More work in this area is needed.

6. Careful attention should be given to recent developments in the evaluation of theory. Ways in which criteria for evaluating specific theories differ from those for evaluating conceptual frameworks are currently being explored. Additionally, sophisticated forms of normative evaluation of theory are being developed. Accelerated efforts to transfer these developments in philosophy into the nursing literature are needed.

REFERENCES

American Nurses' Association. (1980). *Nursing: A social policy statement*. Kansas City, MO: Author.

Arnauld, A. (1964). Translated as *The art of thinking: Port Royal logic*. (J. Dickoff & P. James, Trans.). Indianapolis: Bobbs-Merrill. (Original work published 1662)

Atwood, J. (1977). A grounded theory approach to the study of perimortality care. In M. V. Batey (Ed.), *Communicating nursing research* (Vol. 9). Boulder, CO: Western Interstate Commission for Higher Education.

Bacon, F. (1620). *Novum organon. Part 2. Instauratio magna*. London: J. Billium.

Beckstrand, J. (1980). A critique of several conceptions of practice theory in nursing. *Research in Nursing and Health, 3*, 69–79.

Benoliel, J. Q. (1977). The interaction between theory and research. *Nursing Outlook, 25*, 108–113.

Berkeley, G. (1901). *A treatise concerning the principles of human knowledge* (2nd ed.). London: Oxford University Press. In A. C. Fraser (Ed.), *The works of George Berkeley* (2nd ed.). London: Oxford University Press. (Original work published 1734)

Bircher, A. (1975). On the development and classification of diagnoses. *Nursing Forum, 14*, 10–20.

Bohny, B. (1980). Theory development for a nursing science. *Nursing Forum, 19*, 50–67.

Brodt, D. (1980). A re-examination of the synergistic theory of nursing. *Nursing Forum, 14*, 85–93.

Chinn, P., & Jacobs, M. (1983). *Theory and nursing*. St. Louis: Mosby.

Chrisman, M., & Riehl, J. (1974). The systems-developmental stress model. In J. P. Riehl & C. Roy (Eds.), *Conceptual models for nursing practice* (pp. 247–266). New York: Appleton-Century-Crofts.

Dallmayr, F., & McCarthy, T. (Eds.). (1977). *Understanding and social inquiry*. South Bend, IN: University of Notre Dame Press.

Descartes, R. C. (1644). *Principia philosophiae*. Holland: Elzeulrs.

Dickoff, J., & James, P. (1968). A theory of theories: A position paper. *Nursing Research, 17,* 197–203.

Dickoff, J., James, P., & Wiedenbach, E. (1968). Theory in a practice discipline: Part 2. Practice-oriented research. *Nursing Research, 17,* 545–554.

Diers, D. (1979). *Research in nursing practice*. Philadelphia: Lippincott.

Donaldson, S., & Crowley, D. (1978). The discipline of nursing. *Nursing Outlook, 26,* 113–120.

Douglas, D., & Murphy, E. (1981). Nursing process, nursing diagnosis, and emerging taxonomies. In J. C. McCloskey & H. K. Grace (Eds.), *Current issues in nursing*. Boston: Blackwell.

Duffy, M., & Muhlenkamp, A. F. (1974). A framework for theory analysis. *Nursing Outlook, 22,* 570–574.

Durkheim, E. (1950). *The rules of sociological method* (S. A. Solovay & J. H. Mueller, Trans.). Glencoe, CA: Free Press, 1950. (Original work published 1895)

Ellis, R. (1968). Characteristics of significant theories. *Nursing Research, 17,* 217–222.

Fawcett, J. (1975). The family as a living open system: An emerging conceptual framework for nursing. *International Nursing Review, 22,* 113–116.

Fawcett, J. (1980). A framework for analysis and evaluation of conceptual models. *Nurse Educator, 5*(6), 10–14.

Fawcett, J. (1984). *Analysis and evaluation of conceptual models in nursing*. Philadelphia: F. A. Davis.

Feyerabend, P. (1970). Against method: Outlines of an anarctistic theory of knowledge. In M. Radner & S. Winokur (Eds.), *Minnesota studies in the philosophy of science* (Vol. 4, pp. 17–130). Minneapolis: University of Minnesota Press.

Fitzpatrick, J. J., & Whall, A. L. (Eds.). (1983). *Conceptual models of nursing*. Bowie, MD: Brady.

Forsyth, G. (1980). Analysis of the concept of empathy. *Advances in Nursing Science*. 2(2), 33–42.

Galligan, A. C. (1979). Using Roy's concept of adaptation to care for young children. *MCN: The American Journal of Maternal Child Nursing, 4,* 24–28.

Glaser, B., & Strauss, A. (1967). *The discovery of grounded theory: Strategies for qualitative research*. Chicago: Aldine.

Goodman, N. (1955). *Fact, fiction, and forecast*. Cambridge, MA: Harvard University Press.

Gordon, M. (1982). Historical perspectives: The National Conference Group for Classification of Nursing Diagnoses. In M. J. Kim & D. A. Moritz (Eds.), *Classification of nursing diagnosis: Proceedings of the Third and Fourth National Conferences*. New York: McGraw-Hill.

Gordon, M., & Sweeney, M. A. (1979). Methodological problems and issues in identifying and standardizing nursing diagnosis. *Advances in Nursing Science, 2*(1), 1–15.

Gortner, S. R. (1984). Scientific basis of nursing. In American Academy of Nursing Proceedings. Kansas City, MO: Author.

Griffin, A. P. (1980). Philosophy and nursing. *Journal of Advanced Nursing, 5,* 261–272.

Hanson, N. R. (1958). *Patterns of discovery*. Cambridge, MA: Cambridge University Press.

Hardy, M. (1974). Theories: Components, developments, evaluation. *Nursing Research, 23,* 100–107.

Hempel, C. (1970). On the standard conception of theories. In M. Radner & S. Winokur (Eds.), *Minnesota studies in the philosophy of science* (Vol. 4, pp. 142–163). Minneapolis: University of Minnesota Press.

Hume, D. (1739–1740). *A treatise of human nature*. London: John Noon.

Jacobson, M. (1981, June). *A semantic differential comparison of five nursing theories: A quantitative approach to theory evaluation*. Paper presented at the Fourth Annual Conference on Theory Development in Nursing, Clemson University College of Nursing, Clemson, SC.

Jacox, A. (1974). Theory construction in nursing: An overview. *Nursing Research, 23,* 4–13.

Jacox, A. (1984). Toward the development of a science of nursing. In M. Kravitz & J. Laurin (Eds.), *Nursing research: A base for practice: Proceedings of the Ninth National Conference* (pp. 15–25). Montreal, Quebec: McGill University.

Johnson, D. (1974). Development of theory: A requisite for nursing as a primary health profession. *Nursing Research, 23,* 372–377.

King, I. M. (1981). *A theory for nursing: Systems, concepts, process*. New York: Wiley.

Kritek, P. (1982). The generation and classification of nursing diagnoses: Toward a theory of nursing. In M. J. Kim & D. A. Moritz (Eds.), *Classification of nursing diagnosis: Proceedings of the Third and Fourth National Conferences* (pp. 18–29). New York: McGraw-Hill.

Kuhn, T. (1970). *The structure of scientific revolutions* (2nd ed.). New York: Holt, Rinehart & Winston.

Lakatos, I. (1970). Falsification and the methodology of scientific research programs. In I. Lakatos & A. Musgrave (Eds.), *Criticism and the growth of scientific knowledge* (pp. 91–196). Cambridge, MA: Cambridge University Press.

Laudan, L. (1978). *Progress and its problems: Toward a theory of scientific growth*. Berkeley: University of California Press.

Levine, M. (1971). Holistic nursing. *Nursing Clinics of North America, 6,* 253–264.

Levison, A. (1974). *Knowledge and society: An introduction to the philosophy of the social sciences*. Indianapolis, IN: Pegasus.

Locke, J. (1690). *Essay concerning human understanding*. London: Thomas Basset.

Mathwig, G. (1969). Nursing science. *Dialog, 3*(1), 9–14.

Merton, R. (1968). *Social theory and social structure*. New York: Free Press.

Munhall, P. L. (1982). Nursing philosophy and nursing research: In apposition or opposition? *Nursing Research, 31,* 176–180.

National League for Nursing. (1958). *Concepts of the behavioral sciences in basic nursing education*. New York: Author.

National League for Nursing. (1978). *Theory development: What, why, how?* New York: Author.

Neuman, B. (1982). *The Neuman systems model: Application to nursing education and practice*. Norwalk, CT: Appleton-Century-Crofts.

Norris, C. M. (1982). *Concept clarification in nursing*. Rockville, MD: Aspen.

Nursing Theories Conference Group. (1980). *Nursing theories: The base for professional practice*. Englewood Cliffs, NJ: Prentice-Hall.

Orem, D. (1980). *Nursing: Concepts of practice*. New York: McGraw-Hill.

O'Toole, A. W. (1981). When the practical becomes theoretical . . . relationship between practice, theory and research in psychiatric nursing. *Journal of Psychosocial Nursing, 19,* 11–19.

Parse, R. R. (1981). *Man—living—health: A theory of nursing*. New York: Wiley.

Paterson, J. G. (1971). From a philosophy of clinical nursing to a method of nursology. *Nursing Research, 20,* 143–146.

Paterson, J. G., & Zderad, L. (1976). *Humanistic nursing*. New York: Wiley.

Peirce, C. S. (1931–1958). *Collected works* (Vols. 1–8). In C. Hartshorne, P. Weiss, & A. Burks (Eds.). Cambridge, MA: Harvard University Press.

Peplau, H. (1957). Therapeutic concepts. *The League exchange* (No. 26, Section B). New York: National League for Nursing.

Peplau, H. (1968). Operational definitions and nursing practice (pp. 12–16). In L. T. Zderad & H. C. Belcher (Eds.), *Developing behavioral concepts in nursing*. Atlanta: Southern Regional Education Board.

Peplau, H. (1983). Videotaped interview with H. Peplau, Madison, NJ.

Popper, K. (1959). *The logic of scientific discovery*. London: Hutchinson.

Popper, K. (1965). *Conjectures and refutations: The growth of scientific knowledge* (2nd ed.). New York: Basic Books.

Putt, A. (1978). *General systems theory applied to nursing*. Boston, MA: Little, Brown.

Riehl, J., & Roy, C. (1980). *Conceptual models for nursing practice* (2nd ed.). New York: Appleton-Century-Crofts.

Rogers, M. (1970). *An introduction to the theoretical basis of nursing*. Philadelphia: F. A. Davis.

Rogers, M. (1982). Development of a new knowledge base for nursing. In M. J. Kim & D. A. Moritz (Eds.). *Classification of nursing diagnoses: Proceedings of the Third and Fourth National Conferences* (pp. 247–249). New York: McGraw-Hill.

Roy, C. (1976). *Introduction to nursing: An adaptation model*. Englewood Cliffs, NJ: Prentice-Hall.

Shapere, D. (1983). *Reason and the search for knowledge*. Dordrecht, Holland: Reidel.

Shapere, D. (in press). *The concept of observation in science and philosophy*. New York: Oxford.

Silva, M., & Rothbart, D. (1984). An analysis of changing trends in philosophy of science on nursing theory development and testing. *Advances in Nursing Science, 6*(2), 1–13.

Sokal, R. (1974). Classification: Purposes, principles, progress, prospects. *Science, 185,* 1115–1127.

Sokal, R., & Sheath, P. (1963). *Principles of numerical taxonomy*. San Francisco: W. H. Freeman.

Stevens, B. (1979). *Nursing theory: Analysis, application and evaluation*. Boston: Little, Brown.

Suppe, F. (1972). What's wrong with the received view on the structure of scientific theories? *Philosophy of Science, 39,* 1–19.

Suppe, F. (1974a). Some philosophical problems in biological speciation and taxonomy. In J. Wojciechowski (Ed.), *Conceptual basis of the classification of knowledge* (pp. 190–243). Munich: Verlag Dokumentation.

Suppe, F. (1974b). Theories and phenomena. In W. Leinfellner & E. Kohler (Eds.), *Developments in the methodology of social science*. Dordrecht, Holland: Reidel.

Suppe, F. (1976). Theoretical laws. In M. Przlecki, K. Szaniawski, & R. Wojekki (Eds.), *Formal methods of the methodology of science* (pp. 274–287). Wroclaw, Poland: Ossolineum.

Suppe, F. (1977). *The structure of scientific theories* (2nd ed.). Urbana: University of Illinois Press.

Suppe, F. (1978). [Review of B. Zeigler, *Theory of modelling and simulation*]. *International Journal of General Systems, 4,* 127–131.

Suppe, F. (1981). The Bell and Weinberg Study: Future priorities for research on homosexuality. In N. Koertte (Ed.), *Nature and causes of homosexuality* (pp. 69–97). New York: Haworth.

Suppe, F. (1982). Implications of recent developments in philosophy of science for nursing theory. In *Proceedings of the Fifth Biennial Eastern Conference on Nursing Research* (pp. 10–16). Baltimore: University of Maryland School of Nursing.

Suppe, F. (in press). General systems theory and the development of nursing theory. *Research in Nursing and Health.*

Thibodeau, J. A. (1983). *Nursing models: Analysis and evaluation*. Monterey, CA: Wadsworth.

Toumlin, S. (1972). *Human understanding* (Vol. 1). Princeton, NJ: Princeton University Press.

Wald, F., & Leonard, R. (1964). Towards development of nursing practice theory. *Nursing Research, 13,* 309–313.

Walker, L. O., & Avant, K. O. (1983). *Strategies for theory construction in nursing*. Norwalk, CT: Appleton-Century-Crofts.

Webster, G., Jacox, A., & Baldwin, B. (1981). Nursing theory and the ghost of the received view. In J. C. McCloskey & H. K. Grace (Eds.), *Current issues in nursing* (pp. 26–35). Boston, MA: Blackwell.

Weber, C. M. (1947). *The theory of social and economic organization*. (A. M. Henderson & T. Parsons, Trans.). New York: Free Press. (Original work published 1925).

Wooldridge, P. J., Schmitt, M. H., Skipper, J., & Leonard, R. C. (1983). *Behavioral science and nursing theory*. St. Louis: Mosby.

Yura, H. & Torres, G. (1975). Today's conceptual frameworks within baccalaureate nursing programs. In National League for Nursing, *Faculty, curriculum development. Part 3. Conceptual framework: its meaning and function* (pp. 17–25). New York: National League for Nursing.

Zbilut, J. (1980). Holistic nursing: The transcendental factor. *Nursing Forum, 14,* 45–49.

Zderad, L. T., & Belcher, H. C. (Eds.). (1968). *Developing behavioral concepts in nursing*. Atlanta, GA: Southern Regional Education Board.

Index

ORDER FORM

Save 10% on Volume 4 with this coupon

___Check here to order the ANNUAL REVIEW OF NURSING RESEARCH, Volume 4, 1986, at a 10% discount. You will receive an invoice requesting pre-payment.

Save 10% on all future volumes with a continuation order

___Check here to place your continuation order for the ANNUAL REVIEW OF NURSING RESEARCH. You will receive a pre-payment invoice with a 10% discount upon publication of each new volume, beginning with Volume 4, 1986. You may pay for prompt shipment or cancel with no obligation.

Name ____

Institution____

Address ____

City/State/Zip ____

Examination copies are available to instructors "on approval" only. Write on institutional letterhead, noting course, level, present text, and expected enrollment. (Include $1.60 for postage and handling). Prices slightly higher overseas. Prices subject to change.

Mail this coupon to:
SPRINGER PUBLISHING COMPANY
536 Broadway, New York, N.Y. 10012

ORDER FORM